This book comes with access to more content online.

Take practice tests,
and study with flashcards!

Register your book or ebook at
www.dummies.com/go/getaccess.

Select your product, and then follow the prompts
to validate your purchase.

You'll receive an email with your PIN and instructions.

NCLEX-RN

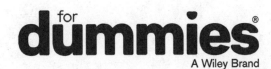

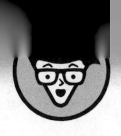

NCLEX-RN

2nd Edition with Online Practice

by Rhoda L. Sommer, RN, MSN Ed
and
Patrick R. Coonan EdD, RN, CNAA

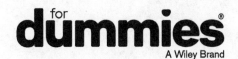

for
dummies®
A Wiley Brand

NCLEX-RN For Dummies®, 2nd Edition with Online Practice

Published by: **John Wiley & Sons, Inc.**, 111 River Street, Hoboken, NJ 07030-5774, www.wiley.com

Copyright © 2020 by John Wiley & Sons, Inc., Hoboken, New Jersey

Media and software compilation copyright © 2020 by John Wiley & Sons, Inc. All rights reserved.

Published simultaneously in Canada

For general information on our other products and services, please contact our Customer Care Department within the U.S. at 877-762-2974, outside the U.S. at 317-572-3993, or fax 317-572-4002. For technical support, please visit https://hub.wiley.com/community/support/dummies.

Wiley publishes in a variety of print and electronic formats and by print-on-demand. Some material included with standard print versions of this book may not be included in e-books or in print-on-demand. If this book refers to media such as a CD or DVD that is not included in the version you purchased, you may download this material at http://booksupport.wiley.com. For more information about Wiley products, visit www.wiley.com.

Library of Congress Control Number: 2020941814

ISBN: 978-1-119-69282-9 (pbk)

ISBN: 978-1-119-69280-5 (ebk); ISBN 978-1-119-69269-0 (ebk)

Manufactured in the United States of America

SKY10020617_082720

Contents at a Glance

Table of Contents

Introduction

Welcome to *NCLEX-RN For Dummies*. Don't worry, you're definitely not dumb for picking up this book. Like millions of other future nurses worldwide, you want straightforward advice and information without having to carry around 4,000-question test prep books. Trust me, you don't want to tackle the NCLEX-RN without understanding how the test is put together and what it's really all about.

The NCLEX-RN is one important test. Clearly, you need a readable, concise, structured resource to help you tackle the exam. You've come to the right place. *NCLEX-RN For Dummies* puts everything you need to know to conquer the exam at your fingertips. I give you a complete review of concepts covered on the test and provide insight on how to avoid the pitfalls that the test developers have designed to test your knowledge. And I do all this in an enjoyable, easy-to-understand way.

I take NCLEX-RN test prep one step farther by guiding you through some of the more difficult areas of the exam and sharing techniques for answering questions when you don't know the answers. I even cover what you need to do throughout the exam process, from registration to test day, and how you become licensed in a state of your choice in the United States or its territories. I also share information about compact or multistate nursing licensing. If you're coming from an international school to practice nursing in the United States, I tell you what you need to do, too.

You may have heard horror stories about the NCLEX-RN, perhaps about how you have to take it on a computer or how the questions get more difficult as you go along. Yes, the NCLEX-RN is no walk in the park, but it's not the hardest test you're ever going to take.

The NCLEX-RN measures minimal competency and your clinical judgment, and the fact that you've graduated from nursing school is an indication that you've attained minimal knowledge competency already. From there, the NCLEX-RN expects you to be able to read carefully and quickly and then apply what you know from your nursing program classes to the situation presented in the question. You already have the nursing knowledge you need to succeed on the NCLEX-RN — you just have to apply your critical thinking skills to each situation to come up with the right answers. This book helps you refine those skills and apply them to the questions on the examination. Reading through this book and doing the practice questions (and I provide a lot of them both in the book and online) can give you a pretty good idea of what you'll face on test day.

About This Book

I suspect you aren't eagerly anticipating sitting for the NCLEX-RN, and you probably aren't looking forward to studying for it, either. The good news is that you already know everything you need to know for this exam, so studying is just identifying and sharpening your weak areas. What I do in this book is give you some points to concentrate on. I make the preparation process easier for you by breaking down the information you need to know into easy-to-process bites.

Each chapter of *NCLEX-RN For Dummies* includes sample questions that illustrate just how the NCLEX-RN tests particular concepts. I want you to be comfortable with the way the NCLEX-RN phrases questions and expresses answer choices, so the sample questions read just like actual test questions. This book also gives you access to two practice exams: The exam that appears in the book is complete with answers and rationales, and the exam online presents the questions in a manner similar to the actual exam. (I provide the answers and rationales for these questions, too.) Each of the practice exams contains 250 questions.

There's no silver bullet for passing this exam, but you can start out on the right foot by considering my advice for how to study and relax before you go in for the test. Time is of the essence when taking the NCLEX-RN, so I provide techniques for answering particular kinds of questions in the shortest amount of time. I also show you how to quickly eliminate incorrect answers and make educated guesses. The key to success on the test is harnessing your ability to draw upon the knowledge you picked up in school and think through the questions and answers. Knowing what the question is asking and then picking the right answer is the key to success, and this book helps you do just that.

Sounds simple, doesn't it? Actually, it *is* simple; it's all in how you approach the exam. With so many review books on the market and so many questions to prepare for, you may be asking yourself, "What's the best way to review for this exam?" Well, the best way is to follow my advice and work through the chapters in this book. Focusing on the topics I cover and reviewing the sample questions and answers should leave you feeling completely prepared to tackle the exam.

Doctor is a broad term encompassing a variety of disciplines and degrees. For simplicity, I use *doctor* throughout this book to refer to a client's medical provider, who may be a physician, a nurse practitioner, and so on.

Foolish Assumptions

While writing this book, I made a few assumptions about you — namely, who you are and why you picked up this book. I assume that

>> You've graduated from nursing school and are seriously considering taking the NCLEX-RN soon. (In fact, the sooner you take it after graduation, the better!)

>> You aren't a dummy; you graduated from nursing school, which is a huge accomplishment in itself. You just know little about the NCLEX-RN and want to increase your chances of being successful and passing on the first try.

>> You've picked up this book primarily because you want to practice your chosen profession as soon as possible, and passing the NCLEX-RN is the only way to get there!

Icons Used in This Book

I use icons throughout this book to call your attention to important tidbits of information. Here's the rundown of what each graphic icon highlights:

You guessed it! This icon marks stuff you should remember. It's also information that you should review if you find yourself with a few extra minutes of study time.

This icon marks useful bits of information that may come in handy when you study for or take the NCLEX-RN.

EXAMPLE

This icon identifies questions resembling those on the actual NCLEX-RN.

WARNING

The Warning icon alerts you to potentially dangerous situations.

Beyond the Book

In addition to what you're reading right now, this book comes with a free access-anywhere Cheat Sheet that includes tips to help you prepare for the NCLEX-RN. To get this Cheat Sheet, simply go to www.dummies.com and type **NCLEX-RN For Dummies Cheat Sheet** in the Search box.

You also get access to two full-length online practice tests (the one in this book and a unique one) and hundreds of flashcards. To gain access to the online practice, all you have to do is register. Just follow these simple steps:

1. Register your book or ebook at Dummies.com to get your PIN. Go to www.dummies.com/go/getaccess.

2. Select your product from the drop-down list on that page.

3. Follow the prompts to validate your product, and then check your email for a confirmation message that includes your PIN and instructions for logging in.

If you do not receive this email within two hours, please check your spam folder before contacting us through our Technical Support website at http://support.wiley.com or by phone at 877-762-2974.

Now you're ready to go! You can come back to the practice material as often as you want — simply log on with the username and password you created during your initial login. No need to enter the access code a second time.

Your registration is good for one year from the day you activate your PIN.

TIP

As this book goes to press, the worldwide COVID-19 pandemic has necessitated some temporary changes in how the NCLEX-RN is administered. Check out the Downloads tab on the NCLEX-RN page at dummies.com for a resource outlining those changes.

Where to Go from Here

If you bought this book or are thinking about it, you must be planning to take the NCLEX-RN. But just buying this book doesn't help you much if it just sits on your bookshelf gathering dust. To get the full benefit, you have to open it up, read it, and work through the sample questions.

Everyone has different strengths and weaknesses, so this book is designed to be read in a way that best suits you. For example, if you feel that you know everything about how to take the NCLEX-RN, from how it's designed to how to tackle questions, then you can skip to Part 2 and the chapters that address client needs. If you're very comfortable with client needs and are an excellent caregiver but are unsure about the test, then you're better off focusing on Part 1. To get the most out of the book as a study tool, I suggest that you take a more thorough approach to the subject and read the whole thing. But regardless of your overall approach, this book is designed in a way that allows you to skim through the sections that you know a lot about (perhaps hitting just the example questions) and focus on sections about which you're not as confident.

If you're considering taking the test for a trial run before you crack this book and really start studying, I recommend against it. Taking the test without studying first is just a waste of your time and money. To get the most out of your NCLEX-RN experience, review all the client needs, know what the test is looking for, and then take the practice examinations. The practice exams show you which areas are your strengths and which areas you need to focus your attention on. I suggest you take the one in the book first, see which areas are your weakest, brush up on those areas, and then proceed online for the other practice exam.

In the end, how you use this book is up to you. You're the one taking the test, and you're the one who has to decide what you study and how much time you set aside to do so.

1

Demystifying the Complexity of the NCLEX-RN

Chapter **1**

Meet the NCLEX-RN: Your Ticket to Getting a License

Congratulations! You graduated from nursing school and you're almost ready to start practicing as a "real nurse." Only one thing stands in your way: the NCLEX-RN, which is prepared and administered by the National Council of State Boards of Nursing (NCSBN) to every nursing school graduate in the 50 United States, the District of Columbia, and five U.S. territories (American Samoa, Guam, the Northern Mariana Islands, Puerto Rico, and the U.S. Virgin Islands).

A passing grade on this exam is your ticket to a new career; without it, you can't practice nursing. From your current vantage point, passing the NCLEX-RN may look like a huge obstacle — one you may be afraid you can't overcome.

Take heart! I'm here to give you the confidence and knowledge you need to conquer the NCLEX-RN. In this chapter, I familiarize you with the test plan, talk about computer adaptive testing, and share what the NCLEX-RN really wants from you. I also tell you how to identify the correct answers to test questions by recognizing keywords and figuring out what the question is asking and give you an idea of what to expect after the exam.

The Big Deal behind the Big Exam

REMEMBER

The NCLEX-RN has only one objective: to determine whether you can safely operate as an entry-level nurse in the state in which you've chosen to practice. It isn't a test of your IQ or how fast you can start an IV. It is looking at your clinical judgment: Do you know what to do in clinical situations? In other words, can you think critically? The NCLEX-RN doesn't predict how successful your nursing career will be or whether you'll become a nurse leader. All you have to do is demonstrate that you have the clinical knowledge and judgment necessary to provide safe and effective care necessary to meet the needs of the types of clients you'll encounter in the healthcare workplace. And in order to get your license, you must pass the test.

NCLEX-RN: THE NEXT GENERATION

You may have heard of the Next Generation NCLEX (NGN), a new version of the exam the NCSBN is developing in an attempt to better test the complexities of clinical judgment new nurses encounter. As part of this process, some candidates receive an extra, completely voluntary section on new question types at the end of their NCLEX exam. You can read more about the NGN at www.ncsbn.org/next-generation-nclex.htm.

Sometimes students think that the NCLEX-RN is a certification examination; it's not. A certification examination is one that certifies a certain body of knowledge by an organization that's accredited to do so. In the case of the NCLEX-RN, you're tested on your ability to practice as a nurse. When you pass, you're issued a license by the state, and once you're licensed, you can go out and get the job of your dreams.

REMEMBER

Here's a little-known secret: If you graduated from a school of nursing, you *can* pass the NCLEX-RN. Nursing schools are evaluated on how well their graduates perform on the exam, so they're reluctant to graduate students who can't demonstrate potential for success on the NCLEX-RN. So if you graduated, you have what it takes. Kudos!

The NCLEX-RN is much less complicated than most exams you've taken in school, less difficult than most of your clinical rotations, and far less time-consuming than all the papers you've written, care plans you've devised, and other requirements you met in order to even be eligible to take this test.

The NCSBN actually conducts a study every three years to determine what entry-level nurses do, what responsibilities they're given, where they work, and what type of care is required to meet the needs of the client. In this way, the council can tailor the test questions to reflect what new nurses actually experience in their first jobs.

TIP

The people who write the NCLEX-RN questions are looking for basic safety, competent decision-making, and logical prioritizing. Keep those topics foremost in your mind!

You Must Remember This: Nursing Basics to Know by Heart

If nursing were just inputting data and outputting care plans, computers could replace live people. But nursing is much more than applying the nursing process to a disease process; it involves the care, feeding, and nurturing of people. The NCSBN, in its somewhat convoluted way, has broken these principles down into what it calls *integrated processes*. (Yes, it's a fancy name for something basic, but after years of nursing school, you should be used to that.) What these four integrated processes — caring, communication, documentation, and teaching — boil down to is really very simple:

>> **Caring:** Caring puts people above equipment or paperwork. Look at your patient before you look at machines, lab results, or even nursing processes. See the person first.

>> **Communication:** Therapeutic communication skills help you immeasurably in dealing with everyone from your patients to lab technicians. Never underestimate the power of effective communication while working as a nurse; failure to communicate well may not only harm your

patient but also make your life miserable. (Check out Chapter 8 for more on therapeutic communication.)

>> **Documentation:** Documenting care given and the patient's response to it is both a legal requirement and one of the major communication methods between healthcare workers.

>> **Teaching:** As a nurse, you teach patients, their caretakers, and other team members every day.

You can be a good technical nurse without integrating these concepts into your nursing care, but nursing is more than curing sick people; it's caring for them, communicating with them, and teaching them.

REMEMBER

The four integrated processes appear on the NCLEX-RN in the form of practical applications. Keeping in mind all the theories and practices that you know from nursing school, you should recognize the following themes in exam questions:

>> Patient safety is always a top priority.

>> Remembering the client's ABCs (airway, breathing, circulation) is essential.

>> Physiological needs should be met before other needs.

>> Doing what it takes to meet patient needs comes before other tasks.

>> A thorough assessment is necessary before undertaking other steps of the nursing process.

>> Part of the first step in the nursing process is assessing the patient's emotional status.

>> Assess the patient's readiness to learn before designing a teaching program.

>> Denial and disbelieving are generally the first responses to news of a loss or anticipated loss.

>> Nurses must deliver care in a nonjudgmental manner.

The NCLEX-RN — Not Your Average CAT Scan!

At some point in nursing school, you learned what a CAT scan is, right? Well, the NCLEX-RN is a CAT exam, but that doesn't mean what you think. In this case, CAT stands for *computerized adaptive testing.*

The NCLEX-RN is no longer a paper-and-pencil exam. Instead, the test is administered on computers, which allow for more reliable test results because the questions can be targeted to your ability (as judged by your answer to each question). Therefore, not everyone gets the same test. The test items that you see are specifically chosen based on the answer you give to the preceding question. Using your most recent response, the testing program searches the item bank for a question that has a degree of difficulty that's equal to your ability. This process goes on until you answer enough questions to make it clear that your ability is either above or below the passing standard. This question process is why some people get 75 questions and pass and others get 75 questions and fail. So the length of your exam is *not* a predictor of a pass or fail result — don't even waste your time trying to predict whether you've passed or failed!

When you take the test, you get anywhere from 75 to 265 questions, all presented in random order. Of these questions, 15 are considered experimental items and are *not* scored because the NCLEX-RN people use them to determine whether they want to subject future test takers to those questions, depending on how you do on them. The NCLEX-RN scores only questions that have been tested for reliability, so some of the questions you get may not actually impact your score. Don't panic if you get a question that you can't seem to grasp; it may just be one of the experimental items. On the other hand, don't assume that every difficult question is an experimental one and disregard it by taking an uneducated guess.

Questions appear one at a time on your computer screen. You can view each question as long as you like, but you can't go back to previous questions. You also can't skip questions. After you choose your answer, you're asked to confirm your choice by pressing the <NEXT> button. You can't go on until you confirm your answer, but you can review the question and change your answer as many times as you like before you submit it.

REMEMBER

Another logistical issue to keep in mind come exam day is that the test is timed. You have up to six hours to complete the NCLEX-RN, with two prescheduled breaks that you may either take or opt out of. (One minute per question is more than enough time to complete the exam ahead of the six-hour limit, so don't panic.) If you do run out of time for the test, the good news is that you still might pass! That's because the test is evaluated by whether you were above the passing standard for the last 60 questions. So missing a question or two but staying above the passing standard down the stretch means you still pass!

The computer tells you when your scheduled breaks begin, but you may break for as long as you like. From my own experience and that of all the nursing professionals I know, I urge you to take your breaks — don't just sit at the computer. Leave the room and do deep breathing exercises, or just take a walk around the test center outside the testing area. During the breaks, don't review your answers with other candidates or check your notes; you're not allowed to do either, and doing so anyway will definitely increase everyone's anxiety because you'll all be convinced that another person was right!

Thinking the NCLEX-RN Way

Students who take the NCLEX-RN often say that it's the hardest test they've ever taken. Is this a logical statement? The NCLEX-RN is primarily made up of multiple-choice and select-all-that-apply questions based on nursing knowledge, and it tests your ability to make clinical decisions based on information provided. Sound familiar? The NCLEX-RN really isn't that different from many other tests that you've already taken and *passed*.

REMEMBER

Primarily isn't the same as *entirely*. The NCLEX features other nontraditional types of questions, such as hot spot and case study, which I cover in Chapter 3.

The following sections give you an overview of some question-answering strategies and example questions to practice on. You can read more about these topics, including the keywords technique I use throughout, in Chapter 4.

Getting to the root of the question

The NCLEX-RN primarily consists of application questions that, when you get right down to it, simply ask, "What would you do in a certain situation?" Most of the situations presented on the NCLEX-RN could really happen, and you're asked to solve problems using a technique called *critical thinking*. Critical thinking is just a buzzword for making a decision based on observing, identifying the problem, deciding what's most important, recovering past knowledge (what you learned in school), and applying that knowledge to the situation presented. That doesn't sound so hard, does it?

TIP

The questions ask only about the particular situation presented. Most students' biggest mistake is adding information that isn't necessary or even appropriate to the questions. Remember, answer only the question that appears on the screen, using only the information you're given. Don't add anything!

The following is an example of a typical critical-thinking question. The answer explanation that follows it walks you through the answer process:

EXAMPLE

A nurse is discussing long-term care with the parents of a child with a ventriculoperitoneal shunt. Which of the following should be included to prevent complications from the shunt?

(1) Restrict all childhood activities.

(2) Have the child wear a protective helmet.

(3) Any signs of illness must receive immediate attention.

(4) Avoid placing the child in a side-lying position.

Use keywords to figure out what the question is truly asking. In this case, the keywords are *long-term care, child with ventriculoperitoneal shunt,* and *should be included to prevent complications from the shunt.* In this situation, the nurse is discussing long-term care, so the correct answer is something that needs to be done in order to maintain the child at an optimal level of function. Which of the choices is most likely to do that? Restricting all activities couldn't possibly maintain optimal function in a child. A protective helmet doesn't protect a ventriculoperitoneal shunt because it's an internal device. Reporting any signs of illness for medical attention is a must because a ventriculoperitoneal shunt can become infected. Avoiding side-lying positioning is a short-term intervention in the recovery period, not in the discharge plan.

So which of the choices answers the question? Of course, it's Choice (3). Even if you don't know what a ventriculoperitoneal shunt is, you can come to this answer by thinking the NCLEX-RN way. Read the question and ask yourself, "What's the main point of the question, and what knowledge do I need to use to choose the best answer?" By focusing on long-term care and what's best for a child, you can eliminate the wrong answers.

Navigating the grand inquisition, or the integrated exam

No matter what answers you have in your head, you may see something totally unexpected on the exam. The questions may be very different from the ones that you're used to getting in nursing school. You need to become "test wise" for the NCLEX-RN, which means that you need to know how to navigate through complex information.

Tests in nursing involve complex information that has not only depth but also breadth. In addition to its own body of knowledge, nursing draws from a variety of disciplines. The content tested on the NCLEX-RN is what I call *integrated,* which means that it isn't divided into separate categories, such as medical, surgical, psychiatric, pediatric, and obstetric nursing. It isn't even limited to nursing classes — you may see questions about chemistry, biology, and all the other courses you took as a student. Questions on the exam may include a combination of these disciplines, as in this example:

EXAMPLE

A pregnant woman presents in the emergency room with complaints of severe headache for two days, some episodes of double vision, and an observation that her rings have become tight lately. She has a history of hypertension and is on a sodium-restricted diet. Which of the following assessments would the nurse report to the physician immediately?

(1) BP 130/88

(2) Proteinuria 2+ on dipstick

(3) Fetal heart rate of 146 with good variability

(4) 2+ nonpitting edema of the feet

Look for keywords: *pregnant woman, complaints of severe headache for two days, double vision, rings have become tight, history of hypertension, sodium-restricted diet,* and *which of the following assessments would the nurse report to the physician.* This question is integrated because it tests your knowledge of different systems. Could the pregnancy be affecting the hypertension? Could the hypertension affect the pregnancy? The answer to those questions is "yes." So which assessment finding is the most abnormal? Or, in other words, which finding needs immediate medical attention?

Choice (1) isn't an abnormal finding based on standard normal blood pressure values in adults of 100/70 to 140/90. Choice (2) is abnormal because urine should never contain protein; it's an indication that the renal function is impaired. Choice (3) is normal; fetal heart rates range from 120 to 160 beats per minute. And as for Choice (4), nonpitting edema of the feet in pregnancy is a common discomfort related to increased pressure on the venous return by the growing uterus.

With this information gathered from thoroughly examining each answer option, you can easily decide which finding should be reported to the physician. Choice (2) is correct because it indicates abnormal renal function needing immediate evaluation and treatment. Isn't this easy? Or at least easier than you thought it was going to be?

Regardless of the primary diagnosis of this patient, the abnormal finding impacts her well-being the same way. Don't let the fact that questions contain integrated content distract you from what you already know!

Avoiding test-taking missteps

REMEMBER

Sometimes, a question pops up that looks like one you've seen already. It may be because several questions address similar symptoms, diseases, or problems and yet address different aspects of nursing care. Also, an experimental (unscored) item may have content similar to an operational (scored) item. Don't assume that a similar question indicates that you answered the first one incorrectly. Always answer each question as if it were the only question on the test; pay no mind to previous questions.

Try not to go into the examination with any preconceived notions about what you'll see on it. You need to use proper test-taking techniques (the ones you pick up in this book) throughout the entire examination. In my experience, most nursing students are able to easily reduce the number of possible answer options to two. But contrary to popular belief, you will only find one correct answer for each multiple-choice question on the examination. You need to use everything that you've taken away from your nursing program — including effective study and test-taking techniques and a positive mental attitude — to conquer the multiple-choice exam.

Chapter 15 has information on other popular misconceptions about the NCLEX.

Finding the real question behind the long scenario

You get settled in your seat and log onto the test; everything's looking good, you're feeling good, and you get the following question:

EXAMPLE

A paraplegic client with a T10 injury from a skiing accident, as well as other trauma-related problems, is recovering from the injuries and getting ready to transfer from the acute care unit to a rehabilitation unit. When a nurse offers to assist in getting ready for the move, the client throws the suitcase on the floor and says, "You nurses around here don't want to help me with anything." Which of the following responses is the most appropriate for the nurse to give?

(1) "You know I want to help you; I offered."

(2) "I'll pick these things up for you and come back later."

(3) "You seem pretty angry today. Going to rehabilitation may be scary for you."

(4) "When you get to rehabilitation, they won't let you behave like a spoiled brat."

You read this question, and you're ready to get out of your seat and leave the testing facility immediately. But you shouldn't panic. Although this question has multiple sentences and this patient appears to have multiple issues, you can apply a methodology to finding the real question hidden under all this detail. (Throughout this book, I guide you through dissecting this type of question in order to find out what you're really being asked.)

Yes, the client has many things going on, but the key is what the client is saying. As you take this question apart, you should always focus on the feelings that are underlying a particular action. The keywords for this question are *paraplegic, ready for transfer, rehab unit,* and *"You nurses around here don't want to help me with anything."* Choices (1) and (4) are confrontational and inappropriate coming from a nurse. Although offering to pick up the client's belongings, Choice (2), is a nice thing to do, it doesn't address the situation, and it reveals the nurse's assumption that the patient can't pick the things up. So the correct answer is Choice (3). The trauma and the T10 injury have nothing to do with the correct answer except to tell you the patient may have a serious back injury.

REMEMBER

Although I can't guarantee that you won't see a question like this one right off the bat, the questions should start out rather simple and get increasingly more difficult as you go through the exam. As you prove your ability to answer more-difficult questions, you get increasingly challenging ones until the computer decides that you have a minimal competency for nursing and doesn't present any more questions.

Keeping your cool when answering select-all-that-apply questions

Select-all-that-apply questions tend to throw students into a panic. Really, they're basically the same as multiple-choice questions; the difference is any number of the facts you know about the subject may appear in the list. You already know the information; just mark what you know and ignore the rest. Make a list on your white board and use it to answer the question. Head to Chapter 4 to read about select-all-that-apply questions.

Here's a simple example:

EXAMPLE

Which of the following actions or conditions may be a secondary cause of lung cancer? Select all that apply.

(1) Genetics

(2) Occupational exposures

(3) Smoking a pipe

(4) Smoking cigarettes

Keywords are *actions or conditions* and *secondary cause of lung cancer*. The correct answers are Choices (1), (2), and (3). As many as 90 percent of clients with lung cancer smoke cigarettes or have smoked them in the past, making cigarette smoking the number one cause of the disease. So Choice (4) isn't a secondary cause. The other answers may in fact cause lung cancer.

When All Is Said and Done

You're sitting at a computer taking an exam when all of the sudden, the computer goes blank. (And no, it's not a power failure.) What do you do? Stay calm and don't panic. The test shuts off automatically *without warning* when you've answered enough questions to determine your ability to provide safe basic care for patients. A screen appears stating that "Your test is concluded." You're then required to answer several exit questions, which are just multiple-choice questions about your examination experience. They don't count toward your results.

After you leave the not-so-horrific chamber of testing horrors, you get to sit on pins and needles for two to six weeks until the state board of nursing mails your results to you. Every computer exam is scored twice — once by the computer testing center and again after it's transmitted to Pearson professional centers. I highly recommend that you put your books aside when you get home from the exam, go outside and play, and let your mind roam free (at least of the exam) for the next few weeks. There's no sense worrying when you can't light a fire under the nursing board anyway.

You can't become licensed until you get the official mailed results. But if you're afraid you'll go crazy waiting to find out whether you passed, you may be able to get an early look at your results unofficially. Pearson offers a Quick Results service in some states that gives you your early results in two business days (for a minimal cost). If your state posts new licensees on its website, you also may be able to find out there. Otherwise, you just have to wait for the mailed results.

Hey, nurse? Yeah, you!

If you passed the exam, you're officially a registered nurse — congratulations! Now comes the fun part . . . you can go out and get a real job. Because this book is about taking the exam, I don't get into how to go out and get the job. (You'll have to find another book to help you do that.) But I want to be the first to offer congratulations and wish you a long and happy career as an RN.

So, you failed — it's not the end of the world

You may not want to read this particular section right now, but you probably should so that you know what happens if you fail the NCELX-RN exam. When you have to tell your family, friends, supervisor, and co-workers that you didn't pass the licensing examination, you may feel like you're the only person who ever failed this test in the entire world. I assure you, you're not alone. If you were, I wouldn't have an NCLEX tutoring business.

If you fail the exam, you receive a diagnostic profile from the NCSBN that tells you how many questions you answered on the examination. (The more questions you answered, the closer you came to meeting the passing standard; see the section "The NCLEX-RN — Not Your Average CAT Scan!" earlier in this chapter for details on how the computer adaptive test measures your competency.) The diagnostic profile helps you identify your strengths and weakness so that you know where to concentrate your study habits when you prepare to take the examination again. However, it doesn't give you the questions you missed or by how much you missed the passing mark.

Many people who fail the first time are disheartened enough to ask, "Should I take the test again?" Absolutely! You've completed your education to become a registered nurse, so don't throw away all that work and planning. Think back to the stages of grieving — that's exactly what you're going through. After you get through the stages of grieving, you're ready to go back and take the exam again. After all, you really want to be a nurse!

You can't retake the examination for 45 days. So schedule your next attempt, and allow yourself enough time to prepare for it. Then figure out why you failed this round. Although it may involve painful self-examination, you need to know why you failed so that you can establish a plan for success the next time. You should prepare differently this time because, well, obviously your old plan didn't work. You need to start fresh with a new plan of action.

REMEMBER

You get only so many tries to pass the exam – for example, Indiana allows three failed attempts before you're required to pursue remediation. A remedy could include taking an accredited NCLEX-RN prep program or refresher course. With a written letter of completion from that program and a 95% pass rate guarantee sent to the board of nursing, you should then be able to take the NCLEX-RN again.

The good thing about retaking the test is that you've already seen it — and that's a major advantage! You know exactly what to prepare for. The computer (clever machine that it is) remembers what questions you were given before, so you won't receive any of the same questions, but the content and style of the questions and the types of answer choices don't change. So you shouldn't have any surprises the second time. (*Note:* The machine just knows which questions you had the last time. It does not specifically give you the content you missed previously to make you fail again.)

Second-time test takers sometimes have test anxiety when going back the second time. Remember, having a good study plan and knowing the content is a way to work around anxiety, but you may also want to come up with an anxiety test plan. What will you do if you become anxious and need to relax — make sure you're wearing a calming scent? Practice deep-breathing exercises? Something else?

REMEMBER

There's no substitute for mastering nursing content. Go through your review books again, and become expert in reading the questions and being able to effectively answer what's being asked. Practice your test-taking strategies, too. (Throughout this book, I give you strategies to help you succeed whether it's your first test or not. Chapter 4 is a good place to start.)

As you gear up for your next attempt at the NCLEX-RN, follow this simple advice. It may seem obvious, but it will help you be more relaxed when you take the exam again:

>> Choose to take the test at the time of the day when you're most alert.

>> Choose a familiar testing site.

>> Accept the earplugs that are offered at the testing site.

>> Take your breaks.

>> If you become distracted or fatigued during the test, take a break.

>> Plan on spending six hours for testing; if you get out early, it's a pleasant surprise.

>> Always keep a positive attitude; say to yourself, "I *will* pass the NCLEX-RN."

Chapter **2**

Preparing for T-Day: Paperwork and Whatnot

As if taking the NCLEX-RN doesn't give you enough things to worry over, you also have to think about the logistics of the exam — the paperwork required just to be allowed to take the test, the fees you have to fork over (even though it may seem fairer to have someone pay you to take the test), and the potential for sudden changes to your test-taking plans (like what happens if you break out in chickenpox the morning of the exam).

One important point to note before you apply for the exam is that you must have graduated with a nursing degree in order to take it (such as an ASN or BSN). If you still have one more course to take, you must complete it before you can file for your application; otherwise, your application will be rejected. The board of nursing doesn't care that you're only two basket weaving credits short of graduation; no diploma, no boards. If you have transfer credits from another school, make sure that they've all been accepted and applied to your academic record. In fact, it's a good idea to sit down with your advisor one last time before your last semester to make sure that everything really is in order for graduation.

In this chapter, I walk you through the application process, tell you how to find a scheduling center, and explain what you need to know to get to that scheduled exam.

How Long Should I Wait after I Graduate? Deciding When to Test

How soon after graduation you take the exam is up to you, with some caveats. Some eager-beaver types want to take the test 14 minutes after graduation, while others are still dragging their feet 14 months from graduation. Each state has its own rules — of course! — about how long after graduation you need to wait before taking the test, but most states require you to wait 45 days. Refer to Appendix A for specific testing information about your state.

TIP

I suggest that you take the exam as soon as you graduate if possible because all that information you crammed into your brain is still fresh. Many students wait months before taking the exam because they feel that they aren't prepared. But the longer you procrastinate, the more you have to study, and the less chance you have of passing on your first try. Most nursing schools provide review courses, so if you're a recent graduate, you've probably honed your test-taking skills in the last few years, and your test-taking ability is at its peak. And the sooner you pass the NCLEX-RN, the sooner you can start work, start helping people, and buy yourself that new fancy car — or pay off your student loans!

REMEMBER

That being said, if you aren't getting the scores the NCLEX prep course you're taking suggests, plan to take more time. No school, family member, or faculty member can tell when you're ready just because everyone else is taking it. Everyone else isn't you. Don't even let a potential new job tell you when to take the test.

Of course, if you've delayed getting transcripts, sending in your fees, and paying your campus parking tickets, you may find yourself taking your test later rather than sooner. You must take the exam while your Authorization to Test (ATT) is valid, so the clock starts ticking after you get your ATT. (For more on the ATT, see "Scheduling the Time and Place" later in this chapter.) Check your calendar for weddings, births (presumably you'll know whether you or your partner will be giving birth any time soon; you're almost a nurse, for heaven's sake!), vacations, moving plans, and other personal events and factors that may delay your taking the exam after you have your ATT in hand.

TIP

Plan to take the exam before you get too involved in a new job as a graduate nurse. Job requirements usually take up a significant amount of your time, especially when you're a new employee. Accepting a position but not starting the job until you actually take the exam may be in your best interest. In this period of acute nursing shortages, healthcare agencies want people to start working right away, but your best bet may be to take the time to study for the exam first. Get it over with, and then start the job with a clear focus on beginning your new career.

REMEMBER

Each state determines the requirements for graduate nurses pending licensure. If you're working as a new graduate nurse, you must be aware of the state rules governing your practice. Check with your local state board for requirements for new graduates and to find out whether you can get a temporary permit in the state in which you choose to work.

Applying to Take the NCLEX-RN

Applying to take the NCLEX-RN may be easy or hard, depending on the size of your nursing school and how much help it can offer you in filling out your paperwork. At some schools, you may just be handed the paperwork in your last semester and told to take care of it; in others, the whole class may go over the paperwork together. (Send your nursing instructors flowers if that's the kind of program you're in.) In order to take the NCLEX-RN, you need to apply to two places: your state board of nursing for licensure and Pearson VUE, the company that contracts with nursing boards to administer the test.

Completing the application process

REMEMBER

Every state has its own application and way to apply. Depending on the state, you may be able to apply online only, on paper only, or through either method. Know your state (see Appendix A for information on each state).

Here's how the application process works.

1. **Apply to your nursing board either online or on paper.**

   Every state charges a fee with this application.

2. **Meet the requirements of your board of nursing (BON) or Nursing Regulatory Board (NRB), as it appears on some state websites.**

   Some states require a school transcript as proof you've completed the program; flip to the later section "Tying up academic loose ends" for more on that process. You also need to get your criminal history done and your fingerprints taken to be eligible to take the test. States differ in how they take care of this process.

3. **Register with Pearson VUE.**

   Pearson VUE sends you your ATT. Then you can schedule your test either online or by phone (check out "Scheduling the Time and Place" later in this chapter for more on the scheduling process).

You can complete your application to Pearson VUE over the phone by dialing 1-866-49-NCLEX. Have a credit card handy (Visa, MasterCard, or American Express) to pay your fees immediately. If you'd rather not talk to a live person, you can register online. Get your credit card out and go to the NCLEX-RN candidate website at www.vue.com/nclex.

If you need to contact Pearson by mail, the general address and email address are

NCLEX-RN Examination Program
Pearson Professional Testing
5601 Green Valley Drive
Bloomington, MN 55437-1099
Email: vuepearsonprofessionaltesting@vue.com

Paying your dues

There's no such thing as a free lunch . . . or a free nursing license! The cost of a license varies from state to state, but the examination fee for the NCLEX-RN is $200. (Yep, you read that correctly — you have to pay a license fee and a test fee.) Appendix A lists the fees for each state. You know that your money has been received and your credit cards accepted when you receive a card from your state board of nursing stating that all your information has been received and you're ready to go. If you don't hear from the state board in a reasonable amount of time (and three hours isn't a reasonable amount of time), call to make sure that your application was received.

Hitting a bump: Potential problems with the licensure application

Problems are inevitable. Life is full of them. So don't be surprised to experience a glitch or two when you're trying to get your paperwork all filled in, sent, and processed. Many problems arise when people (this may mean you) don't read the instructions — all the instructions. In your rush to complete application paperwork and get it out of your house and out of your sight, don't overlook some major requirement; correcting the error can hold you up even more.

Tying up academic loose ends

Some states require that your permanent transcript be mailed with your application. You can get an official sealed student copy of your transcript from your school's registrar, but you can't always get it the same day you request it, so put in the request before you actually need the transcript. (I emphasize the point of an official sealed student copy because a licensing agency may not accept an opened unofficial transcript. You can't just copy your grades for the last three years of classes and send them in.)

If your school has closed since you've left and you still need a transcript, find out who the school transferred the responsibility of dealing with its transcripts for past graduates to and contact that organization. All states have a State Board of Education; if needed, you can contact it if you need assistance in getting your transcript.

You can also avoid problems with your application by making sure that you've met all the requirements for graduation. Some students truly do get all the way to the end of their senior years and start planning graduation parties and inviting friends and family to the big event just to find out that they've been ill-advised and still need to take those infamous electives or that one math course that they put off for two or three years. If you think this misstep doesn't happen to otherwise intelligent people, think again!

Have you been delinquent during your college years? If so, pay up! If you owe any library fines or have any unpaid parking tickets, your school can delay the release of your permanent transcript and delay your application for NCLEX-RN testing. In fact, the school can refuse to let you graduate at all! Think this scenario sounds far-fetched? It isn't. You often see long lines of fuming seniors paying off their parking tickets so they can collect their caps and gowns. To be sure it doesn't happen to you, check with the registrar, library, and security office to find out whether you have any outstanding fines and fees. And start looking under your bed for those books you misplaced freshman year!

I can't emphasize this point enough: Take care of all the little details way before graduation week arrives. Know your state board of nursing's exact requirements; some state boards require a statement from your nursing school saying that you met all the requirements needed for graduation. You don't want to be running around looking for someone to write this statement the week after graduation when your campus resembles a ghost town. Taking care of these things is up to you; most nursing programs want to see their students take and pass the NCLEX-RN and can give you some information about paperwork and the whole process, but don't count on someone else to do the application work for you. Be proactive!

Working around personal issues

Suppose you just met the person of your dreams, and that person wants to move out of state. You just applied for licensure in the state you went to school in, and now you're moving halfway across the country. How do you handle this one? It's actually quite simple: You apply for a license in the new state, which costs you more money because you forfeit your original application fee paid to the state you're currently in. Ain't love grand?

Refer to Appendix A to check on the requirements for the other states. Then call or write the board of nursing for the state you're heading to and request a new candidate application for licensure. (You're getting pretty good at this application process, aren't you?) After you pass the NCLEX-RN, you receive your nursing license from the state where you applied for licensure no matter where you actually took the test. If you and your newfound love want to live like nomads for a few years, you can apply for licensure in multiple states, and you will, in fact, receive licenses in multiple states after you pass the exam. For a fee, of course!

TIP

Some states have introduced what's called a *compact state license.* For a fee this program allows you to hold a license in your home state (the state on your driver's license) and also practice in other participating states. Compact state licensing is now available in 33 states and growing. (Appendix A tells you which states are compact states.) This licensing is especially helpful for military families who are required to relocate often. It also helps in case you're involved with telehealth covering more than one state.

Scheduling the Time and Place

After you submit all your application materials and everything is in order, Pearson VUE sends you a document called the Authorization to Test (ATT) via email. The ATT comes to you by email; be sure to check that email account frequently. You can't schedule your test until you receive this form.

REMEMBER

The ATT contains your assigned candidate number, which you need to know when scheduling your exam. Your ATT is valid only for a specific period of time, which is determined by the state board of nursing where you choose to be licensed.

Although you can take your NCLEX-RN any day of the week, you can't just walk into your nearest university and ask to take it. The Pearson VUE Corporation administers the NCLEX-RN for the National Council of State Boards of Nursing (NCSBN) at many sites around the country as well as internationally. You'll receive a list of testing centers with your ATT, but if you don't want to wait, you can access the most up-to-date and complete list of centers in the U.S. and international locations at www.pearsonvue.com/nclex.

Most states have multiple testing locations where you can take the exam, but because of small demand for testing sites, the following states and territories offer only one testing site:

>> Alaska

>> American Samoa

>> District of Columbia

>> Guam

>> Hawaii

>> Idaho

>> The Northern Mariana Islands

>> New Hampshire

>> New Mexico

>> Puerto Rico

>> Rhode Island

>> U.S. Virgin Islands

>> Vermont

TIP

For complete information on the most frequently asked questions regarding the NCLEX-RN and testing sites, go to https://www.ncsbn.org/nclex-faqs.htm. Testing locations are subject to change, and additional locations are added frequently, so checking this website often for the most convenient testing site for you is in your best interest.

You can schedule your NCLEX-RN on the web at www.pearsonvue.com/nclex or over the phone:

>> For testing in the United States, call 1-800-274-3444.

>> For testing in American Samoa and the Northern Mariana Islands, call 684-633-1222.

>> For testing in Guam, call 671-735-7407.

If you require any type of special accommodation, such as for a disability, you must schedule your examination over the phone by speaking with an exam program coordinator in NCLEX-RN candidate services. Understand that testing dates with such accommodations may be harder to find, especially if you need to reschedule.

You need to have your ATT with you when you show up to take the exam, so recording your testing details on it simply keeps all important information in one place. After you schedule your exam, you'll also receive confirmation of your scheduled date and time.

You must take the NCLEX-RN before your ATT expires. When studying and taking practice tests, don't forget your ATT end date. If you choose not — or forget — to take the test during this period (I don't know why you wouldn't, but I'm sure you have your reasons), you have to reapply to take the exam when you're ready and pay those testing fees all over again! You also have to observe 45-day wait just as if you'd failed the test.

Planning Ahead for the Big Day

If you live miles from civilization, you may have to travel a significant distance to take the NCLEX-RN. Don't combine your trip with a vacation or any other social activities, and, if possible, don't take anybody with you on this trip. They may distract you and make you lose your focus for the exam.

Don't go to the test with a friend who's also taking it; that's sure poison. One of you will finish first, leading the other to walk out as well, thinking "Surely I should be finished, too." I've seen many students fail for this reason alone. Taking the NCLEX-RN is like being born and dying — you have to do it by yourself.

I suggest that you run through this checklist before you go to take the exam, wherever it may be:

>> Determine how long you'll take to get there and how long you're going to stay.

>> Make your travel reservations and arrive the day before you're scheduled to take your exam.

>> If you're driving, plug the address into your phone or GPS or get appropriate directions from your local travel organization.

>> Confirm your hotel reservations, if applicable.

>> If you're going straight from your house to the testing site, minimize distractions in the house so you can focus strictly on the exam. If you have small children, arrange for them to stay with friends or family the night before the exam.

>> Wear layered clothing and be ready to peel like an onion. It gets hot in those centers.

» Bring your ATT.

» Bring one picture ID (and make sure the picture looks like you!) that also includes your signature. Otherwise a second ID with your signature is required.

» Don't test on an empty stomach! Bring along a healthy snack or something to chew on before the test or during breaks to help you keep your focus and burn off some nervous energy!

Plan to arrive at the test center at least 30 minutes before your scheduled test time. If you're late, you may lose your opportunity to take the NCLEX in that session. When you check in, the routine is as follows:

1. **Present your ATT.**

2. **Show one form of identification.**

   Your first and last names must exactly match the first and last names on the ATT; otherwise, you have to bring legal name change documentation to the center on the day of the test. Your ID must be government issued and not expired with your name, a recent photograph, and a signature. If the ID doesn't meet these requirements, you may be turned away.

3. **Sign in digitally.**

4. **Take a palm vein scan.**

   A palm vein scan requires placing your hand on a scanner which takes a picture of your veins. This scan allows you to access the center if you leave and need to enter again to finish the test.

5. **Get your picture taken.**

   Note that you can't wear your coat and hat while taking the picture.

6. **Place all your belongings in a locker outside the testing room.**

   Things not allowed in the room include purses, bags, wallets, watches, large jewelry, lip balm, coats, hats, food or drink, gum or candy, scarves, or gloves. I've known students who couldn't even take in tissues when they had a cold.

   You must put all electronics in a Pearson VUE sealable bag and leave them alone for the time you're there, even while on a break. Reading notes or a book or accessing your electronic device is grounds for dismissal from the site. You don't want to lose your chance to take the test and pass.

After you check in, you'll head into a room with 10 to 20 computers placed along the perimeter. You get your own desk and an adjustable chair, and dividers separate the desks so that you can't see the person sitting next to you. The room also has an observation window where the proctor can monitor the testing, and video cameras and sound centers on the walls monitor each candidate. Sounds relaxing already, doesn't it?

TIP

If you're easily distracted, ask for a set of earplugs. You won't be the first!

Because the Pearson testing centers offer tests for more than just the NCLEX-RN, you may find yourself seated next to someone taking an SAT exam or an exam for licensing in some other profession. In other words, you may feel very alone, but this isolation may help you by allowing you to focus and concentrate on your exam.

Help, My Car Won't Start! Rescheduling the Test

Planning well can prevent a lot of problems, but it can't prevent all problems. If you live in the Northeast and are planning to take your exam in the middle of February, when you know you may wake up to a blizzard, consider sleeping in your car in the testing center parking lot the night before. Just kidding — you shouldn't really go that far. The police may pick you up, and then where would you be? But seriously, what if you wake up the week of test day with a horrifying rash or break your leg rushing down the stairs?

To reschedule your exam, you must notify Pearson VUE 24 hours prior to your scheduled appointment. You can't reschedule on the day of the exam. So if you think you're coming down with the flu or someone in the family may die during the next few hours, reschedule. You should also reschedule if you have extreme nerves or test anxiety in the days leading up to the test. The odds are against you on passing in that condition.

My advice is to be mindful of when your 24-hour cutoff is. Pay attention to the weather forecasts and reschedule if you're unsure that you can get there at the proper time. Plan for the unexpected. You don't want to come up to the day and time of the test and not be able to get there.

If you miss your appointment, you forfeit your testing fees and must reapply to both the state board of nursing and Pearson VUE to schedule a new date. Have contingency plans for every possible foreseeable problem, but don't worry about things you have no control over. Rescheduling isn't the end of the world.

REMEMBER

If you're not facing an emergency and simply need to reschedule your test, don't call the test center directly. Instead, call Pearson VUE, which handles all scheduling related matters.

Chapter **3**

The NCLEX-RN Blueprint

Wouldn't you just love to know what's really on the NCLEX-RN? Well, today's your lucky day because that's what this chapter's all about. I can't give you a copy of the test, but I can review the exam content. I tell you what topics the exam covers so that you don't find yourself studying obscure scenarios that will never, ever be on the exam and explain how those topics break down percentage-wise on the test. This chapter also covers the concept of alternate questions: what they are, how they're worded, and what their purpose is (besides giving you one more thing to worry about).

Considering the Four Main Categories of Client Needs

The people who make up the NCLEX-RN like everything to be neatly organized, so they take a list of topics to be covered on the test and break each topic down into categories and subcategories. The test consists of four categories of topics with subcategories: safe and effective care, health promotion and maintenance, psychosocial integrity, and physiological integrity. Each of these categories are classified as a "client need." Two of these client needs have subcategories. The idea is that all your patients' needs fit into one of the categories listed in the following sections, whether it's a need for pain medication or a need for a chocolate milkshake. Understanding the categories gives you a good idea of how this test is constructed and what areas questions come from. I guarantee that you'll see questions from each of these general areas on the exam.

As if categories and subcategories weren't enough, the following processes are integrated throughout:

>> Nursing process

>> Caring, Communication, and documentation

>> Teaching and Learning Culture and Spirituality

The client needs categories exist to cover and test you on just about any nursing problem, action, or intervention from the cradle to the grave. The following sections break down the categories, with the most common topics related to each listed below the subcategory titles.

I wrote this book's chapters to correspond to the different client needs categories. I urge you to complete each of the chapters on client needs and identify your weak areas so that you can put in extra study in those areas. To study up on any of the areas listed in the following sections, just flip to the corresponding chapter.

Not sure what to focus on? On the content side, the four categories and their subcategories comprise certain percentages of questions addressing each topic on the exam. They're all pretty close percentage-wise, but a few sections are a bit more heavily weighted, so you may want to spend more time reviewing them. The breakdown appears in Table 3-1.

TABLE 3-1 **Percentage Breakdown of NCLEX-RN Content**

Client needs category	Subcategories	Percentage of Test
Safe and Effective care Enviroment	Management of care	17–23%
Safe and Effective care Enviroment	Safety and infection control	9–15%
Health promotion and maintenance	N/A	6–12%
Psychosocial integrity	N/A	6–12%
Physiological integrity	Basic care and comfort	6–12%
Physiological integrity	Pharmacological and parenteral therapy	12–18%
Physiological integrity	Reduction of risk potential	9–15%
Physiological integrity	Physiological adaptation	11–17%

Client need #1: Safe and effective care environment

The first client need, safe and effective care, includes nursing care that addresses anything that falls under management of care and safety and infection control.

Management of care (Chapter 5) covers

>> Advance directives/self-determination and life planning

>> Advocacy

>> Assignment, delegations, and supervision

>> Case management

>> Client rights

>> Collaboration with the multidisciplinary team

>> Concepts of management

>> Confidentiality/information security

>> Continuity of care

>> Establishing priorities

» Ethical practice

» Informed consent

» Information technology

» Legal rights and responsibilities

» Performance improvement

» Referrals

Safety and infection control (Chapter 6) covers

» Accident prevention/error/injury prevention

» Emergency response plan

» Ergonomic principles

» Handling hazardous and infectious materials

» Home safety

» Reporting of the incident event/irregular occurrence/variance

» Safe use of equipment

» Security plan

» Standard precautions/transmission-based precautions/surgical asepsis

» Use of restraints and safety devices

Here's an example question that falls under this first client need category:

EXAMPLE

The nurse is making an assignment for the unlicensed assistive personnel (UAP) who has been floated to the unit for the shift. Which of the following assignments would be appropriate for a UAP?

(1) A 62-year-old with a fractured hip, four days post-op

(2) A 75-year-old admitted three hours ago with intermittent chest pain

(3) A 49-year-old, one day post-op bowel resection, NPO with a nasogastric tube

(4) A 50-year-old who is being discharged

The correct answer is Choice (1). Keywords are *assignment, for unlicensed assistive personnel (UAP), floated,* and *appropriate assignment.* (Check out Chapter 4 for how to zero in on keywords.) What do you remember about delegation? What are the rules of how to delegate patient assignments? The UAP can perform all activities of daily living, which include bathing, feeding, mobilizing, toileting, and basic comfort. The LPN can provide all the activities of daily living as well as skills that require sterile techniques, medication administration, invasive procedures, and treatments. The RN can do all the activities of daily living, all the skills, and all the assessments and teaching. Knowing about delegation makes it really easy to determine the correct answer. The UAP can't be assigned any patient who requires skilled care, assessment, or teaching. Therefore, the most appropriate patient to assign to the UAP is the most stable patient who doesn't need any medications, assessment, treatments, or teaching.

REMEMBER

Any patient who's being admitted or discharged must always be assigned to the RN.

Client need #2: Health promotion and maintenance

The second client need, health promotion and maintenance, includes all things pertaining to the health in a person's life — prevention and care out of the hospital and all things concerning a normal pregnancy and delivery, among other things.

Health promotion and maintenance (Chapter 7) covers

- Aging process
- Ante/intra/postpartum and newborn care
- Developmental stages and transitions
- Health promotion/disease prevention
- Health screening
- Family Planning
- High-risk behaviors
- Human sexuality
- Immunizations
- Lifestyle choices
- Principles of teaching and learning
- Self-care
- Techniques of physical assessment

Questions in this category may be worded like so:

EXAMPLE

The mother of a 2-month-old brings her baby to the well baby clinic for his first health assessment. Which of the following would be appropriate anticipatory guidance for the nurse to present to the mother?

(1) "Start using your car seat as soon as he can hold his head steady."

(2) "Begin adding cereal to his formula."

(3) "Expect him to begin to go for longer periods in between feedings."

(4) "Consider taking him to play groups for additional stimulation."

The correct answer is Choice (3). The keywords here are *2-month-old*, *well baby clinic*, *first health assessment*, and *appropriate anticipatory guidance for mother.* By 2 months of age, babies' stomachs have grown enough to accommodate larger feedings, which allow them to go for longer stretches before needing refueling. A 2-month-old should already be using a car seat. Cereal isn't added until the child is at least 4 months old (around the same time that teeth erupt), and a 2-month-old is only interested in his primary caregivers.

Client need #3: Psychosocial integrity

The psychosocial integrity category tests your knowledge of culture, health practices, mental health disorders, addictions, crisis theory, and the foundations of mental health nursing. This section is all about feelings and emotions and how to get the client to express them to be therapeutic.

Psychosocial integrity (Chapter 8) covers

>> Abuse/neglect

>> Behavioral interventions

>> Coping mechanisms

>> Crisis intervention

>> Cultural awareness/cultural influences on health

>> End of life care

>> Family dynamics

>> Grief and loss

>> Mental health concepts

>> Religious and spiritual influences on health

>> Sensory/perceptual alterations

>> Stress management

>> Substance use and dependencies

>> Support systems

>> Therapeutic communications

>> Therapeutic environment

The following is an example of a question addressing this client need:

EXAMPLE

A nurse is providing information to the family of an alcoholic patient. The nurse encourages the wife of the patient to attend an Al-Anon support group. The wife states that it's difficult for her to face other people because she is embarrassed by her husband's behavior. What would the nurse most appropriately tell a wife to help alleviate some of her concern?

(1) She doesn't need to tell anybody her name or other identifying information.

(2) She won't know any members of the support group.

(3) The members of the group have all experienced the same problem.

(4) The group is always led by a nurse, physician, or other healthcare provider.

The correct answer is Choice (3). Keywords to look at are *wife of alcoholic patient, attending Al-Anon meetings, embarrassed by husband's behavior,* and *most appropriate to alleviate some of her concerns.* This question relates to supporting the client's wife during an embarrassing event. Al-Anon is a support group for spouses and friends of alcoholics or addicts of any kind. Support groups are based on the premise that people who have experienced a problem are able to help others with the same problem. Choice (2) is wrong because the nurse can't be sure that the spouse won't know anybody in the group. Although Choice (1) may be correct, it's not the most appropriate response to give to the wife of this patient. Choice (4) is incorrect because, although a nurse or other healthcare professional may be asked to speak at a group meeting, the members of the support group usually lead it themselves.

Client need #4: Physiological integrity

The last client need, physiological integrity, includes four different subcategory client needs: basic care and comfort, pharmacological and parenteral therapies, reduction of risk potential, and physiological adaptation. *Basic care and comfort* addresses the knowledge, skills, and ability required to provide comfort and assistance to the client in the performance of activities of daily living. *Pharmacological and parenteral therapies* address the knowledge, skills, and ability required to administer medication and other intravenous therapies. *Reduction of risk potential* addresses the knowledge, skills, and ability required to prevent complications or health problems related to the client's condition or any other prescribed treatment or procedures. Physiological adaptation addresses the ability to provide care to clients with acute, chronic, or life-threatening conditions.

In the category of physiological integrity, you'll encounter questions from the following subcategories:

» Basic care and comfort (Chapter 9) covers
  - Assistive devices
  - Elimination
  - Mobility/immobility
  - Non-pharmacological comfort interventions
  - Nutrition and oral hydration
  - Personal hygiene
  - Rest and sleep

» Pharmacological and parenteral therapies (Chapter 10) covers
  - Adverse effects/contraindications/side effects/interactions
  - Blood and blood products
  - Central venous access devices
  - Dosage calculation
  - Expected outcomes/effects
  - Intravenous therapy
  - Medication administration
  - Parenteral/intravenous fluids
  - Pharmacological pain management
  - Total parenteral nutrition

» Reduction of risk potential (Chapter 11) covers
  - Changes/abnormalities in vital signs
  - Diagnostic tests
  - Laboratory values

- Monitoring conscious sedation
- Potential for alterations in body systems
- Potential for complications of diagnostic tests/treatments/procedures
- Potential for complications from surgical procedures and health alterations
- System specific assessments
- Therapeutic procedures

» Physiological adaptation (Chapter 12) covers

- Alterations in body systems
- Fluid and electrolyte imbalances
- Hemodynamics
- Illness management
- Medical emergencies
- Pathophysiology
- Unexpected response to therapies

The following is an example question addressing the physiological integrity client need:

EXAMPLE

Which of the following would the nurse expect to be interventions for a client with acute kidney disease? Select all that apply.

❑ **(1)** I&O every two hours for color and characteristics

❑ **(2)** Sodium bicarbonate to be used if acidosis occurs

❑ **(3)** Monitor for wheezing, rhonchi, and *edema,* which is an indication of fluid retention and overload

❑ **(4)** Daily weight

❑ **(5)** Monitor urinalysis for hematuria, casts, specific gravity, and glucose levels

The correct answers are Choices (2), (3), and (4). Keywords are *nurse expect, interventions,* and *acute kidney disease.* This question addresses the subcategory of physiological adaptation. Because it asks which interventions would be expected for acute kidney disease, Choice (1) is incorrect; it has the nurse monitoring I&O every two hours, when the monitoring should actually occur every hour. Choice (2) is correct because you'd monitor for acidosis and treat with sodium bicarbonate. Choice (3) is correct because wheezing, rhonchi, and edema are all signs of fluid overload. Choice (4) is correct because taking daily weights to check for weight gain — a sign of fluid overload if greater than 2 pounds in 24 hours — is appropriate for this condition. Choice (5) is incorrect. You'd monitor urinalysis for all but the glucose in acute kidney disease.

Check out the later section "Select all that apply" for more information on questions with more than one correct answer.

TIP

DECIDING WHETHER TO JOIN A REVIEW COURSE

Whatever you do to invest in your success in passing the NCLEX-RN is worth it. For some students, review books are really helpful. For others, it's investing in live review classes. You're most likely to be successful when you know what works for you and utilize it. If that means paying $500 for a review course (that's the average cost), well, it's money well spent, and your first paycheck as a nurse will be all the proof you need.

Review courses for the NCLEX-RN are very popular. Although no law says that you have to take a class to pass the NCLEX-RN, doing so definitely can't hurt your study efforts. You can choose from all types of review courses to help you focus on the knowledge and strategies essential for passing the nursing boards.

In order to pick the course that will help you the most, first figure out what type of learner you are. (Various websites, such as vark-learn.com, can help you determine your learning preference.) Do you need to be in a classroom setting with an instructor? Do the live review classes fit into your schedule? Do you have the discipline to take an online review course? Choosing a review course just because all your friends are taking it isn't the best way to make this decision!

Live review courses, which put you in the same room as a real live instructor, not a video, are offered throughout the year. In these courses, the instructors follow lesson plans that teach you to apply your nursing knowledge to answering exam questions. Some courses may teach you specific strategies to help you arrive at the correct answer. Some courses guarantee your money back if you fail the boards; of course, this approach is kind of like betting against yourself, but if it gives you peace of mind, why not?

If you don't think you need live interaction, look into online review courses that allow you to take them anytime and anywhere. If you need flexibility and months of online access to questions and nursing content, you may find this type of review beneficial. Another computer-based option is home study programs; these programs review the nursing content extremely well in addition to providing tests to determine your strengths and weaknesses.

Another option is an NCLEX tutor, who can give you access to an answer directly. Live or online classes typically have many students, and the instructor may or may not answer your exact question. But meeting with a tutor one-on-one lets you ask as many questions as you want and get them answered.

Queuing Up Question Types

The NCLEX-RN examination includes cognitive-level questions. Cognitive questions on the NCLEX-RN are based on Bloom's Taxonomy (no, not taxidermy — taxonomy), which is a classification of three educational domains. They're the three areas — cognitive (knowledge), affective (attitude), and psychomotor (skills) — that are important in learning. Questions on the NCLEX-RN test your knowledge, comprehension, and ability to apply and analyze information.

REMEMBER

Bloom's cognitive level breaks down into six subcategories, two of which, application and analysis, constitute most of the questions on the NCLEX-RN. You must have the ability and knowledge to analyze and apply the information provided in the questions because when you pass the NCLEX-RN, you must have the ability, skills, and knowledge to be a safe and effective nurse at the entry-level RN position. No one expects you, as a new nurse, to have the abilities to analyze situations and apply solutions that a 20-year nursing veteran (nicknamed "Sarge," of course) has. These questions aren't intended to test the ability of an experienced nurse but rather a nurse who will begin practice after graduation.

STUDY GROUPS: ARE THEY HELPFUL?

The answer to this question is different for everyone, and you probably already have an idea of whether study groups work for you based on your experience in nursing school. In general, however, an NCLEX-RN study group works best if

- It's a small group whose members work well together.

- Everyone prepares themselves before coming to the group and then uses the group setting to review with each other.

- Group members come prepared with questions to ask the group.

Although teaching others is a great way to reinforce the material, study groups aren't right for everyone. If you find that you get more accomplished at home by yourself, or if you try a group and find that everyone else just slows your progress down, then a study group may not be right for you.

TIP

With any kind of question, use keywords to ensure that you're picking the correct answer; see Chapter 4.

Putting knowledge into action: Application questions

The application questions test your ability to recall your hard-earned knowledge from nursing school and apply it to the test questions. Remember, in a few months, you'll be using these skills on real, live people!

Here are two examples of application questions:

EXAMPLE

The nurse is caring for a patient who is a Jehovah's Witness. The patient is scheduled for surgery at 6 a.m. tomorrow. Understanding this patient's religious preference, the nurse will document which of the following in the patient's medical record?

(1) Patient refuses surgery. Physician notified.

(2) Patient refuses administration of blood products. Physician notified.

(3) Patient consents to be NPO throughout the night.

(4) Patient consents to have vital signs taken after surgery.

The correct answer is Choice (2). Keywords are *Jehovah's Witness, scheduled for surgery, patient's religious preference,* and *document.* In this example, you must know the health beliefs of this religious group (Jehovah's Witness) and then apply your knowledge to the question scenario (scheduled for surgery, document in medical record). For Jehovah's Witnesses, administration of blood and blood products is forbidden, and followers may avoid food prepared with or containing blood. With this knowledge, you can eliminate the other answer options as not in conflict with the group's religious beliefs.

A patient has just been brought to the emergency department by ambulance. The patient has stated that he has been vomiting a large amount of blood for several days. Which of the following actions would be the nurse's first priority?

(1) Take vital signs.

(2) Give the patient a drink of water.

(3) Give an antiemetic.

(4) Schedule the patient for surgery immediately.

The correct answer is Choice (1). The keywords here are *vomiting a large amount of blood, several days,* and *nurse's first priority.* In this example, you must know about blood loss and then apply the information to the question scenario. Knowing that blood loss can cause all types of problems, you must first assess vital signs to determine patient stability and assess for symptoms of shock.

Becoming an assessor: Evaluation questions

The function of the evaluation questions is to check your ability to evaluate information given about a certain situation. You have to be able to break down the information provided, such as labs and medications being given. Do the medications make the labs abnormal? If so, what action would the nurse take?

EXAMPLE

The nurse is giving digoxin to a patient with heart failure. Which of the following would show a therapeutic effect of digoxin for this patient?

(1) Increased pitting edema on lower extremities

(2) Decreased crackles in lungs

(3) A pulse of 84 beats/minute

(4) A potassium level of 3.1

The correct answer is Choice (2). Keywords are *digoxin, heart failure,* and *therapeutic effect of digoxin.* Decreased crackles in the lungs would show that digoxin has increased contraction of the heart and the blood is moving around the body correctly and not pooling in any area, such as the lungs or tissues. All the other answers show that the heart failure is still a problem and the digoxin isn't being therapeutically effective.

Slipping into Sherlock's shoes: Analysis questions

The function of analysis questions on the NCLEX-RN is to see whether you can analyze, compare, calculate, differentiate, or discriminate. These questions test your ability to break a given situation down into components in order to gain a better understanding of the situation. Analysis questions require that you interpret data, which involves a high level of critical thinking.

The following are two examples of analysis questions:

EXAMPLE

A nurse is reviewing a patient's laboratory report and notes that the patient's lithium level is 2.0 mEq/L. The nurse interprets this level as

(1) Normal level

(2) Below the normal range

(3) Above the normal range

(4) Needing to be repeated in two weeks

The correct answer is Choice (3). Keywords are *laboratory report, lithium level, 2.0*, and *interprets as*. In this example, you must be able to analyze the results of the lithium level. Severe toxicity can occur when drug levels exceed 1.5 to 2 mEq/L and may lead to coma, goiter, and renal toxicity. Lithium is contraindicated in cardiovascular, kidney, and liver disease.

EXAMPLE

A patient has just been diagnosed with an abdominal aortic aneurysm. The nurse knows that which of the following findings will be found during the assessment?

(1) Systolic bruit over the area of the mass

(2) Diastolic bruit over the area of the mass

(3) Nonpulsatile mass

(4) No findings will be found

Keywords here are *abdominal aortic aneurysm* and *findings found during assessment*. The correct answer is Choice (1). In this example, you must be able to differentiate the symptoms listed. In other words, you need to know the signs, symptoms, and assessment findings of an abdominal aortic aneurysm in order to answer this question correctly.

Getting creative: Synthesizing and creating questions

The function of synthesizing and creating questions is to see whether you can create or synthesize a plan of care for a particular patient with certain conditions. These questions test your knowledge of outcomes of the conditions.

EXAMPLE

A 52-year-old type-2 diabetic comes to the healthcare provider's office after several days of high glucose in the morning. The doctor suspects the Somogyi effect; the nurse would expect which of the following orders?

(1) Increased evening insulin to NPH 16 units and 4 units of regular insulin

(2) Increased snack prior to bedtime

(3) Increased morning insulin to NPH 24 units and 4 units of regular insulin

(4) Decreased morning insulin to NPH 10 units and no regular insulin

Choice (2) is the correct answer. Keywords are *52-year-old, type-2 diabetic, high glucose level in morning, Somogyi effect*, and *following orders*. This question addresses the outcome and planning care for a patient suffering from the *Somogyi effect*, where nighttime insulin is too effective at lowering blood sugar, leading the body to overcompensate at raising it. The patient needs to increase caloric intake at bedtime. Choice (1) increases the likelihood of hypoglycemia in the night. Choices (3) and (4) don't address the hypoglycemic periods during the night and between 2 a.m. and 3 a.m., respectively.

Exercising individuality: Alternate test questions

Alternate test questions were introduced on the April 2003 NCLEX-RN. An alternate question is a question that veers away from the typical, four multiple-choice item format. These types include, select all that apply, hot spot, fill-in-the-blank, drag and drop, chart/exhibit, audio, and case study questions. The multiple-choice questions are also still there.

KNOWING WHAT'S NORMAL, AND OTHER LAST-MINUTE TIPS

In order to do well on the NCLEX-RN, you need to know what's normal. If you know what's normal, identifying what's abnormal is very simple. Throughout this book, I review normal results, including those from lab and blood tests as well as from other kinds of tests. Review normal results and know them cold when you walk through the door.

Here are a few more quick tips to help you through the examination:

- The exam isn't based on nursing in the real world. Don't worry about things such as limited time and resources that you may have encountered in your clinical rotations; they don't exist in NCLEX-RN questions.

- You may use your real-world experience to help you visualize the patient described in the test question, but your answers must come from what you've learned in textbooks.

- When in doubt, always select the textbook answer.

- Patients always come first; equipment is always a secondary concern.

- Don't be quick to call the physician. The people who write this exam want to know what you would do in the situation, not what the doctor would do. With that being said, if you can do nothing for the patient and they need help, call the doctor.

- Don't look for the correct response; rather, eliminate all the wrong answers.

- Always focus on the patient, not the nurse. After all, nursing is about taking care of patients.

- Know the scope of nursing responsibilities and appropriate delegation criteria.

- Think, think, think before answering; the obvious isn't always right.

- The NCLEX-RN is all about caring for patients and establishing priorities.

- Don't cram! This test isn't about recall and memorization. Knowing more facts doesn't necessarily mean that you'll get more right answers.

Alternate questions are worded in a variety of ways and require different actions than standard-format questions. Knowing how to break down multiple-choice questions and pick the best answer isn't enough; alternate questions require you to really know your stuff! I give you some common examples in the following sections.

Select all that apply

Select all that apply are multiple-choice questions that may have more than one correct response. You don't have to prioritize the answer options because the question tells you to choose all the correct answers, whether that's one, some, or all of the choices.

The following are two select-all-that-apply questions:

EXAMPLE

The nurse is documenting a note in the medical record prior to the end of her shift. Which of the following are examples of appropriate documentation? Select all that apply.

- ❑ **(1)** Input nursing assessment/care into the computer.
- ❑ **(2)** Leave blank spaces.
- ❑ **(3)** Time and date your entries.
- ❑ **(4)** Change documentation of another healthcare professional.
- ❑ **(5)** Document treatments after completion with outcome.
- ❑ **(6)** Document client responses to procedures.

The correct answers are Choices (1), (3), (5), and (6). The keywords in the question are *documenting, examples of,* and *appropriate.* Rephrase the question in your own words to focus on these terms: Which of the following is the appropriate way to document in a medical record? That automatically eliminates Choices (2) and (4) because both are inappropriate documentation measures.

EXAMPLE

A nurse is preparing a poster for an educational session discussing factors associated with breast cancer. From the list below, select the risk factors for breast cancer that the nurse should consider putting on the poster. Select all that apply.

- ❑ **(1)** Age greater than 40
- ❑ **(2)** Family history of breast cancer
- ❑ **(3)** Early menopause
- ❑ **(4)** Previous cancer of the breast, uterus, or ovaries
- ❑ **(5)** First child born before the age of 30
- ❑ **(6)** High-dose radiation exposure to the chest
- ❑ **(7)** Early menarche
- ❑ **(8)** Multiparity

The risks for breast cancer include Choices (1), (2), (4), (5), (6), and (7). Keywords are *factors associated with breast cancer.* All of the options *except* early menopause and multiparity are risk factors.

Hot spot

This type of alternate question asks you to identify an area on a graph or picture by clicking the mouse on the correct location(s).

The following are examples of this type of question:

EXAMPLE

A nurse is shopping at a department store. The nurse observes an elderly man collapse on the floor. The nurse is going to defibrillate the elderly man by placing the paddles in which positions? (Indicate on Figure 3-1.)

As Figure 3-2 shows, Paddle A belongs at the third intercostal space to the right of the sternum, and Paddle B belongs at the fifth intercostals space on the left midaxillary line.

EXAMPLE

The nursing instructor is demonstrating to the student nurses how to take a radial pulse. Identify the area where the nursing instructor should place the tips of her first two fingers. (Indicate on Figure 3-3.)

As Figure 3-4 shows, to take a radial pulse, your first two fingertips go on the patient's wrist.

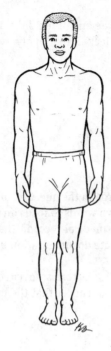

FIGURE 3-1: Locate where to place the defibrillator paddles to help this man.

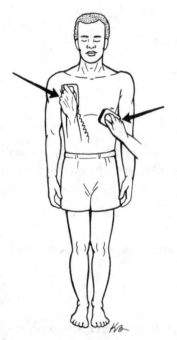

FIGURE 3-2: Place the defibrillator paddles as indicated.

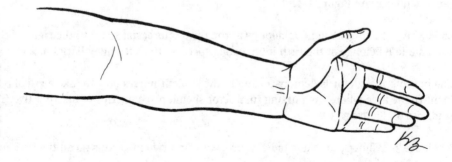

FIGURE 3-3: Locate where the fingers should be placed to take a radial pulse.

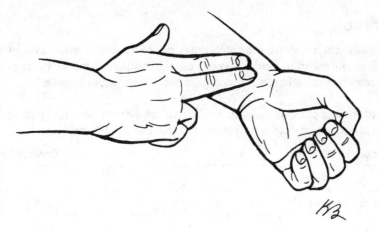

FIGURE 3-4:
For a radial
pulse, place
the fingers
as indicated.

Fill-in-the-blank

This type of alternate question asks you to do just what it says — fill in the blank. More specifically, you're given specific information about a patient, and instead of choosing an answer, you have to provide the answer yourself.

Fill-in-the-blank questions don't appear often on the official test, and when they do, they tend to require basic knowledge recall, basic calculations (a calculator feature is provided), or one-word answers. Fill-in-the-blank questions usually are some of the easier questions on the exam; you likely will see only one or two on test day.

The following examples give you an idea of what fill-in-the-blank questions are like on the NCLEX-RN:

EXAMPLE

The patient is on intake and output for the first three days postoperatively. What is the total intake for Day 1 considering all the following items?

Orange juice 60 cc

Water 20 cc

IV fluid 1,000 cc

Ham-and-cheese sandwich

Type the total intake in the following box. ☐

The correct answer is 1,080 cc. (You don't count the sandwich because it's a solid.) So you'd type the appropriate response in the box provided. Keywords here are *intake and output, total intake,* and *considering all of the following items.*

EXAMPLE

A patient is started on phenelzine for the treatment of depression. A food tray containing yogurt, tossed salad, crackers, and oatmeal cookies is delivered to the patient. Which food item should the nurse remove from the patient's tray?

Type the food item to be removed in the following box. ☐

The correct answer is yogurt. Keywords are *phenelzine, depression, food item to be replaced, yogurt, tossed salad, crackers,* and *oatmeal cookies.* Phenelzine is an MAO (monoamine oxidase) inhibitor. Patients on these types of drugs should avoid foods high in tyramine; these types of food include yogurt, cheese, cold cuts and processed meats, red wine, and fruits such as avocados, raisins, and figs.

Drag-and-drop

Drag-and-drop questions are usually for procedures the nurse would follow in a given situation. In this type of alternate question, you're asked to use the computer's mouse to drag answers from one side of the screen to the other in chronological order. Here's an example:

EXAMPLE

The nurse is preparing to place a nasogastric tube (NG) on a newly admitted patient. Place the actions listed below in priority order for placing the NG. Use all options.

Unordered Options	Ordered Options
Position client in high Fowler's.	
Secure the tube to the nose of the client with adhesive tape.	
Explain the procedure.	
When the tube comes to the back of the throat, have the client swallow or drink water.	
Lubricate the tip of the tube with water-soluble lubricant.	

The correct chronological order is

1. Position client in high Fowler's.
2. Explain the procedure.
3. Lubricate the tip of the tube with water-soluble lubricant.
4. When the tube comes to the back of the throat, have the client swallow or drink water.
5. Secure the tube to the nose of the client with adhesive tape.

Chart/exhibit

In this alternate format question type, you're presented with a nursing issue and a chart/exhibit containing info you need to answer the question. To read the information presented in the exhibit, you click on the chart/exhibit button at the bottom of the screen and then click each tab.

In the following example question, clicking Tab 1 would flash "complaints of dizziness upon standing" on the screen, clicking Tab 2 would flash "assessment of weak, irregular, and thready pulse and shallow, ineffective respiration" on the screen, and clicking Tab 3 would flash "medications taking are digoxin, furosemide, and docusate sodium" on the screen.

EXAMPLE

Tab 1	Tab 2	Tab 3
complaints of dizziness upon standing	assessment of weak, irregular, and thready pulse and shallow, ineffective respiration	medications taking are digoxin, furosemide, and docusate sodium

Which of the following conditions is the patient experiencing?

(1) hypokalemia

(2) hyponatremia

(3) hyperkalemia

(4) hypernatremia

The correct answer is Choice (1). Keywords are *complaints of dizziness; weak irregular and thready pulse and shallow, ineffective respiration; digoxin, furosemide, and docusate sodium;* and *condition is the patient experiencing.* The complaint of dizzy could be orthostatic hypertension which is a symptom of hypokalemia. The weak, irregular pulse and shallow, ineffective respirations are signs of hypokalemia. The furosemide depletes potassium.

Audio

In this alternate format question, you get a question that corresponds to some accompanying audio. For example, you may hear a clip of some lung sounds and then have to answer a question about an action you'd take for that lung sound.

EXAMPLE

The nurse is auscultating the lung sounds on an asthma client. Listen to the audio. Which adventitious lung sound does the nurse hear?

(1) Stridor

(2) Wheezes

(3) Crackles

(4) Rhonchi

When faced with an audio question, be sure you know what the question is asking for specifically before you listen to the clip. For example, this question asks for the sound made by an asthmatic client. That person would have constricted bronchioles which would make wheezing sounds like a musical note during inspiration and expiration.

Case study

Case study questions give you a scenario with information that you must base your answers on. Case study questions include more background information in the question section than other question types. The answers can be either multiple choice or select-all-that-apply. With more text to wade through, it's important to quickly find the keywords and eliminate distracting details that aren't important to answering the question.

Here's a case study question using select-all-that-apply answering:

EXAMPLE

A 58-year-old male is admitted to the emergency room with a blood sugar level of 640 mg/dL. The nurse assesses the patient for the following: fruity breath, Kussmaul respirations, and lethargy. Family arrives and tells the nurse that the patient was just recently diagnosed with type 2 diabetes mellitus and hasn't been following the recommended diet or medication regime. Which of the following interventions would be the nurse's next best steps in this situation? Select all that apply.

(1) Giving glucagon IV

(2) Starting an IV of D5W at 150 ml/hour

(3) Starting an IV infusion of regular insulin

(4) Starting an IV of normal saline at 150 ml/hour

(5) Drawing an ABG

The correct answers are Choices (3) and (4). Keywords are *58-year-old, blood sugar level of 640 mg/dL, fruity breath, Kussmaul respirations, lethargy, type 2 diabetes, hasn't been following diet and medication regime,* and *top two priorities.* Choice (3) addresses the problem of bringing down high blood glucose. Choice (4) deals with the fact the patient is dehydrated from all of the diuresis and urinating. The patient has lost fluids and needs normal saline to replenish the fluid loss. Choice (1), giving glucagon, makes the blood sugar rise, not come down. Choice (2) gives more glucose, and the patient already has too much. Drawing an ABG, Choice (5), isn't a priority in this situation.

Chapter **4**

Buffing Up: Study Tips and Test-Taking Strategies

I f you feel well prepared to take the NCLEX-RN, congratulations! The majority of test takers dread the NCLEX-RN to a degree usually reserved for dental appointments. After all, you can't work as an RN until you pass it.

Fortunately, it doesn't have to be that way. The NCLEX-RN is somewhat predictable; the test questions are worded to test specific knowledge — no trick questions. Knowing how to study and what to look for in the questions increases your chance of passing on the first try, and reviewing as many test questions as possible gives you the best idea of what to expect. The secret to passing the NCLEX-RN is doing lots of practice questions, and throughout this book, I give you all the questions your heart could desire!

In this chapter, I cover a lot of ground to make sure you get no surprises when you sit down to take the NCLEX-RN. I help you get in gear by outlining a study schedule and telling you how to tailor it to your needs. I also show you how to identify your weaknesses (subject-wise, that is), how to use your textbooks without getting bogged down, and how to study well for the NCLEX-RN by homing in on the general concepts that you absolutely must know to succeed.

This chapter also gets to the specifics of test questions, explaining how to break a question into its parts to get at its real point, how to think critically about all the components, and how to effectively prioritize answer options when more than one is right (which you should expect to be the case on this test because, unfortunately, few medical situations are ever black and white). I also share some strategies for eliminating wrong answers and guessing wisely when you really don't have a clue about the right answer.

Setting Up an NCLEX-RN Study Schedule

Not long ago you thought the day would never get here, and now it's approaching at lightning speed. Ready or not, test day is coming. Don't let it catch you unaware; being successful on the NCLEX-RN requires careful and effective utilization of your time. A good study schedule actually saves time, decreases your anxiety levels about getting everything done, and saves you from last-minute cramming (which definitely isn't an effective way to study!).

Try to avoid scheduling the test around big dates like getting married, going on vacation, and so on. Your brain will be elsewhere, as it should be. As soon as you know your test date, get out your digital or paper planner and start setting up a daily study schedule and attack plan. Don't have a planner? Run to the nearest office supply store or app store on your phone and get one that breaks each day down into hourly increments. Follow these general steps:

1. **Enter the date of the test on the calendar and determine how many days you have to study.**

2. **Write down your commitments.**

   Begin with your *fixed* time commitments that occur in the weeks ahead. These items are activities that are essential and unchangeable. (For example, classes, work, family obligations, mealtimes, sleep time, and religious services are all fixed.) Then write in your *flexible* time commitments (hobbies, recreational activities, and the like). Remember that giving yourself a break from studying and doing things you really enjoy is important. If you don't take this time out, you'll drive yourself — and everyone who knows you — crazy.

TIP

   Tell family and friends what events you'll attend, and then be there, in every sense of the word. Leave studying at home and be with them. You need the time away.

3. **Identify time slots in each day when you can study.**

   A rule of thumb is to try to devote a minimum of two to three hours per day to studying. They don't have to be consecutive, as I discuss later in this section. Remember to tell your family that study time is your time, because you want to get this test right the first time!

4. **Divvy up your study topics and record your plans for studying each one.**

   Divide the content on the exam into sections, and determine which areas you feel most prepared for. Plan to study these areas last and begin with the content areas that you're mostly unfamiliar with because you need to devote more time to them.

TIP

If your schedule allows it, devote an entire week to each major topic and completely immerse yourself in that topic for the week. Don't jump around or let anxiety get the better of you. You should spend most of your time doing practice questions, which you can find throughout this book and in the test included with the online material.

As you plan out what you'll study when, keep the following tips in mind to maximize your study potential:

>> **Study at the time of day when you're most alert.** If you're exhausted, the time you spend studying is wasted. If you're a morning person, plan to do the bulk of your studying shortly after you get up. Studying during daylight hours is usually more effective than studying at night, but if you're a night owl, it's okay to hit the books then.

>> **Studying when you have a long block of time available is optimal but not absolutely necessary.** Breaking up your studying into small increments of time can be helpful because it keeps you from procrastinating. So when you're waiting for a doctor's appointment, eating your breakfast, or waiting for a class to start, have a review book handy (preferably this one!).

If you do study for a long stretch, take a break every hour or so to give your brain a rest; it can only absorb information for about an hour at a time. Set alarms for 10 to 15 minutes to tell you when to take a break and when to get back to the books.

>> **Prioritize your study topics.** As I recommend earlier in this section, make a list of your strengths and weaknesses according to the topics on the NCLEX-RN. Start with the most difficult topics (or the ones that you feel the least confident in) and move on to the easier ones. Organizing your study this way helps decrease your anxiety early on because after you master difficult content, you feel more confident about the "easier" material. If you're unsure which areas you're weak in, take the comprehensive tests in the online bonus material that comes with this book and see what areas have the lowest scores. A low score indicates a weak area.

REMEMBER

Your study schedule is a guideline. If you have a family emergency, you need to get a root canal, or your friend needs a shoulder to cry on one night, it's okay to adjust your schedule. Plan a little flexibility into the schedule to allow for life, and don't be discouraged by minor detours as long as you get back on track.

Identifying Your Weak Points and Hitting the Books

As I say throughout this book, the best way to study for the NCLEX-RN is to do lots and lots of practice questions. Don't get discouraged if you get many of them wrong initially; simply reframe the issue as "what do I need to learn?" rather than "what did I miss?"

REMEMBER

The more questions you review, the better you become at answering different styles of questions. (Flip to Chapter 3 for more on the variety of question types you find on the NCLEX-RN.) Also, understanding the rationale behind the answers to all the practice questions you do (not just the ones you answer incorrectly) is vitally important. Answering a question doesn't do you any good unless you study the answer and reasoning behind it; this extra attention helps you identify your weak and strong areas. Be sure to review all the questions in the chapters and take the full-length practice exam in Chapter 13 and the online bonus material — you'll be thankful you did. No matter where you are in the book, review the questions as you get to them.

After you finish a batch of practice questions, go back to your textbooks to review the topics you aren't comfortable with or are unfamiliar with. If you threw out or resold (or possibly burned) your books, check out the following list of some of the most common textbooks used in nursing schools. This list isn't meant to be comprehensive but rather is just a sampling of frequently used books. You should use the textbooks required in your nursing school courses as your primary reference books, but you may find the following sources useful if you don't have them already:

>> **On the fundamentals of nursing:**

- *Fundamentals of Nursing,* 9th Edition, by Patricia Potter and Anne Griffin Perry (Mosby)

- *Fundamentals of Nursing: The Art and Science of Person Centered Care,* 9th Edition, by Carol Taylor, Pamela Lynn, and Priscilla LeMone (Lippincott Williams and Wilkins)

>> **On medical and surgical nursing:**

- *Brunner and Suddarth's Textbook of Medical-Surgical Nursing,* 14th Edition, by Janice L Hinkle, Kerry H. Cheever Brunner, and Doris Smith Suddarth (Lippincott Williams and Wilkins)

- *Medical Surgical Nursing: Assessment and Management of Clinical Problems,* 10th Edition, by Sharon Lewis, Linda Bucher, Margaret Heitkemper, and Mariann Harding (Mosby)

- » **On obstetrics and women's health nursing:** *Maternity Nursing Care,* 2nd Edition, by Lynna Littleton and Joan Engebretson (Cengage Learning)

- » **On pediatric nursing:** *Wong's Nursing Care of Infants and Children,* 11th Edition, by Marilyn Hockenberry and David Wilson (Mosby)

- » **On psychiatric and mental health nursing:** *Principles and Practice of Psychiatric Nursing,* 10th Edition, by Gail Stuart and Michele Laraia (Mosby)

- » **On community health nursing:** *Public Health Nursing Population Centered Health Care in the Community,* 10th Edition, by Marcia Stanhope and Jeanette Lancaster (Mosby)

TIP

Don't fall into the trap of trying to reread entire textbooks — it's not practical and probably won't help you. Use your textbooks as a reference. Instead of trying to cram every last fact about increased intracranial pressure into your brain at the last minute, read only to fill in the gaps in your knowledge of the subject.

REMEMBER

The writers of the NCLEX-RN aren't testing your ability to memorize facts. They're much more interested in your ability to apply your knowledge, analyze a patient situation, and provide safe patient care based on that knowledge. That being said, you can memorize certain "pearls of wisdom" to help you answer certain questions correctly. Throughout this chapter and this book, I highlight some of those pearls.

ENVIRONMENT COUNTS: SETTING UP YOUR STUDY SPACE

All right, so some of my recommendations for your study space may sound unrealistic or simply impossible (like the suggestion that you study in a room free of distractions even though you have two small children and live in a studio apartment). But these guidelines are the ideals for studying; just do the best you can in your circumstances.

- If possible, study at the same time and place each day, preferably a desk equipped with everything you need, including an alarm clock, pencils, pens, pads of paper, a calculator, and reference nursing textbooks. Have everything within your reach.

- Have the study space well lit, organized, and free of clutter.

- Make the room comfortable (but not too comfortable). If the room is too warm, you'll feel sleepy; if it's too cold, you may have difficulty concentrating.

- Free the room of distractions: Put your cellphone on silent (that includes social media), turn off the television, and hang a "Do Not Disturb" sign on the door if necessary.

- When doing practice questions on the computer, focus! Being in close proximity to a computer can tempt you to send messages to friends, check your email, surf the web, and waste time on a host of other computer activities. If you know the computer is your weak spot, use a review book instead.

- Listen to soothing instrumental music. If you must study in a place with noise in the background (such as a dorm room), soft music without words may be the white noise that drowns out everything else.

Remembering Dear Maslow and His Needs

When you're studying for a nursing exam, you can't go wrong if you start with Abraham Maslow, the creator of Maslow's hierarchy of needs, a laundry list of what people need most in life. Maslow will be your best friend when you take the NCLEX-RN.

Maslow's hierarchy has it all. If you follow Maslow, your nursing care will be organized by priority, with the really important things — like the need to be breathing — always at the top of the list.

TIP

Setting priorities is a much bigger part of nursing than it may seem to you right now. Take my word for it: The ability to set priorities not only helps keep your future patients alive but also helps you finish your charting on time. Know Maslow well — and put him first in every situation.

Maslow divided the needs of people into six incremental stages (see Figure 4-1), from most important to least important. Maslow's needs are arranged in the form of a pyramid, with physiological needs (what everyone needs to live) on the bottom, holding everything else up, so to speak. After all, if you can't breathe, you can't have a new house or be a best-selling author because you're dead. Everyone achieves the needs at the bottom of the pyramid, but not everyone achieves the needs at the top.

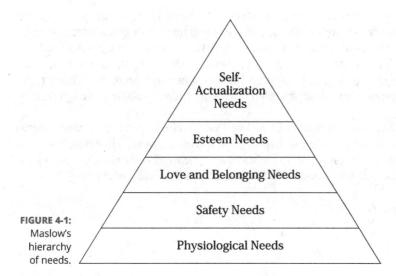

FIGURE 4-1:
Maslow's
hierarchy
of needs.

Notice that all needs are important, but some are way more important than others. This point is essential to remember not only on the exam but also when you're working as a nurse and have to prioritize your six patients' 101 needs in order of importance. For example, giving someone a bed bath is never as important as suctioning someone with a clogged endotracheal tube.

NCLEX-RN questions love to test your ability to prioritize in nursing situations. "What should you do first?" is a question you see frequently on the test. Obviously, you should first do what's most important, and what's most important is found in Maslow's hierarchy at the bottom of the pyramid. Here are some quick guidelines for setting priorities in nursing care:

>> Nurses decide priorities by assessing and analyzing.

>> To assess priority, start with the ABCs — airway, breathing, circulation, or most life-threatening — and Maslow's hierarchy.

>> Priorities can be high, intermediate, or low.

>> Treating potentially life-threatening problems before they become life-threatening is a high priority.

>> Non-life-threatening needs are intermediate priorities.

>> Low-priority needs are needs that aren't related to the patient's diagnosis.

>> Always consider time and resources as laid out in the question.

>> If the patient considers a problem important, then it is.

Applying the Nursing Process in Test Questions

Here's something to remember for the exam: nursing process, nursing process, nursing process; prioritize, prioritize, prioritize. Understanding the nursing process and prioritizing care are the basis of the whole test. Don't leave home without the ability to utilize the nursing process and prioritize accordingly in your sleep.

As important as the nursing process is, some instructors chop it into infinitesimal pieces so that making sense of it is darn near impossible; the process may end up sounding too lofty and complicated to be of any earthly use. But the nursing process is nothing more than a problem-solving technique (although I prefer "mystery-solving," à la Nancy Drew or Sherlock Holmes). It's a step-by-step process that uses a systematic approach. Nurses use this problem-solving technique to identify human response to illness and plan, implement, and evaluate nursing care.

Perhaps it has been months since you graduated and you've mercifully put the nursing process right out of your head to concentrate on items higher on Maslow's hierarchy, like taking a vacation. (Check out the preceding section for more on Maslow's hierarchy of needs.) As a refresher, here are the five steps to the nursing process and the questions at the heart of them:

1. **Assessment:** What's happening here?

2. **Analysis:** What does it mean?

3. **Planning:** What can I do about it?

4. **Implementation:** How do I go about doing what I need to do?

5. **Evaluation:** Did it work?

These steps and the order in which you must do them should become second nature to you. When you look at questions on the NCLEX-RN, always remember that assessment comes before analysis comes before planning and so on. In the following sections, I examine each step and provide related practice questions. (*Note:* In the examples throughout this section, I talk about questions' keywords; you can read more about identifying keywords and using them to help answer the question in the later section "Dissecting the Questions and Finding Keywords.")

REMEMBER

In the past the majority of the questions on the exam were written in the application format; in other words, they tested your ability to analyze information, apply it to a situation, and come up with the answer most likely to keep your patient alive and well — the nursing process in action (surprise!). But recently the NCLEX has changed. Students are encountering more and more select all that apply and priority questions (even 30 or more of each of these types of questions). This change is to more clearly assess your ability to make good clinical judgments.

Assessing the situation

Assessment involves collecting accurate information, making sure that it's correct, and communicating the information properly. Information can be subjective or objective:

>> *Objective data* is information you can actually see and measure, like blood pressure or lab results.

>> *Subjective data* is information you get from the patient, information that may be colored by his feelings or perceptions.

Assessment is nothing more than gathering information, and you collect information by interviewing or observing the patient, looking at past history or performing an exam, evaluating results, and working with other members of the healthcare team.

Assessment questions test your knowledge of information, principles, and skills related to the assessment of the patient. If an assessment action isn't one of the answer options, use the steps of the nursing process as your guide to select your initial or first action. The following are some examples of assessment questions:

>> The nurse should collect which of the following data?

>> Which data should be collected first?

>> Your patient develops chest pain. What data should the nurse collect next?

>> Which resources should be used to collect the information?

Words that indicate an assessment question include the following:

>> Adaptations	>> Notify
>> Assess	>> Observe
>> Check	>> Perceptions
>> Communicate	>> Question
>> Determine	>> Signs and symptoms
>> Identify	>> Sources
>> Inform	>> Stressors
>> Inspect	>> Verbal and nonverbal
>> Monitor	>> Verify

Make sure when reading questions that you have enough information or assessment done to make a diagnosis or perform an intervention. Most wrong answers to assessment questions are wrong because they don't collect enough information or they use information that's inaccurately collected. Some answers are wrong because they contain irrelevant or unverified information. Information can be obtained in a number of ways, including physical examination, interviewing techniques, and reviewing records.

The following are examples of assessment questions:

EXAMPLE

The nurse is caring for patients in a psychiatric clinic. The nurse would be most concerned if which of the following was observed?

(1) An adolescent with self-inflicted lacerations on her arm and legs

(2) An elderly man on antidepressants with a BP of 110/78

(3) An 11-year-old on Ritalin with a pulse of 78

(4) A 10-year-old on lithium with a blood level of 0.50

The correct answer is Choice (1). Keywords in this question are *psychiatric clinic, concerned,* and *observed.* Essentially, the question asks, "Which of the following would be of concern if observed in a psychiatric clinic?" All the options are assessments, so you have to figure out which patient requires immediate attention. The patient with self-inflicted lacerations displays suicidal ideation and carried out a plan to hurt herself, so this patient requires the highest priority and the nurse's concern. The other three patients display normal findings for their respective conditions.

EXAMPLE

When making rounds, a nurse finds the patient on the floor, where it appears he has fallen. What should be the nurse's initial response?

(1) Inspect the patient for injuries.

(2) Transfer the patient back to bed.

(3) Move the patient to a chair.

(4) Report the incident to a supervisor.

The correct answer is Choice (1). Keywords in this question are *finds a patient on the floor* and *initial response.* The *appears he has fallen* isn't important because that's an assumption; the nurse doesn't know objectively how the patient got to the floor. You have to determine what the priority action for finding a patient on the floor is. In an emergency situation, a nurse must first assess the condition of the patient. This assessment is basic to any emergency response by a nurse. Moving a patient before doing a complete assessment can make any injury worse.

After you collect information through assessment, you need to verify that it's accurate. You can verify the information by collecting additional data, questioning orders, obtaining judgments and/or conclusions from other team members when appropriate, and collecting data yourself rather than relying on technology or other people. Verifying data ensures its authenticity and accuracy.

An example of this type of question (verification) follows:

EXAMPLE

The nurse takes a patient's blood pressure and records a diastolic pressure of 118. What should the nurse do first?

(1) Retake a blood pressure.

(2) Take the remaining vital signs.

(3) Notify the nurse in charge.

(4) Notify the physician.

The correct answer is Choice (1). Keywords in this question are *a patient's blood pressure, diastolic pressure of 118,* and *nurse do first.* You don't have enough information to make a decision as to care, so you must get more information or verify. The nurse's first action is to wait and then retake a blood pressure because an error may have been made when she took it the first time. This question tests your ability to recognize that you need to verify information when the results are unexpected or outside the normal range.

Analyzing the situation

Analysis is the second step of the nursing process and the most difficult component. Analysis requires you to validate the information and decide whether it's significant. In other words, what does the information mean, if anything? Analysis questions are challenging because they require you to understand the principles of physiological responses and have the knowledge to interpret the meaning of your findings. You have to draw conclusions about what's going on with your patient by comparing your patient's symptoms to what's considered normal. These questions also require critical thinking in that you need to know why your therapeutic responses will work.

You need to use reasoning to apply knowledge and experience when answering analysis questions. After you initially analyze information, you may need to collect and analyze more information. Analysis questions may look like this:

>> Which data supports the diagnosis of renal colic?

>> Which diagnosis is most appropriate for this patient?

>> The patient with the diagnosis of myocardial infarction is at risk for developing which of the following complications?

Words that indicate that the question is focused on analysis include these:

>> Analysis   >> Organize

>> Categorize   >> Pattern

>> Cluster   >> Problem

>> Contribute   >> Reexamine

>> Decision   >> Reflect

>> Deduction   >> Relevant

>> Diagnosis   >> Significant

>> Formulate   >> Statement

>> Interpret   >> Valid

Wrong answers result when test takers select options that

>> Omit information

>> Analyze data prematurely

>> Make a nursing diagnosis before all significant data has been gathered

Here are two examples of analysis questions:

EXAMPLE

A patient has received a peripherally inserted central catheter (PICC) line. The nurse has explained the advantages of this line over other types of infusion lines. Which statement indicates that the patient may not understand what is being done and needs further teaching?

(1) "This type of catheter is very reliable."

(2) "This doesn't cost as much as other lines."

(3) "I can be given more than one medication through my PICC line."

(4) "This is only for the short term."

The correct answer is Choice (4). Keywords in the question are *PICC, explained the advantages,* and *which statement indicates that the patient may not understand.* You're looking for the wrong answer. At this point you should think about what is the PICC used for? Keeping in mind that PICC lines are intended for long-term use, not short-term use, you can see that Choice (4) indicates a lack of understanding on the patient's part. The other statements are true; PICC lines are reasonable in cost and don't need routine replacement. These catheters are also reliable and can be used for administering many types of medications.

EXAMPLE

Pressure ulcers are most often associated with patients who

(1) Are immobilized

(2) Have psychiatric diagnoses

(3) Experience respiratory distress

(4) Need close supervision for safety

The correct answer is Choice (1). Keywords in the question are *pressure ulcers* and *associated with patients who.* This question tests your ability to recognize a relationship between immobility and the formation of pressure ulcers. Prolonged pressure on the site interferes with cellular oxygenation, which causes cell death, which results in a pressure ulcer. Choices (2), (3), and (4) don't have a direct relationship to the formation of pressure ulcers.

Planning your actions

Planning is the third step of the nursing process, in which you put all the information you've gathered together. You identify goals, project expected outcomes, set priorities, identify interventions, and ensure that the patient's healthcare needs are appropriately met. Planning questions require prioritizing nursing diagnoses, determining goals and outcome criteria for those goals, developing the plan of care, and communicating and documenting the plan.

REMEMBER

Because the NCLEX-RN is a nursing examination, the correct answers most likely involve something included in a nursing care plan rather than a medical plan.

A care-planning question may look like the following:

>> Which outcomes are most important for a patient with a diagnosis of chest pain?

>> Which intervention is most likely to be effective in managing the symptoms of chest pain?

>> Which nursing measures should be included in the plan of care for a patient with asthma?

>> Which teaching strategy would be most appropriate for a patient who is 12 years old?

Words that indicate that a test item focuses on planning include the following:

>> Achieve	>> Desired
>> Anticipate	>> Desired results
>> Arrange	>> Determine
>> Collaborate	>> Develop
>> Coordinate	>> Effective
>> Design	>> Establish

» Expect	» Plan
» Formulate	» Present
» Goal	» Priority
» Modify	» Select
» Outcome	» Strategy

Testing errors occur in planning questions when test takers select answers that

» Don't include the patient in setting goals and priorities

» Establish inappropriate goals

» Misidentify parties

» Contain unrealistic goals

If you select options that reflect inappropriate planning or incomplete plan interventions or that fail to include family members and significant others when appropriate, you're choosing wrong answers. And most important, failure to coordinate or collaborate with other healthcare team members is definitely a wrong answer.

Two examples of planning questions follow:

EXAMPLE

The nurse is planning care. Which of the following is the most appropriate activity for a 5-year-old in traction after a femur fracture?

(1) A televised sports game

(2) Cellphone

(3) Picture books

(4) Crayons and a coloring book

The correct answer is Choice (4). Keywords are *the most appropriate activity,* and *5-year-old,* and *in traction.* Preschool play is simple and creative and includes things that let the child's imagination work. Picture books are appropriate for infants, and adolescents generally appreciate cellphones and sports shows.

EXAMPLE

A patient has just returned from surgery with an IV and has no gag reflex. What is the priority intervention?

(1) Ensure an adequate airway.

(2) Monitor the dressing for drainage.

(3) Check for infiltration.

(4) Monitor vital signs.

The correct answer is Choice (1). The keywords are *just returned from surgery, IV, no gag reflex,* and *priority intervention.* This question is about priority-setting. Priority means the most life-threatening — airway, bleeding, and so on. Even though all these interventions are important, the airway always comes first because oxygenation is essential to maintaining life.

Implementing care

After you figure out what to do, it's time to do it. *Implementation* is the nursing process step in which you carry out your nursing interventions by initiating and completing your planned actions (refer to the preceding section). This part of the nursing process includes such actions as organizing and managing care, counseling and teaching patients, providing planned care, supervising, and coordinating and evaluating the process of the delivery of care. And, of course, don't forget to document everything you do.

You have three types of nursing interventions:

>> **Independent:** These interventions are within the scope of nursing practice and don't require supervision.

>> **Dependent interventions:** These interventions are based on written orders of the physician.

>> **Interdependent interventions:** These interventions are shared with other members of the healthcare team.

REMEMBER

The examination is about nursing, so focus on nursing actions rather than medical action as the priority unless a question asks you which medical order would be anticipated next. Answer any question as if the situation were coming out of your textbook.

The actual question part of an implementation question may be along the lines of the following:

>> Which of the following actions should be implemented immediately?

>> Nursing interventions for this patient include . . .

>> Which of these nursing interventions is a priority for a patient with chest pain?

>> A patient with a diagnosis of asthma complains of shortness of breath. What should the nurse do first?

>> Which of the following situations should be immediately reported to a manager?

Words that indicate the question focuses on implementation include these:

>> Assist	>> Method
>> Change	>> Motivate
>> Counsel	>> Perform
>> Delegate	>> Procedure
>> Dependent	>> Provide
>> Facilitate	>> Reassess
>> Give	>> Referred
>> Implement	>> Strategy
>> Independent	>> Supervise
>> Inform	>> Teach
>> Instruct	>> Technique
>> Interdependent	>> Treatment

Testing errors occur on implementation questions when test takers select answers that

>> Implement actions that are outside the definition of nursing practice

>> Fail to identify and respond to a life-threatening situation

>> Fail to reassess the patient and modify interventions in response to the changing needs of the patient

>> Fail to identify additional assistance required to deliver safe care

>> Show a lack of knowledge necessary to safely implement interventions

>> Don't document a patient's response to care

>> Fail to supervise and evaluate delivery of delegated interventions

Two examples of implementation questions follow:

EXAMPLE

What should the nurse do to provide support for the patient who complains of nausea?

(1) Provide mouth care every hour.

(2) Delay meals until nausea passes.

(3) Position a basin within easy reach.

(4) Explain that nausea will go away with time.

The correct answer is Choice (3). Keywords are *complains of nausea* and *nurse do to provide support for the patient.* Nausea precedes vomiting, so placing the basin within easy reach anticipates an event.

EXAMPLE

The nurse is caring for a post-op patient who has just had a vaginal hysterectomy. What care should be avoided with this patient?

(1) Removing anti-embolism stockings twice a day

(2) Elevating the knee area of the bed

(3) Checking the placement of compression boots

(4) Assisting with the range of motion leg exercises

The correct answer is Choice (2). Keywords are *a post-op patient, vaginal hysterectomy,* and *care should be avoided.* This question asks for the wrong answer, so you need to determine which of the answers the nurse wouldn't do for a patient who'd just had a vaginal hysterectomy. Elevating the knee portion of the Gatch bed decreases circulation to the lower extremities and increases the risk of deep vein thrombosis (DVT). All the other choices are helpful in preventing DVT. Implementing measures that prevent DVT is the treatment of choice.

Evaluating your actions

You look at your patient, see what's going on, analyze your information, come up with a plan to help him, carry it out, and now you come to the final piece — evaluation. Did your plan work? Did you get the results you expected? If not, why? Do you need to change anything? If you're thinking a bit ahead, you can see that this stage leads you back into assessment, analyzing, and so on. That's the nursing process for you; it's a process that you carry out many times in a day. Thoroughly understanding the nursing process is essential not only to success on the NCLEX-RN but also to administering safe and effective nursing care.

As the final step in the nursing process, *evaluation* includes identifying patient responses to care, comparing a patient's actual outcomes to the expected outcomes, analyzing the factors that affected the outcomes, and modifying nursing care plans as necessary.

TIP

The actual question part of an evaluation question may look like the following:

>> Which of these responses indicates that the medication given was effective in treating the patient's chest pain?

>> The patient is taking nitroglycerin for chest pain. Which of these data indicates a side effect of the medication?

>> Which of the following observations indicates that the patient knows how to use his inhaler?

>> Which statement by the unlicensed assistive personnel (UAP) indicates the need for further teaching?

Words that indicate that a question focuses on evaluation include the following:

>> Achieved

>> Compared

>> Compliance

>> Desired

>> Effective

>> Evaluate

>> Expected

>> Failed

>> Ineffective

>> Met

>> Modified

>> Noncompliance

>> Reassess

>> Response

>> Succeeded

Most testing errors occur on evaluation questions when the test taker selects answers that

>> Don't thoroughly reassess the patient after the care is given

>> Fail to understand the significance of new data

>> Come to inappropriate or inaccurate conclusions

Here's an example of an evaluation question:

EXAMPLE

A patient returns to a clinic after having been prescribed a week's worth of antibiotics and is still exhibiting signs of a urinary tract infection. What should the nurse's initial reaction be?

(1) Have the physician write a new antibiotic order.

(2) Obtain a urine specimen for culture and sensitivity.

(3) Determine whether the patient took the medication as ordered.

(4) Make an appointment for the patient to be seen by a physician.

The correct answer is Choice (3). The keywords in this question are *patient returns to a clinic, been prescribed a week's worth of antibiotics, signs of a urinary tract infection,* and *nurse's initial reaction.* This question tests your ability to recognize the need to analyze all the factors that influence the outcome of care. Stating that the client had a week's worth of medication doesn't mean she took it. You're looking for an answer that goes along with medication being taken. Choices (1), (2), and (4) are wrong because they involve intervention without more assessment.

TIPS FOR SUCCESSFUL STUDYING

It's my opinion that you can never have too much advice when it comes to studying for the NCLEX-RN, so here are some more tips to consider:

- **Take a power nap.** A 15-minute nap may be just what you need to keep going.

- **Use flashcards for important information.** When you come across an important point that you aren't familiar with or a question that you can't answer, write it down on a flashcard. Keep the cards with you and flip through them whenever you have some free time in order to reinforce the material. Writing facts down helps many people remember them more easily. You can also find some vocabulary flashcards in the online bonus material that comes with this book.

  Tip: If you're a *kinesthetic* learner (you learn best by doing), use one card for the question and another for the answer. Put matching numbers or letters on the back. When you have more than five or six sets, place all the cards on the table face up. Find the answer to the question and bring the cards together. Your brain will see this action as doing, and you'll learn faster.

- **Set realistic goals and stick to them.** Don't overload your schedule with study sessions, and don't cram each session with so many practice questions that you don't have enough time to really think about each one.

- **Take care of your needs before you sit down to study.** Get a drink, get a snack, use the bathroom, and so on. Too many "field trips" can be disruptive.

Dissecting the Questions and Finding Keywords

Multiple-choice questions hog most of the space on the test because they're objective and efficient and can assess the depth and breadth of your understanding of curriculum content. Therefore, it's extremely important that you know how to break down multiple-choice questions in order to get to the "meat" of what's being asked.

A multiple-choice question is called an objective test question because the perceptions or opinions of another person (the subjective assessment) don't influence the answer. On the NCLEX-RN, the question is followed by four answer options, yet only one answer is correct, even if it asks you for the best option — technically, the "correct" option means the "best" option, which is only one answer. So you either answer the question correctly or incorrectly — it's that simple.

Each item (test question) consists of keywords. You can easily identify keywords by following these steps:

1. **Look for who your client is.**

   This info limits your answer to a specific group, such as infant, Hispanic, preoperative, and so on.

2. **Look for the condition.**

   What is the pathophysiology of the condition? How does the condition affect the client? What medications are used for this condition? What labs are affected by this condition? What complications are related to this condition?

3. **Look for labs, medications, and signs and symptoms.**

   Are these items due to the condition? The complication? Are the medications normally given for the condition?

4. **Look for what the question is looking for.**

   Is the desired answer a nursing action? A diagnosis?

TIP

Always focus on the information in the question and, more specifically, what the question is asking. Avoid reading elements into the question that aren't specifically included in the stem and options ("what if they mean . . ."). That's a rabbit hole you should leave to the rabbits.

Pinpointing the keywords

Many questions are designed to make sure that you're really paying attention and using only the information available, not making snap decisions based on incomplete information. Don't read into the question or add extra parts unless those parts are inherent to what is in the question. For example, if you know the treatment of the condition in the question involves an IV, then an answer could center on an IV even though the question doesn't explicitly mention the IV. When you read the question to yourself, don't think the writers forgot a certain keyword; believe me, they didn't! If something seems to be missing, there's a reason for it. Use only the concrete information that you're given in the question.

The purpose of keywords (the part of the item that contains all the details necessary to answer the question and actually asks the question) is to present the problem in a clear and concise manner. The keywords of a question can be all or some of the words. I teach my students to pick out only the keywords needed to answer the question. I encourage them to put the question in their own words without adding anything to the original question.

Try your hand at identifying the keywords in each of the following examples in order to choose the best answer:

EXAMPLE

The nurse is seeing patients in the psychiatric emergency room. Which of the following patients should the nurse see first?

(1) A 52-year-old male who needs a refill of his Prozac

(2) A 13-year-old male who threatened to stab himself in the school bathroom

(3) An 18-year-old female who has lost 5 pounds in the last month and feels sad

(4) An 89-year-old female who has been experiencing insomnia for three weeks following her son's death in a car accident

The keywords are *psychiatric emergency room* and *see first*. *Psychiatric* limits your answers to this specialty. To determine who requires immediate attention, use Maslow's hierarchy of needs (see the section "Remembering Dear Maslow and His Needs" earlier in this chapter). In the hierarchy, physiological needs come before psychological issues. Prioritize the patients according to Maslow's hierarchy, beginning with the most life-threatening, and you arrive at the correct answer, which is Choice (2).

EXAMPLE

A cab ran onto the sidewalk and went through a storefront. Your charge nurse says that four patients will be arriving in a couple of minutes. When the patients arrive, which of the following patients takes the highest priority?

(1) A patient with a laceration to the left arm

(2) A patient who is feeling anxious

(3) A patient who has a blood pressure of 72/42 and is very restless

(4) A patient who has shortness of breath and vital signs that are within normal limits

Keywords here are *cab ran onto the sidewalk, patients arriving,* and *takes the highest priority?* The correct answer is Choice (3). To determine this use Maslow's hierarchy and remember that physiological needs come first. This patient is going into shock, which you know because you know that the signs and symptoms of shock are hypotension, cool and clammy skin, rapid breathing, weak and rapid pulse, and restlessness.

Putting the keywords in context

When reading the question, pay attention to its polarity. *Polarity* simply means a positive or negative context. An item with a *positive polarity* asks a question relating to something true, and an item with a *negative polarity* asks a question in relation to something false. On the NCLEX-RN, the majority of questions have a positive polarity.

In an item with positive polarity, the answer is a fact and is something that should be implemented. A positively worded keyword wants to know whether you're able to understand, apply, or differentiate correct action. The following question is an example of positive polarity:

EXAMPLE

A patient has a nasogastric (NG) feeding tube. What part of the body requires special hygiene when the tube is in place?

(1) Rectum

(2) Abdomen

(3) Perineal area

(4) Oral cavity

Keywords are *NG feeding tube, part of the body,* and *requires special hygiene.* Putting this into a question using my own words, "What area of the body requires special hygiene due to having a NG tube in place?" it's easier to determine that the correct answer is Choice (4). Patients with nasogastric tubes don't necessarily have to chew. With the lack of chewing, salivation decreases, which causes mucous membranes to dry up. The rectum, abdomen, and perineal area don't need any special treatment related to an NG tube.

A keyword with a negative polarity has a question with a negative statement. You usually see words such as *except* or *not* in a question with negative polarity. Sometimes the words used are a little bit more obscure, such as *contraindicated, not acceptable,* and *avoid.* These questions challenge you to recognize exceptions or interventions that are contraindicated or unacceptable.

The following is a question with negative polarity:

EXAMPLE

A 2-month-old has been admitted to the hospital unit. The parents are at the bedside. The doctor is describing the treatment for tetralogy of Fallot. Which of the following statements would indicate the parents need more teaching?

(1) "A shunt will fix our baby, and we won't have to deal with it again."

(2) "A total repair can occur after our baby is 1 year old."

(3) "The total repair will require a medial sternal incision."

(4) "The shunt isn't a complete fix and only relieves the symptoms for now."

Keywords in this question are *2-month-old*, *tetralogy of Fallot*, and *parents need more teaching*. This question is a negative polarity, so you're looking for an incorrect statement. Choices (2), (3), and (4) are all true statements, but Choice (1) is false. After the shunt is in place, further surgery will need to occur to fix the condition. The correct answer is Choice (1).

Developing Critical-Thinking Strategies

The NCLEX-RN tests your critical-thinking skills, so you need to start thinking about your critical-thinking abilities both in providing nursing care and in inserting yourself into the nursing situations created in each exam question. When providing nursing care, your ability to think critically is called *clinical judgment*. Clinical judgment involves taking your assessment findings, putting them together in a meaningful way, and coming up with some possibilities of what may be going on with the patient. The people who write the NCLEX-RN are very concerned about your clinical judgment. Therefore, you need to fine-tune these skills and apply them to each question on the NCLEX-RN.

Critical thinking involves

>> Using your senses: Observation, smell, hearing, and touch

>> Deciding what's important and what's not

>> Puzzle-solving by looking for patterns and relationships

>> Identifying problems

>> Transferring your knowledge from one situation to another

>> Applying your knowledge

>> Making choices and educated decisions

>> Evaluating intervention based on established criteria

REMEMBER

In order to do well on the examination, you need to know what's normal; doing so helps you know what's abnormal. In Chapter 11, I review normal results, including lab, blood, and other test results.

Knowing the expected outcomes

You spent much of your time in nursing school learning about what could go wrong with patients and their care, and because nurses need to deal with problems and illnesses, this approach to nursing education makes sense. But in order to prove minimal competence on the NCLEX-RN, you must demonstrate an ability to make appropriate nursing judgments that include recognizing both expected and unexpected outcomes.

Expected outcomes are the changes in condition or behavior that you think will occur as a result of nursing care. These outcomes allow you to evaluate whether goals have been met.

TIP

Don't rely on your experience. The NCLEX-RN world isn't the real world, so you need to rely on what your textbooks say.

Suppose that you have an elderly patient with a sudden onset of confusion. Taken by itself, you know that the symptom of confusion in an elderly patient can mean any one of a number of things: hypoxia, electrolyte imbalance, infection, decreased cardiac output, dementia, or increased intracranial pressure. How do you narrow down what's going on with your patient and what's the best intervention? Using good clinical judgment, you look at the whole situation and get the information you need to make an informed decision.

You note that this patient also has a history of chronic obstructive pulmonary disease (COPD), is cyanotic and restless, and has an O_2 saturation of 88%. When you listen to his lungs, you auscultate inspiratory and expiratory wheezes throughout the lung fields. Based on this data, you determine that the patient may be experiencing an exacerbation of his COPD, with resultant hypoxia (low pO_2) and hypercarbia (high pCO_2). You suspect possible respiratory acidosis. The interventions, or outcomes, that you choose are based on this knowledge.

Finding the elusive question topic

An NCLEX-RN question has two parts. One part presents information about a clinical event, topic, concept, or theory. The other part asks you for some kind of response. The response part asks you to choose the best option that answers the question based on information presented by the keywords. (The earlier section "Dissecting the Questions and Finding Keywords" covers keywords.)

In your mind, you need to separate the information presented in the keywords from the response part of the question. In some questions, the information presented in the keywords, both information and response, is very clear. However, other questions may leave you less clear about which is the information part and which is the response part.

The information part of the question in each of these examples is in italics:

Which one of the following *is a patient goal?*

Before administering any medication, what should the nurse do first?

If you were taking the exam on paper, you'd be able to underline the important portion of each question. However, I don't think the computer center would appreciate you making any marks on the screen, so you have to make these "marks" in your head when you take the actual test or write the keywords down on the whiteboard. Just be sure to read what's actually in the question, and don't make assumptions about any of the information presented in the question after pulling out keywords.

When you're reading the options and the correct answer is entirely clear, refer to the words that you mentally underlined as being important in the stem. Compare any information you've analyzed to any of the options and relate the options directly back to what's being asked in the response part of the stem.

When faced with an option that contains the correct information, be sure to examine it closely because it may or may not have anything to do with the information and response parts of the stem.

Making an educated guess

You may come across a question that you have no idea how to answer. For example, you may not know the side effect of a certain medication or know the symptoms of a disease or disorder. Should you guess? Under certain conditions, yes. But make sure it's an educated guess — don't just pick Choice (3) because that's your favorite number.

An *educated guess* is the selection of an option based on partial knowledge, without knowing for certain that it's really a correct answer. After you reduce your final selection to two options (usually because the others just aren't related to the subject), reassess these options in the context of the knowledge that you do have and make an educated guess. One way to make a good educated guess is to utilize Maslow's hierarchy of needs. Making wild guesses, flipping a coin, or choosing your favorite number aren't recommended methods.

This examination is sensitive to how well you answer increasingly difficult questions (see Chapter 15 for an explanation), so making an educated guess on questions when you're reasonably sure about the answer works to your advantage. You're not penalized for making a wrong guess; however, you get additional questions based on the level of difficulty of that question. So you should use your critical-thinking skills and go for it!

TIP

When you make a guess, put your answer back into the question as the answer to see whether it creates a correct statement. For example, say the question asks, "Which of the following labs indicates the client is at risk for a complication from tumor removed from around the pituitary?" and you've settled on the answer choice "specific gravity of 1.003." Now reword the question as a statement including that choice and your reasoning: "The lab of specific gravity of 1.003 indicates diabetes insipidus, which is a complication from a tumor removed from around the pituitary." Yes, that's correct!

Picking the best answer when you're completely clueless

So it's not Colonel Mustard in the ballroom with the knife, but you can get clues from the answer options. Because the NCLEX-RN tests your critical-thinking ability, some questions may address topics that you don't know about. For example, you may face a question that concerns an injury, procedure, or disease process that you're completely unfamiliar with.

REMEMBER

If you're unsure of the answer to a question, don't panic! First, try using your critical-thinking skills to break down the question and see whether you can figure out the answer. When you read the question, ask yourself the following questions:

>> **Who is the client?**

>> **What is the diagnosis or symptom?**

>> **What is the time frame?**

>> **What do I know about this diagnosis or symptom?**

When you're stumped, you may find yourself reading the question and answers three, four, or five times because deep down in your brain you hope that at some point you'll remember seeing this topic in your notes or on some textbook page somewhere within the last two years. Or you're convinced that the proverbial light bulb will go on in your brain and you'll remember something about this topic. In desperation, you believe that hiding somewhere in the question is a clue that can point you to the correct answer.

Does this scenario sound familiar to you? Have you tried this approach on other exams? If so, what usually happens? In my experience, absolutely nothing — no sudden flashes of insight and no miracle recollection of seeing this question elsewhere. So you randomly select an answer choice, any choice, because you have a 25% chance of getting it right. Trust me, this tactic isn't a good way to approach questions that you don't know anything about.

If you find yourself completely lost after carefully reading a question over and over, try these methods to find some clues:

>> **Try not to read the question over and over.** Read the question once and identify the topic by noting the keywords.

>> **Read all the answer choices carefully.** You're not trying to find the correct answer but rather to identify the question topic. This process can lead you to the subject that you should be thinking about to answer the question.

>> **If you read all the options and still aren't any closer to an answer, reword the question using some of the keywords as clues to the subject you've picked up.**

>> **If you're really out of ideas, you can't skip the question — just make an educated guess.**

No matter how much you prepare for this exam, it will contain topics that are completely unfamiliar to you. Reading and carefully considering all answer options for clues will increase your chances of making an educated guess. Remember that you do have the knowledge; after all, you've completed your nursing classes. You just have to remember the basics, calm down, and think!

Here's an example question:

EXAMPLE

How should a nurse advise a client who complains of nausea and abdominal pain and has type 1 diabetes?

(1) "Increase your activity level."

(2) "Eat more foods with sugar."

(3) "Check your blood glucose level every three to four hours."

(4) "Hold your regular dose of insulin."

The correct answer is Choice (3). Keywords for this question are *advise* and *client who complains of nausea and abdominal pain and has type 1 diabetes.* If you read this question and can't identify the topic of the question, start narrowing down what you do know. The keywords give you the action of the nurse, the symptoms the client is complaining of, and the condition the client has. Which topic does the correct action address for a type 1 diabetic?

You know that each option deals with ways the patient can maintain normal blood sugar. Choice (4) decreases the patient's blood glucose level, so the nurse should assess the situation first. The same goes for Choice (2), which increases the patient's blood sugar level. Choice (1) decreases the blood sugar level. Choice (3) is an assessment of the patient and is the only correct answer because Choices (1), (2), and (4) are all patient interventions. As I discuss in the earlier section "Applying the Nursing Process in Test Questions," you must assess before you intervene.

Knowing how to prioritize when all the answers are right

In a prioritization question, all the options may be correct (and often are), and this type of question is a popular one on the NCLEX-RN. With this type of question, you must always read all the responses carefully and consider appropriate therapeutic communication techniques. A common mistake is to look at the first option and choose it without really reading all the other options closely simply because that one looks correct. Your job, though, is to analyze the situation and determine the best answer, which is technically the correct answer. Most importantly, always keep in mind what the question is asking:

>> Which option is the patient's most immediate need, OR

>> Which option should be the nurse's first action

When answering questions about patient needs, remember Maslow's hierarchy (see the section "Remembering Dear Maslow and His Needs" earlier in this chapter). Physiological needs come first, followed by safety and then psychosocial needs. If all the answer options are physiologic needs, use your ABCs (airway, breathing, circulation) or determine which concern is most life-threatening. When answering questions about the nurse's priority action or intervention, use the five steps of the nursing process (assessment, analysis, planning, implementation, evaluation) to figure out priorities. You can read more about implementing the nursing process on the test in the earlier section "Applying the Nursing Process in Test Questions."

The following words, phrases, and questions in the stem of the question should clue you in to the fact that you're dealing with a question about setting priorities:

>> Highest priority

>> Immediate action

>> Most important goal/action/and so on

>> Most essential

>> Primary goal

>> The nurse would initially . . .

>> Which is the best action?

>> Which (need) should be addressed first?

Here are some examples of an NCLEX-RN questions requiring you to set priorities and use your critical-thinking skills:

EXAMPLE

A nurse is reviewing the lab results of a newly admitted 75-year-old patient with a diagnosis of COPD exacerbation and respiratory distress. The patient is confused and agitated. Which lab finding would require the nurse to take immediate action?

(1) Hemoglobin (Hgb) 10.2 g/dl; hematocrit (HCT) 30.4%

(2) Platelet count 100,000

(3) BUN 42; creatinine 3.2

(4) ph 7.10, pCO$_2$ 80, pO$_2$ 45

The correct answer is Choice (4). The keywords are *75-year-old patient, COPD exacerbation and respiratory distress, confused and agitated,* and *lab finding would require the nurse to take immediate action.* The fact that the patient has COPD, coupled with the signs and symptoms, tells you that the problem is respiratory in nature. Although all the lab results are abnormal, the one that requires the nurse's immediate action is the arterial blood gas (ABG) report.

This ABG result indicates acute respiratory acidosis (uncompensated) with hypoxemia. (Normal ABG values are ph 7.35 to 7.45 and pCO$_2$ 35 to 45.) In respiratory acidosis, the patient is hypoventilating (not moving enough air and therefore retaining CO$_2$). This finding is the common acid-base abnormality seen in an acute episode of respiratory distress. The patient's low pO$_2$ (normal is 80 to 100) indicates hypoxemia. Although all the lab findings should be communicated to the physician, the nurse's most immediate action is related to the ABG result indicating hypoxemia (a life-threatening condition). Immediate action is required.

The critical-thinking process for the preceding example goes something like this:

1. I know that COPD is some kind of lung disorder that's prevalent in the elderly.

2. I know that confusion and agitation can be signs of hypoxemia (low pO$_2$) and hypercarbia (high pCO$_2$).

3. I know that this patient's ABG result is abnormal.

4. Therefore, the most life-threatening abnormality must be the ABG result.

EXAMPLE

Which nursing diagnosis assumes the highest priority for a patient admitted with a diagnosis of Guillain-Barré syndrome?

(1) Risk for impaired skin integrity related to immobility

(2) Risk for ineffective breathing pattern related to ascending paralysis

(3) Risk for disuse syndrome related to muscle atrophy

(4) Altered elimination: constipation related to immobility and decreased peristalsis

The correct answer is Choice (2). The keywords for this question are *highest priority* and *Guillain-Barré syndrome.* Although ineffective breathing pattern is a potential (risk for) diagnosis, it's the highest priority in this case. *Guillain-Barré syndrome* is a peripheral neuropathy in which patients experience ascending paralysis. Respiratory muscles can be affected, resulting in respiratory compromise. Nursing measures are directed at early identification of this complication of the syndrome so that patients can receive adequate respiratory support if needed. The wording "assumes the highest priority" tells you that this is a prioritization question: All the options may be correct (indeed, they are), but preventing a compromised airway is a priority (remember your ABCs).

EXAMPLE

A patient with a history of cirrhosis of the liver is admitted to the emergency department with massive bright red hematemesis. The nurse's first priority is to

(1) Initiate two IV lines with 18-gauge catheters

(2) Prepare for endoscopy by performing a gastric lavage with normal saline solution

(3) Perform a focused nursing assessment

(4) Draw blood to be sent to the lab for a type-and-crossmatch test

The keywords for this question are *history of cirrhosis of the liver, massive bright red hematemesis,* and *nurse's first priority.* The correct answer is Choice (3). It's the only option that's an assessment; the other options are all interventions. The patient is experiencing an acute upper gastrointestinal bleed. Although all the options are correct and should be implemented, the nurse must first assess for signs of shock by checking vital signs, urine output, and signs of decreased peripheral perfusion. Remember, in most situations, assessment comes first!

EXAMPLE

A client has had a surgical amputation of his right lower extremity below the knee. Which nursing measure will have the greatest priority in planning his care?

(1) Encouraging the client to verbalize his feelings about the loss of limb

(2) Referring the client to a support group for amputees

(3) Teaching the client about wound care prior to discharge

(4) Using strict sterile technique when changing dressings

The correct answer is Choice (4). The keywords for this question are *amputation of his right lower extremity, nursing measure,* and *greatest priority.* Remember that physiologic needs come first on Maslow's hierarchy. Maintaining strict aseptic technique when changing the dressing helps decrease the incidence of wound infection, a major complication of this surgery. The other needs are psychosocial and knowledge needs and, although important, don't assume as high a priority.

EXAMPLE

A 22-year-old man is brought to the emergency department after sustaining a skull fracture in a motor vehicle accident. Thirty minutes after his admission, the nursing assessment reveals a Glasgow Coma Score decrease from 10 to 5, signs of nuchal rigidity, and changes in mental status. On the basis of the nursing assessment, what is the priority nursing intervention?

(1) Notifying the physician of the client's change in status

(2) Implementing measures to decrease intracranial pressure

(3) Minimizing environmental stimuli

(4) Protecting the client from injury if seizures occur

The keywords for this question are *22-year-old man, sustaining a skull fracture, Glasgow Coma Score decrease from 10 to 5, nuchal rigidity, changes in mental status,* and *priority nursing intervention.* The correct answer is Choice (1). The client is exhibiting signs of an acute deterioration in neurologic status, and the physician must be notified immediately. In this case, the nurse has already completed a focused assessment and identified a potentially life-threatening emergency. The other options are interventions and may be needed, but the priority is to contact the physician.

EXAMPLE

A patient who is receiving a transfusion of packed red blood cells develops chills and a temperature of 101.5 degrees Fahrenheit. The nurse's priority action is to

(1) Slow the transfusion and notify the physician

(2) Stop the transfusion and notify the physician and blood bank

(3) Discontinue the IV catheter

(4) Administer Benadryl 50 mg po as per MD order

The correct answer is Choice (2). The keywords for this question are *transfusion of packed red blood cells, chills and a temperature of 101.5,* and *nurse's priority action.* The patient is experiencing symptoms of either a febrile transfusion reaction or an acute hemolytic reaction. The transfusion must be immediately stopped and the patency of the IV line maintained by infusing normal saline solution. The nurse must notify the physician immediately, and the blood bank should also be notified. Discontinuing the IV is incorrect because you need IV access in a patient with an acute hemolytic reaction.

Avoiding Test Question Pitfalls

Although NCLEX-RN questions may seem designed to trip you up and make you feel like a fool, that's not the case. The questions make sure you have the critical-thinking skills you need to be a safe nurse, and that involves making sense out of information that's sometimes confusing and difficult to evaluate. They're really testing your ability to "see through" the distractors (wrong answers). Enter: questions that test your ability to get all the facts and evaluate them properly.

Don't read into the question

Reading into questions is a major pitfall. You can easily read into a question and get the wrong answer because you're looking for something that's not there. How can you avoid this pitfall in test taking?

>> Read the question thoroughly and carefully while asking yourself, "What is the question specifically asking me?" Use keywords to help you figure out the topic of the question.

>> Be alert to important terms and phrases as well as true and false response questions.

>> Focus only on information in the question — no more, no less. Avoid asking yourself, "What if they're looking for this?" or "Do they really mean that?"

>> Read and consider every option presented.

>> Use all your nursing knowledge, your clinical experiences structured by your instructor, the test-taking skills that you acquired in nursing school, and the strategies covered in this chapter to settle on the correct answer.

TIP

When reading the question and the answer options, use the process of elimination. Reread the question, and determine what the question is asking specifically. It may be helpful for you to whisper the question to yourself, but this approach could get you into trouble, especially if you have a "stage whisper" — you know, one that people can hear across the room. But sometimes hearing a question out loud helps you internalize the answers, and the question becomes clearer.

If you're faced with questions that require you to fill in a blank, focus on all the information requested and reread it. What is the question specifically asking? If the question requires you to do a medication calculation, recheck your work and calculation with the pull-down calculator to verify your answer before moving on to the next question.

Read the whole question and reword it

Sometimes you look at a question and just can't seem to get what it's asking. In these cases, looking at the question from a different angle may be helpful. Follow these simple steps to put the question in other words:

1. Read the question carefully, reading all the words.

No speed-reading or skimming like you did in your cramming days!

2. Look for hints in the question from keywords.

Keywords such as *first, most,* and *initial* are favorites for priority-setting questions.

3. Change the words around to make the sentence more simple and complete.

Turn it into a statement to see whether it's true.

TIP

The phrase "further teaching is necessary" indicates that the answer contains incorrect information. And the phrase "client/caregiver understands the teaching" indicates that the answer contains correct information.

The following is an example of a question related to normal patient findings that requires you to reword the question in order to determine the answer:

EXAMPLE

A patient is brought into an emergency department complaining of chest pressure. His blood pressure is 160/98 with a pulse of 94 and respirations of 22. A nurse administers nitroglycerin 0.4 mg sublingual as ordered. Reevaluation in five minutes reveals that the patient's blood pressure is 100/72 with a pulse of 94 and respirations of 20. What should the nurse do next?

(1) Note that the patient has become hypotensive and obtain an order to administer fluid.

(2) Place the patient in semi-Fowler's position and administer oxygen at 4 L per minute.

(3) Administer a second dose of nitroglycerin.

(4) Document the results and continue to monitor the patient.

The correct answer is Choice (4). The keywords here are *complaining of chest pressure, blood pressure is 160/98, pulse of 94 and respirations of 22, nurse administers nitroglycerin, reevaluation in five minutes, blood pressure is 100/72 with a pulse of 94 and respirations of 20,* and *nurse do next.* If you were to reword this question, it would say, "What do you do for a patient who has a normal response to nitroglycerin?" The key to this question is knowing what the normal response to nitroglycerin is and understanding how the medication works. Because the findings are normal, the other interventions aren't necessary.

Eliminate wrong answers

When answering questions, use the process of elimination and look for similar answer options. Any options that include the same idea are incorrect, and you can eliminate them. Usually, the option that's different from the others is the correct response.

Here's an example of a question in which you can use the process of elimination to arrive at the correct answer:

EXAMPLE

A nurse is assigned to care for a group of patients. Reviewing the patients' medical records, the nurse determines that one of her patients is at risk for excess fluid volumes. Which patient is it?

(1) The client with an ileostomy

(2) A client on diuretics

(3) A client on continuous gastric suctioning

(4) A client in renal failure

Keywords in this question are *risk for excess fluid volumes* and *which patient?* The correct answer is Choice (4). This client is the only one with a condition that involves retaining water. All the other clients are losing water. You need to know the pathophysiology of each of these clients' conditions in order to treat them accordingly.

REMEMBER

Eliminate options that contain absolute words, which tend to make an option incorrect. Absolute words include the following:

>> All

>> Always

>> Every

>> Most

>> Never

>> None

>> Only

Try not to predict answers

Many people try to predict the answer before reading the entire question. Follow these tips to avoid this pitfall:

>> When you first read the question, if an obvious answer comes to mind, restrain yourself from looking for it in the answer choices.

>> Read each option twice.

>> Use the spacebar on the keyboard to highlight each choice as you consider it. For each answer option, say to yourself "Yes, this answers the question," "No, this doesn't answer the question," or "Maybe this answers the question."

>> If you have an immediate preference for an option on a multiple-choice question, read all the choices to be sure that your choice is the only "yes" answer. If you have only one "yes" answer at that point, then you've successfully eliminated the other three distractors.

>> If you identify more than one "yes" option for a single multiple-choice item, then evaluate the other options in terms of which is more "yes" than "maybe." If you can't determine which is a "yes," then choose the strongest "maybe."

TIP

Always choose the answer that has the highest probability of being a "yes." Review all options critically, and if you see options that are opposites, know one of them is probably the "yes" answer.

2

Testing Your Knowledge of Client Needs

Handle patients' rights and care. Understand your legal obligations.

Work to prevent injuries, accidents, and infections and know what to do when they happen anyway. Be ready for disasters and emergencies.

Monitor growth, development, health, and wellness. Implement care plans and maintain cultural sensitivity.

Get a handle on how people behave and help clients through abuse, grieving, and crises.

Apply the basics, such as hygiene, sleep, and mobility. Brush up on complementary therapies and nonpharmacologic approaches.

Medicate patients properly through a variety of methods.

Focus on typical lab tests and results. Perform proper conscious sedation.

Understand how the balance (and imbalance) of body fluids relates to health.

Chapter 5

Management of Care

According to studies done by the National Council of State Boards of Nursing, the nurse's role in patient care has changed drastically over the years. The nurse in today's healthcare setting is responsible for managing all aspects of the patient's care: legal, ethical, information, security, and referrals. Nurses have to know how to maintain clients' rights; uphold laws and regulations; coordinate with the rest of the healthcare team and other stakeholders; provide individualized, cost-effective care; and support patients' independence. And that's not just for the NCLEX but also for real-world practice on the facility floor.

This chapter delves into the variety of plates nurses have to be able to keep spinning and provides sample exam questions on these topics so you're ready for both the test and what comes next.

First Things First: Knowing Your Patient's Rights

Nurses are frequently faced with matters that may or may not be related to direct patient care, such as dealing with death and dying issues and healthcare decisions when the patient can't make them. When faced with this kind of situation, the following documents convey the patient's desires and dictate whether a nurse is permitted to take care of the patient at all:

» **Advance directives:** What the patient wants to be done for their health in the event that he or she is unable to make those decisions.

» **Client rights, also known as the Patients' Bill of Rights:** Reflects the patient's acceptance to participate in care with an emphasis on his or her autonomy. A hospital can't violate these rights, which include the client's right to be able to refuse treatment or medications and so forth. This document sets up the relationships between the client, system, and providers.

Although most NCLEX-RN questions that address these guidelines don't specifically state the guideline itself, you must choose the answer that reflects your knowledge of these guidelines. Most of the time, these types of questions may seem to be asking you to begin a treatment or procedure when what you really should do is first ensure that patient's rights are being respected.

The following sections discuss important patient rights.

You must heed prearranged treatment options

An *advance directive* is a document signed by a competent person giving direction to healthcare providers about that person's treatment choices in certain circumstances. The two types of advance directives are

» **Durable power of attorney for healthcare:** Also referred to simply as *durable power;* allows a person to name a patient advocate to act for the patient and carry out the patient's wishes. The patient advocate helps the patient work with others who have an effect on the patient's health, including doctors, nurses, insurance companies, case managers, and lawyers.

» **Living will:** Allows a person to state his or her wishes in writing but doesn't name a patient advocate.

When a patient picks an advocate: Durable power of attorney for healthcare/medical

A durable power of attorney for healthcare is a legal document that allows a patient to name anyone at least 18 years old to be an advocate and make healthcare decisions for the patient. The patient may pick a family member, friend, or any other trusted person. A durable power can accept or refuse any treatment for the patient; if the patient wants his or her advocate to be able to refuse any treatment, then this permission must be stated specifically in the durable power document. A durable power goes into effect only when the patient is unable to make decisions for himself or herself.

A question related to advance directives may look like the following:

A nurse is caring for an 86-year-old man who has been in the intensive care unit for two weeks. The patient is on a ventilator after having a cerebral vascular accident (CVA). The doctors and nurses on the unit are discussing whether a feeding tube should be inserted into the patient. During the discussion, which of the following statements made by the nurse would be most appropriate?

(1) "I will insert the tube as soon as the doctor's order is written."

(2) "I will check the chart to see if the patient has an advance directive."

(3) "We should call a meeting with the patient's family first."

(4) "I will call the patient's daughter and ask her what she wants us to do."

The keywords for this question are *86-year-old man, on a ventilator, CVA, feeding tube should be inserted,* and *statements made by the nurse would be most appropriate?* The correct answer is Choice (2). The patient is on a ventilator, so he can't tell the healthcare workers his wishes. If the patient can't speak for himself, the nurse must know whether he has an advance directive in his chart before starting any treatment that requires consent or agreement on the part of the patient.

When a nurse has to be the patient advocate

Nurses can advocate for patients at any time, and they often do in that they take the patient's concerns and help change the care plan to allow the patient to get what he or she needs. Nurses need to ensure that the patient knows the treatment options and respect the patient's choice after the decision is made. They also must educate the other staff under them as to the client's rights and the staff's responsibilities to the client. As a patient advocate, a nurse may work with social workers, those in the chain of command at work, and interpreters to ensure the client understands the information given.

The following is an example of a question related to patient advocacy:

EXAMPLE

An infant is in need of an IV. The child's mother is very upset and worried because the last time the child needed an IV, several attempts were made before the insertion was successful. Which of the following actions taken by the nurse would address the mother's concerns?

(1) Assuring the mother that this time it will go better

(2) Staying with the child during the procedure

(3) Calling the IV team to ensure that the most experienced person inserts the IV

(4) Letting the doctor know that the mother is worried

Keywords for this question are *infant, in need of IV, mother is very upset and worried, last time the child needed an IV, several attempts were made before the insertion was successful,* and *actions taken by the nurse would address the mother's concerns.* The correct answer is Choice (3). As a patient advocate, the nurse is charged with providing the most effective care and addressing the patient's concerns. Making statements that the nurse can't support isn't appropriate, and just supporting the patient's concern isn't taking steps to address the problem.

All lips must remain sealed

Patients share personal information with nurses. You have a duty as a nurse to respect the patient's trust and keep this information private by restricting others' access to the information. Furthermore, creating a trusting environment by respecting patient privacy can encourage the patient to be as honest as possible during the time in which you care for him or her. When the nurse and the medical team know all that's affecting the patient's well-being, they can provide the best care.

Questions related to patient privacy may resemble this:

EXAMPLE

The nurse is caring for an emergency room patient who was in a motor vehicle accident and is now in X-ray. A phone call regarding the patient is transferred to the nurse. When the nurse answers, a woman on the phone states she's the patient's wife and wants to know what happened and how her husband is doing. Which of the following responses by the nurse would be most appropriate?

(1) "I know you're upset, but I can't give out information regarding any patient over the phone."

(2) "I'll transfer you to the doctor so that he can explain the extent of the injuries."

(3) "The patient is currently in X-ray and is doing well."

(4) "The patient will call you himself when he gets back from the X-ray."

The correct answer is Choice (1). The keywords for this question are *emergency room patient, motor vehicle accident, in X-ray, woman on the phone states she's the patient's wife,* and *which of the following responses by the nurse would be most appropriate?* Although refusing to answer the questions of a worried family member may seem heartless, sometimes the caller really isn't a family member; it may be an insurance agent, lawyer, or someone who may use the information to harm the patient.

Respecting a client's confidentiality ensures that the patient receives safe care. In this case, the nurse can tell the patient that his wife called, but telling the wife that the patient will call her when he gets back from X-ray reveals too much information. Other healthcare providers are bound to the same confidentiality clauses as nurses and aren't permitted to share patient information either.

Information and technology changes

Healthcare has moved right along with all the changes in technology. These changes call for the nurse to follow more security procedures. Gone are the days of paper charts in hospitals and looking through long stacks of paper health history. This information is now accessible online.

But this technology has created more things to be aware of, such as passwords for accessing patient charts and protocols for totally closing down computers prior to leaving them. Figuring out how to document in an electronic health record (EHR) brings new challenges for the nurse when dealing with doctors' orders and charting.

Here is an example of an NCLEX question related to these technological concerns:

EXAMPLE

After a busy morning, the nurse is finally charting online in the hallway for her care of a client in room 204. The hallway is full of visitors for her new patient just a few steps away. An emergency light comes on in another room. Which of the following actions should the nurse do next?

(1) Minimize the screen and go help the emergency client

(2) Turn the screen around toward the wall

(3) Leave the computer as it is and go

(4) Close all screens prior to answering the emergency call light

Keywords in this question are *charting online in the hallway, hallway is full of visitors, emergency light comes on,* and *which of the following actions should the nurse do next?* The correct answer is Choice (4). The nurse needs to close the computer screens and protect the information from any visitors walking past. The other options leave visitors — or anyone — able to view the client's information.

Nothing happens without informed consent

Informed consent is the client's agreement, based upon an appreciation and understanding of the facts and implications of any actions or outcomes, to have his or her body touched by someone else, period; it's only valid if a patient is in possession of all his or her faculties and not mentally impaired at the time of consenting. Impairments include sleep, intoxication, and being under the influence of drugs or other health problems that interfere with judgment.

The healthcare provider is responsible for informing the patient about the risks and benefits of the procedure or surgery. The nurse serves as a witness and is responsible for ensuring that the patient or patient's designated advocate signs the consent. The nurse also ensures that the person signing the consent understands what's happening and that all of his or her questions are appropriately addressed.

There are times, however, when informed consent can't be obtained. For example, when a patient is unconscious and needs emergency surgery to save her life and her advocate can't be reached. In such a case, the client is taken directly to surgery.

The following question is an example of exam questions related to informed consent:

EXAMPLE

A doctor comes out of the room of a patient who is going to have a lumbar laminectomy. The doctor hands the nurse the signed consent form. Which of the following would make the nurse question the reliability of the consent?

(1) The patient doesn't ask the nurse any questions afterward.

(2) The patient was given a sedative 30 minutes prior to the doctor's visit.

(3) The patient doesn't speak fluent English but is accompanied by an interpreter.

(4) The patient's wife was present when he signed the consent.

The correct answer is Choice (2). Keywords for this question are *lumbar laminectomy, doctor, hands the nurse the signed consent,* and *nurse question the reliability of the consent.* What conditions from the answer choices may make the nurse doubt the obtained consent? You know that anything that impairs a patient's judgment invalidates a consent form, and the sedative in Choice (2) may do just that. None of the other options impair judgment.

Ethical decisions don't require your opinion

Ethical practice involves recognizing when decisions have ethical components, knowing how your personal values and beliefs affect ethical decisions, and making ethical decisions despite your personal feelings about the choice. You need to be able to evaluate the outcomes of interventions designed to promote ethical practices. This practice encourages nurses to practice in a way that is consistent with the code of ethics for nurses.

The following example question is related to ethical practice:

EXAMPLE

A nurse is caring for a postpartum patient. The nurse provides discharge teaching for the patient and reviews birth control options with the patient. The patient then asks the nurse, "Which birth control method is best?" The nurse's best response would be

(1) "Which birth control method do you feel most comfortable with?"

(2) "Oral contraceptives like the pill are the best birth control method."

(3) "Personally, I find the diaphragm most useful."

(4) "Condoms work best at preventing sexually transmitted infections."

Keywords for this question are *postpartum patient; discharge teaching; birth control options; asks the nurse, "Which birth control method is best?";* and *the nurse's best response.* The best reply from the nurse is therapeutic and requires the patient to provide her feelings and thoughts about the topic at hand. The correct answer is Choice (1). Even though this response may seem vague, the nurse is allowing the patient to choose the method that's best for her. *Best* is a subjective word, and therefore the best method is the one that's best for the patient. You may be thinking, "But isn't the pill best? Or even a condom?" If the question were to ask which method were the most *effective,* then those answers would be more appropriate because effectiveness is measurable. Giving a patient a personal opinion is always wrong.

REMEMBER

The answer to this question turns the question back to the patient, which is a common strategy when helping patients make decisions.

Rallying the Troops: Managing Care

Most students find answering questions regarding the management of patient care confusing and difficult, mostly because those questions require a clear understanding of the roles and responsibilities of other healthcare workers. Many nursing students are so busy trying to keep the sterile field intact that they have no idea who else is responsible for providing care to the patient and don't even think about being the one to oversee it. When you put these considerations together, NCLEX-RN questions that reflect your knowledge of care management can easily seem overwhelming.

This section looks at the different responsibilities a nurse has with patient care management and includes examples of related questions that may appear on the exam.

Assuring the quality of patient care

Patient care policies and procedures follow strict guidelines that are determined by governing bodies to ensure that all care that patients receive is equal and fair. *Quality assurance* is a set of procedures designed to ensure that medical professionals adhere to quality standards and processes and that the care a patient receives meets or exceeds the required technical and performance requirements. Quality assurance requires all hospitals and patient care facilities to develop standards of practice and policies that maintain high quality care and meet accreditation guidelines. Some of the ways in which hospitals and patient care facilities maintain high quality care include the following:

>> Providing therapeutic communication

>> Maintaining confidentiality — reviewing a breach if it occurs and putting into place policies or practices that prevent another breach

>> Knowing a patient's care needs and advance directives

>> Evaluating client goals

>> Preventing injury by reviewing all incidents that caused injury or no injury

One of the ways in which nurses consistently maintain quality care is by following *critical pathways* (also known as *care plans*) that identify care strategies and expected outcomes for patients with specific health issues. Critical pathways include all aspects of patient care, from admission to discharge, and they ensure continuity of care when different nurses take care of the same patient. In order to achieve the expected outcomes for the patient, the nurse must follow the critical pathway, evaluate whether goals are being achieved, and, if they aren't being achieved, know how to modify the care. The patient and family need to be made aware of the plan and be in agreement with the goals and outcomes. Nurses also use critical pathways to provide patient education and to address discharge plans.

The following two questions address quality assurance issues:

EXAMPLE

A patient who is one day postoperative is supposed to ambulate today. When the nurse gets the patient out of bed, he becomes dizzy. What is the best nursing action to take?

(1) Assist the patient back to the bed and reevaluate his condition.

(2) Try to get the patient into a chair.

(3) Call the doctor and ask to have the order changed to bed rest.

(4) Have the patient do some deep breathing to avoid feeling dizzy.

The keywords for this question are *one day postoperative, ambulate today, gets the patient out of bed, he becomes dizzy,* and *best nursing action to take.* Reworded, this question asks, "Which action is the best nursing action for a patient who gets out of bed and becomes dizzy?" The correct answer is Choice (1). Returning the patient to bed and reevaluating is the first step in maintaining patient safety, which is a quality assurance requirement. (On the exam, you may have a question that appears to address one topic but really includes all aspects of client safety.) Getting the patient into a chair may cause injury if the patient continues to feel dizzy, and having the patient do deep breathing may cause increased dizziness from hyperventilation. Although calling the doctor may be appropriate, it isn't the first action to take.

TIP

If you only pick up one new piece of information before you take the NCLEX-RN, make it this: Patient safety is always a priority, so when you encounter an exam question with an answer option that involves safety, choose that answer!

EXAMPLE

A patient is receiving a blood transfusion of packed red blood cells (PRBCs). The nurse instructs the patient on signs and symptoms to report. The patient calls the nurse back to the room after a few minutes and states that he feels itchy. Which is the best action for the nurse to take?

(1) Stop the transfusion.

(2) Take a set of vital signs.

(3) Obtain a urine specimen.

(4) Notify the physician.

The correct answer is Choice (1). Keywords for this question are *transfusion of packed red blood cells, instructs the patient on signs and symptoms to report, calls the nurse back to the room after few minutes, feels itchy,* and *best action for the nurse to take.* The correct answer is Choice (1). Procedures such as blood transfusions follow specific protocols that reflect standards of practice. When a patient begins to complain about physical symptoms during a blood transfusion, the nurse should prevent further injury by stopping the infusion. The other actions are appropriate, but none are the best action because they don't prevent further injury.

Prioritizing when your hands are full: Group care

Determining priorities for care is one of the most difficult aspects of the NCLEX-RN. The exam includes test questions that require the establishment of priorities and coordination and the delegation of client care responsibilities. When prioritizing group care, you need to look at each client in the group and assess his or her individual needs; only then can you decide whose needs are most urgent and how much caring for each patient will take. To determine priority, look at who is in the most life-threatening condition or is the most unstable.

Questions about prioritizing group care may look like this:

EXAMPLE

A nurse has been assigned to care for multiple patients. Which patient would the nurse assess first?

(1) A patient requesting pain medications three days postoperatively for abdominal surgery

(2) A patient ready for discharge

(3) A patient requiring routine dressing changes

(4) A patient receiving oxygen who is breathing normally but had difficulty on the previous shift

The correct answer is Choice (4). This question's keywords are *multiple patients* and *which patient would the nurse assess first?* Choice (4) is correct because in the previous shift the patient complained of difficulty breathing. Inability to breathe would be life threatening if it exists. The other patients are stable. Don't fall for the distractors.

Tailoring care for each patient: Case management

Case management is a form of patient care management that usually requires organizing and coordinating resources and services in response to individual healthcare needs. The goals of case management are

>> To center high-quality services around the patient's needs

>> To foster patient self-managed care and to help maintain independence (for example, by providing discharge instructions)

>> To maximize efficient and cost-effective use of health resources (what would be the most effective but cost the least)

Case management involves collaboration, comprehensive assessment, developing a plan, monitoring the plan, and evaluating the plan of care and use of resources. These days, nurses are becoming more and more involved in client case management, so it's an area that the NCLEX-RN wants to be sure you understand.

The nurse is the best person to be involved in the management of a case because the nurse is the one who's on the front lines with the patient. The nurse spends the most time with the patient, does the most comprehensive assessment of the patient and his or her needs (for example, O_2, suction machine, and so on), and has the most knowledge of the patient.

Other healthcare providers come to the nurse to ask about assessment findings, patient responses, patient concerns, and whether the patient is meeting patient-centered outcomes. When it comes to case management issues, informing other healthcare providers of changes in the patient's condition, such as by updating the care plan, is the nurse's responsibility.

The following three questions are related to case management:

EXAMPLE

While ambulating a 73-year-old patient with rheumatoid arthritis, the nurse notes edema of the lower extremities, diminished pedal pulses, and cool skin on the left leg. Which action should the nurse take next?

(1) Put the patient on strict bed rest.

(2) Elevate the patient's leg.

(3) Place a warm compress on the affected area.

(4) Notify the patient's doctor.

Keywords for this question are *73-year-old patient, rheumatoid arthritis, edema of lower the extremities, diminished pedal pulses, cool skin on the left leg,* and *which action should the nurse take next?* The correct answer is Choice (2). Use the symptoms and age of the patient to decide the answer. Edema, diminished pedal pulses, and cool skin are all signs of poor circulation. Elevation of the extremity helps reduce edema while the nurse notifies the doctor.

Putting the patient on bed rest and applying a warm compress aren't independent nursing judgments because the activity level and the application of heat or cold require doctor orders. Notifying the physician is an appropriate action, but it shouldn't be the first one taken. After notifying the physician, the nurse must be prepared to report complete assessment findings and nursing interventions that have been implemented to address the problem. The physician then orders care that's within the medical domain.

The nurse enters the room of a 42-year-old woman who has just been diagnosed with adrenocortical insufficiency (Addison's disease). Which of the following assessment findings should be reported to the physician immediately?

(1) A blood pressure of 106/68

(2) Blood glucose of 48

(3) A bronze color to the skin

(4) Bleeding gums

The correct answer is Choice (2). The keywords in this question are *42-year-old woman, diagnosed with adrenocortical insufficiency,* and *assessment findings should be reported.* Adrenocortical insufficiency signs and symptoms are dehydration, dizziness, fainting, fatigue, lightheadedness, loss of appetite, low blood pressure, low blood sugar, and electrolyte imbalances. Management of this patient requires the nurse to know which assessment finding requires immediate attention. Although patients with Addison's disease tend to run lower BPs and have bronze skin tones and gum disease, the blood glucose finding requires something to be done to prevent further decompensation. This case is an example of how the management of patient care requires the nurse to know when (and whom) to call for help.

An 82-year-old woman is being discharged home after a colostomy placement for colon cancer. She lives alone and has some limited visual fields due to macular degeneration. Which of the following interventions by the nurse would ensure the patient makes a smooth transition to caring for her colostomy at home?

(1) Teaching the patient's daughter how to care for the colostomy

(2) Explaining to the physician that the patient isn't ready to go home

(3) Contacting the hospital's home-care department to see what services are available

(4) Discussing nursing home options with the patient and her family

Keywords for this question are *an 82-year-old woman, discharged home after a colostomy placement, lives alone, some limited visual fields, macular degeneration, interventions by the nurse,* and *ensure the patient makes a smooth transition to caring for colostomy at home.* So which intervention keeps the patient caring for her colostomy at home the most? The correct answer is Choice (3).

Remember, it's all about the patient's independence in caring for herself. Nurses must know what services are available to patients in order to ensure that discharges home are safe. The patient may need more teaching and follow-up assessments in the home before other options are discussed. Because the patient lives alone, teaching the daughter to care for the colostomy may not ensure daily care, and delaying the discharge isn't necessary when the patient can be managed at home with assistance from a home-care nurse.

Collaborating with other medical team members

One of the most important things to remember about managing patient care is that you know what's happening with the patient better than any other person on the healthcare team. As I note in the preceding section, your assessment findings are the first and often most complete assessments, so you must manage the team. The manager of any team has to know what each of the team members is able to do and coordinate how all the members achieve the team's goal.

In a healthcare scenario, the patient's needs are the focus of the team. The nurse is the team manager, and other team members may include physicians; nurse practitioners; occupational, respiratory, and physical therapists; and social workers, child life specialists, and other people who have specific functions in making sure that the patient receives appropriate and safe care. Collaboration usually includes planning care that allows all the other team members to be able to work with the patient in optimal conditions.

This example question relates to the nurse's management of patient care:

EXAMPLE

The nurse is caring for a 6-year-old who's scheduled to have a tonsillectomy. The child is very afraid of needles and tells the nurse that he won't allow anyone to stick him with a needle. The doctor has ordered that an IV be started. Which of the following actions would be most useful in helping the child cope with his fears?

(1) Explaining the procedure

(2) Having the child work with the child life specialist

(3) Offering a reward for good behavior

(4) Avoiding discussion of the procedure until it's time to start the IV

The correct answer is Choice (2). The keywords for this question are *6-year-old, scheduled to have a tonsillectomy, afraid of needles, won't allow anyone to stick him with a needle, ordered that an IV be started,* and *most useful in helping the child cope with his fears.* The child is afraid and needs to be able to express his feelings. Which answer allows the 6-year-old to do so? Utilizing the child life specialist to use play as therapy can help a young child express his fears about a situation or procedure. Explaining the procedure may not address the child's fears; rewards are useful, but they don't help the child cope with fears. Avoidance is never a therapeutic way to deal with any situation.

Getting others to lend a hand: Delegation

The *delegation* process, which is giving a task or assignment to someone else to complete, is the most common management area that you come across as a nurse. As a nurse these days, you don't have to provide all the care a patient needs simply because he or she is your assigned patient — you can get some help. In fact, you have the legal responsibility to practice within the legal scope of practice and to delegate to others within their legal scope of practice.

Delegation isn't as hard as you think. You can rely on delegation guidelines that are consistent for every patient situation to help you make the appropriate delegation decisions when necessary. Here are the rules:

» **Never delegate patient assessment, patient teaching, or evaluation.** These tasks are always and forever the responsibility of the RN.

» **Delegate tasks that follow standard procedures, such as taking vital signs.** Unlicensed assistive personnel (UAP) can do vital signs, give baths, ambulate patients, take weights, empty catheters, deal with meal intake, and feed patients who have no risk of aspiration. But they can't give medications, insert catheters, insert nasogatric (NG) tube, or read labs or take orders.

>> **Delegate tasks for stable patients with expected outcomes.** Licensed practical nurses (LPNs) can take care of chronic conditions such as COPD, hypertension, and so on as long as the patient isn't in an exacerbation. LPNs can give per mouth (PO), intramuscular (IM), and subcutaneous medications, and IV fluids. But they generally can't give IV push medications or IVPB antibiotics. LPNs can insert catheters and NGs, but after surgery, the LPN can't assess the NG if a problem has occurred and the patient is unstable.

Stick to these simple rules, and you can't go wrong. The remaining challenge is figuring out what patients need to meet delegation criteria. With every patient, ask yourself the following three questions. If the answer to any of the questions is "yes," you can't delegate.

>> Does this patient need an assessment?

>> Does this patient need to be taught something?

>> Is this patient most likely to become unstable?

When delegating, you must communicate which tasks need to be completed and give a time frame for reporting back any concerns. You're responsible for evaluating the care given by others and their ability to perform the tasks assigned.

The following questions address delegation:

EXAMPLE

The nurse is planning care for a patient who's hospitalized after an acute myocardial infarction. The patient is on a telemetry monitor and has an IV infusing into his left hand. Which of the following duties can't be assigned to unlicensed assistive personnel?

(1) Taking an EKG (electrocardiogram)

(2) Interpreting an EKG reading

(3) Replacing the electrodes from the telemetry monitor

(4) Removing the electrodes from the telemetry monitor

The keywords for this question are *planning care, acute myocardial infarction, on a telemetry monitor, IV infusing,* and *duties can't be assigned to unlicensed assistive personnel.* Reworded, the question looks like "Which of the following can you not assign to unlicensed assistive personnel because it's out of their scope of practice?" The correct answer is Choice (2). Interpreting an EKG reading is an assessment and requires judgment and critical thinking, so it's an RN responsibility. The other duties follow a prescribed set of standard procedures and are the same for any patient. You can delegate them because they don't require judgment, only knowledge of the task.

EXAMPLE

The nurse is getting ready to begin caring for a group of patients. Which of the following patients should not be assigned to the LPN?

(1) A 36-year-old woman whose status is postmastectomy

(2) A 49-year-old man who will be getting out of bed following a knee replacement

(3) A 62-year-old woman who has just been admitted for a spinal fusion

(4) A 91-year-old man who's on oxygen and requires Q two hour turning and positioning

Keywords for this question are *a group of patients, should not be assigned,* and *LPN.* Which patient should the RN not give to the LPN because the needs are out of his or her scope of practice? The correct answer is Choice (3). Remember, LPNs take care of stable clients. Who is stable? Who requires teaching? Who requires an assessment? In this case, all the patients are stable even though some have had surgery. The woman who has just been admitted requires an admission assessment and possible pre-op teaching, so the nurse shouldn't delegate her care to the LPN.

EXAMPLE

The nurse is making the daily assignment of the unlicensed assistive personnel. Which of the following would be the most appropriate assignment for unlicensed assistive personnel?

(1) Feeding a patient who has difficulty swallowing

(2) Performing glucose monitoring for the diabetic patients

(3) Going over discharge instructions with a patient with a colostomy

(4) Changing a dressing on a decubitus ulcer stage 3

Keywords for this question are *daily assignment*, *most appropriate*, and *unlicensed assistive personnel*. Which of the assignments can a UAP do within his or her scope of practice? The correct answer is Choice (2). Glucose monitoring is a procedure with specific guidelines, and collecting the data doesn't require judgment or critical thinking. Interpretation of the glucose results is the responsibility of the nurse, but a unlicensed assistive personnel can handle the test safely. The other patients in this scenario require either assessment or teaching and should remain the assignment of the registered nurse.

Recognizing Legal Rights and Nursing Responsibilities

Today's healthcare system presents many ethical and legal dilemmas for nurses. Nurses are legally accountable for all the care they provide and even for the care they don't provide. A nurse must understand some aspects of civil law (also known as the law of torts) in order to ensure that a patient's legal rights are maintained. An understanding of torts as they apply to healthcare can help you keep that license that you work so hard to obtain.

» **Unintentional tort:** Unintentional tort can be negligence or malpractice. Both negligence and malpractice can be intentional or accidental failures to meet the standard of care. *Malpractice* is a type of professional negligence that occurs when the nurse fails to meet a standard of care and that failure may end up injuring the patient. For example, a nurse forgets to give a dose of insulin to a diabetic patient, and the patient ends up in diabetic ketoacidosis.

» **Intentional tort:** A willful act that violates another person's rights. To qualify as an intentional tort, the act doesn't have to cause injury to the patient. The three types of intentional torts are

• **Assault:** Threatening the patient. For example, saying "If you don't eat, I'll put this NG down and feed you that way" constitutes assault.

• **Battery:** Striking the victim, knocking the victim down, or otherwise doing violence to the victim. Touching a client without his or her consent is battery even if no injury occurs.

• **False imprisonment:** Intentionally restraining another by physical force or the threat of physical force without privilege or authority. For example, restraining a patient who's agitated without first obtaining a physician's order for restraints is false imprisonment.

» **Quasi-intentional tort:** An act involving communication that may violate a person's privacy or civil rights or adversely affect his or her reputation. This kind of tort includes breach of confidentiality as defined by

• **Defamation of character:** A false statement about someone, either written or oral, that leads to harm. For example, a patient's friend overhears an unlicensed hospital employee imply that the patient is having an affair with his doctor. The family friend relays this unfounded information to the patient's wife, who then sues for divorce.

• **Slander:** An oral defamation of character with the intention to hurt someone's reputation.

- **Libel:** Slander in writing. For example, a nurse documents in a chart that a patient is using drugs without verifying the information.

- **Invasion of privacy:** Violation of the client's right to keep information private. For example, the nurse answers a phone call from someone who claims to be a patient's relative and gives confidential information regarding the patient's diagnosis over the phone; it turns out that the caller was from an insurance company.

Other legal issues nurses need to be aware of include the following:

>> **The client has the right to refuse treatment and medications.** Knowing this fact, and what do when this situation occurs, is part of the responsibilities of the nurse.

>> **Nurses are responsible for managing a client's valuables according to facility policy.**

>> **Nurses need to know when and what to report in cases of assaults, injuries caused by animals, child or elder abuse, or communicable disease, as well as unsafe/illegal practices by other healthcare workers.**

On the NCLEX-RN, questions that involve knowledge of legal responsibilities may resemble the following:

EXAMPLE

A nurse is having lunch in public with another nurse who works in the same clinic. They're discussing a patient who was treated for a sexually transmitted infection earlier in the day. The patient's husband is sitting at the next table and overhears their conversation. Which tort are the nurses guilty of?

(1) Slander

(2) Defamation of character

(3) Assault

(4) Invasion of privacy

The keywords in this question are *having lunch in public, discussing a patient who was treated for a sexually transmitted infection, the patient's husband is sitting at the next table,* and *which tort are the nurses guilty of?* The important fact here is that the husband hears the conversation at lunch in a public place, so others there may hear also. That makes the correct answer Choice (4). The nurses' conversation is an invasion of privacy because they violated the patient's right to keep information private. Slander intentionally hurts someone's reputation using false oral statements; defamation of character intentionally hurts someone's reputation using false statements (either oral or written), and assault involves the threat of physical contact.

EXAMPLE

A patient who's scheduled for a biopsy in the morning signs the consent form but then changes his mind about having the procedure. What is the most appropriate action taken by the nurse?

(1) Attempting to convince the patient that the procedure is necessary

(2) Explaining to the patient that, without the procedure, he may not be able to receive treatment for his condition

(3) Calling the physician to report the patient's decision and documenting the action

(4) Telling the patient that the consent form is a legally binding document and must be honored

Keywords in this question are *scheduled for a biopsy, signs the consent, changes his mind,* and *most appropriate action taken by the nurse.* So if the client has decided against having the biopsy and tells the nurse, what action should the nurse take next? The correct answer is Choice (3). Informing the physician of the patient's decision is important because the physician is part of the collaborative team and is responsible for directing the patient's medical plan. Choices (1) and (4) — convincing the patient to have the procedure and telling him that the consent form is a binding legal document — aren't therapeutic and don't help him make an informed decision. Telling the patient that he may not be able to receive treatment if he doesn't have the procedure is punitive.

Knowing Where to Get the Support You Need

The people behind the NCLEX-RN don't just want to be sure that you're able to make safe patient care decisions and follow all legal and ethical guidelines when managing patient care situations. They also want to know that you, as a new nurse, know how to get what you need to be able to perform all your new skills and responsibilities. The following sections cover some of the ways nurses accomplish that task.

Keeping up with education and training

All nurses must adhere to policies and standards that are set in writing. Nurses also are involved in evaluating and revising these policies and standards and therefore must continue to educate themselves on new research findings and new ways of practicing nursing even after they leave nursing school. This area is known as *continuing education* or *staff development*. As a new nurse, you continue to learn things that improve your skills and critical thinking.

Most hospitals and patient care facilities expect all the nursing staff to participate in facility-based education programs that ensure that everyone follows all safety protocols. The following sections break down some of these areas of training.

CPR

Nurses also must demonstrate competency in national safety standards such as cardiopulmonary resuscitation (CPR). Keeping current on approved CPR steps (which are updated regularly with small changes) so you can maintain CPR certification is required for nursing practice positions. Be sure you're also aware of how the steps are different for administering CPR to infants and children.

The following question is related to CPR:

EXAMPLE

The nurse enters a patient's room and finds the patient unresponsive. Which of the following actions should the nurse take immediately?

(1) Call for help.

(2) Shake the patient and shout, "Are you okay?"

(3) Place the patient in a supine position.

(4) Start rescue breathing.

The correct answer is Choice (2). Keywords for this question are *finds the patient unresponsive, actions,* and *nurse take immediately.* You must establish true unresponsiveness before starting any of the cardiopulmonary protocols. The other options are part of the CPR protocol.

Emergencies

Knowing the standard protocols that nurses must follow is important not only because they appear on the NCLEX-RN but also because they're expected in practice. Nurses also are expected to respond to specific situations that constitute emergencies. This action is known as disaster planning. Nurses have specific roles in disaster management with regard to patient safety, and you're expected to participate in safety drills and to know how to ensure safety on the units. The nurse's responsibilities in a disaster or emergency situation include

>> Handling hazardous and infectious materials

>> Considering and protecting patient safety

>> Prioritizing patient needs for groups of clients

>> Assessing mental health

>> Performing crisis management

Here's a question that addresses disaster planning:

EXAMPLE

The nurse comes on duty at 8 a.m. After she receives reports and begins to organize care for her select group of patients, the fire alarm begins to ring. Which action taken by the nurse indicates that the nurse is aware of fire safety?

(1) Close all doors on the unit.

(2) Begin to move patients for evacuation.

(3) Leave the unit to get help.

(4) Instruct all visitors to leave the building.

Keywords for this question are *fire alarm begins to ring, action taken by the nurse,* and *aware of fire safety.* The correct answer is Choice (1). Remember RACE when answering similar test questions:

>> **R**escue patient

>> **A**ctivate alarm

>> **C**ontain fire (or **C**lose doors on the unit)

>> **E**xtinguish

In the example question the alarm already has been activated, so the nurse correctly moves to the next step in the process — she closes all doors to prevent fire or smoke from spreading. Hospital administration decides when to move patients for evacuation, leaving the unit qualifies as abandonment, and instructing visitors to leave may complicate rescue efforts. Choice (3) of leaving the unit is not a part of RACE, even to go get help. It's not rescuing, containing, or extinquishing the fire.

REMEMBER

Much of what is expected of nurses in providing a safe and effective environment requires not only knowledge of specific nursing functions but also knowledge of other disciplines and how they contribute to the safe choices made in nursing care.

Expecting adequate supervision

All new nurses should expect adequate supervision from their superiors. Managers are responsible for the actions of their staff members and must see to it that they grow and have success. Adequate supervision includes the following:

>> Providing clear direction for what's to be done and how to report back

>> Following up on care given by others to ensure care and tasks are done correctly and in a timely manner

>> Providing educational instruction for those who need to improve on the care they're giving or tasks they're undertaking

Questions related to nursing supervision may look like this:

EXAMPLE

The nurse manager on your unit is an excellent role model. She actively encourages participation in the unit's decision-making process and helps everyone improve their skills. This manager is effectively functioning in what role?

(1) Manager

(2) Autocrat

(3) Leader

(4) Authority

The correct answer is Choice (3). Keywords for this question are *excellent role model, encourages participation, unit's decision-making process, helps everyone improve, effectively functioning,* and *what role.* A leader influences the success of a unit by being an excellent role model while guiding and facilitating staff growth. Managers may have formal power, but a leader exhibits these additional qualities. An autocrat just tells you what to do, and authority is conveyed by the position someone holds.

Making referrals

Although some NCLEX-RN preparation books tell you not to refer to anyone, I say if you can't do anything for a patient, refer the patient to someone who can help. An example would be a patient who needs help with activities of daily living (ADLs). Nurses are limited in helping patients regain independence, so referring to occupational therapy by getting an MD order is the most appropriate step for the nurse in this case.

EXAMPLE

A CVA patient is struggling to walk to the restroom without help. The nurse assists the patient while he's in the hospital. The nurse worries how this patient will manage these needs at home. Which of the following represents the most appropriate action by the nurse?

(1) Tell the patient to keep working on it at home and he'll soon be able to do it smoothly

(2) Tell the family to find the patient a nursing facility

(3) Tell the patient he needs a wheelchair

(4) Ask the doctor for an occupational therapy (OT) order to help provide the patient assistance

The keywords for this question are *struggling to walk to the restroom without help, how this patient will manage these needs at home,* and *most appropriate action by the nurse.* The correct answer is Choice (4). The doctor can provide the order for an occupational therapist to see the patient and determine if something could help him be more independent. Telling the patient he just needs to practice, finding a nursing facility, and getting a wheelchair don't promote independence.

Chapter **6**

Safety and Infection Control

I f you remember no other nursing principle for the NCLEX-RN, remember that safety always comes first. Safety is the second tier of Maslow's hierarchy of needs, and it needs to be addressed as soon as the basic physiologic needs are met. When you pass the NCLEX-RN, you're assumed to have the ability, skills, and knowledge to be a safe and effective nurse at the entry-level RN position. That means that, among other things, you're expected to keep your patient from falling out of bed and also to know that giving him a medication he's known to be allergic to is a big mistake.

Safety and infection control is a subcategory of the client needs section of the exam. This area focuses on maintaining environmental safety and preventing accidents. Environmental safety — fire safety, electrical safety, safe radiation therapy, and proper disposal of infectious wastes — is the first consideration for preventing accidents and injuries. The client needs portion of the NCLEX-RN also tests your knowledge of the proper use of restraints and nursing actions that should be taken in the event of a disaster, of biological and chemical warfare agents, and of infant abduction. In this chapter, I address all these elements of the client needs section as well as how to protect patients from infection and how to document any incidents that do occur.

Preventing Accidents and Injuries

Keeping your patients safe is your first responsibility. That doesn't just mean giving them the correct medications at the correct times (although careful medication dispensing certainly is a part of being a safe practitioner). It also means preventing accidents, maintaining a safe environment with equipment, and knowing what to do in case of a disaster or fire. If you're working in a home environment, part of your job is assisting clients and families to identify environmental hazards in the home and educating them about accident prevention. In today's disaster-conscious world, you also may need to educate families and patients on what to do at home in case of a natural disaster or emergency (see the section "Disaster Planning and Emergency Response" for more).

In the following sections, I look at the most common areas that can lead to accidents and safety hazards. As well as giving good patient care, you also must protect your patients when they're in your care.

REMEMBER

EXAMPLE

If you get a safety question, remember that human needs come before mechanical needs. An example of a safety question follows:

A nurse is caring for a patient with chronic renal failure who just completed a hemodialysis treatment. On assessment, the nurse notes that the patient's temperature is 101.5 degrees Fahrenheit. Which of the following is the initial nursing action?

(1) Monitor all vital signs.

(2) Monitor the shunt site.

(3) Monitor the IV tubing.

(4) Monitor the machine for contamination.

The keywords for this question are *chronic renal failure, hemodialysis, temperature is 101.5*, and *initial nursing action*. The correct answer is Choice (1) because it's the only one that focuses on the patient first and not on mechanical needs. This answer demonstrates that you have the ability to ensure patient safety. For example, if monitoring shows that the patient's temperature remains elevated, you should suspect sepsis.

Using electrical equipment safely

REMEMBER

Following facility procedures is important when using various kinds of equipment. If the equipment is unfamiliar to you, contact the staff development department, a biomedical department, or your supervisor for information regarding the use of that particular equipment. Don't try to figure out something unfamiliar by yourself! Be sure to read any available manufacturer's literature or attend any in-service education given regarding the operation of equipment that you're not used to working with.

If you're working with a piece of equipment that you suspect is malfunctioning, meaning that it doesn't do what it's supposed to do consistently or correctly, it makes unusual noises, or it gives off unusual smells or extreme temperatures, then heed the following:

>> Don't try to repair it.

>> Remove the equipment from the patient's environment immediately.

>> Replace it immediately.

>> Contact maintenance or the appropriate department so that the faulty equipment can be checked, repaired, and safely put back to work.

Hospitals are full of electrical equipment, and many medical folk are so used to seeing it that they often don't give it the respect it deserves. Electricity can be dangerous! When working with electrical equipment, nurses need to follow these safeguards:

>> Electrical equipment must be kept in good working order.

>> Electrical equipment needs be grounded. Always use equipment with a three-pronged plug.

>> Any electrical equipment that a client brings into the healthcare facility must be inspected for safety before use. Check with your nursing supervisor for the correct process for your facility.

>> Check exposed electrical cords and outlets for frayed or damaged wires.

>> Avoid overloading any circuits.

>> Read all the warning labels on equipment, and never operate unfamiliar equipment.

>> Use safety extension cords only when necessary, and never run electrical wiring under carpets.

>> Never use electrical appliances near sinks, bathtubs, or other water sources.

>> Always disconnect the plug from the outlet before cleaning equipment or appliances.

>> If a client receives an electrical shock, turn off the electricity before touching the client.

Questions related to safe equipment use may look like this:

EXAMPLE

A homecare nurse performs a home safety assessment and sees that a client is using a space heater. Which of the following instructions should the nurse provide to the client regarding the use of the space heater?

(1) A space heater shouldn't be used in an apartment.

(2) A space heater needs to be placed at least three feet away from anything that can burn.

(3) A space heater should be shut off at night.

(4) A space heater should be kept on a low setting at all times.

Keywords for this question are *home safety assessment*, *space heater*, and *which of the following instructions should the nurse provide to the client regarding the use of space heater*. The correct answer is Choice (2). Space heaters need to be used appropriately because they present a great risk of fire. A space heater should be placed at least three feet from anything that can burn. Turning off a space heater at night defeats the purpose of having one, and using it on a low setting doesn't reduce the risk of fire. Space heaters can be used in apartments if there's ample space and the user follows safety precautions.

Keeping clients from falling

One of the most common injury-related causes of hospital incident reports is patient — and staff — falls. Sensory loss (such as hearing and vision loss) can cause accidents, so assess patients for diminished senses. Developmental age can also have specific issues that can cause a fall. Although some tumbles aren't preventable, you can take a number of measures to help prevent your patients from falling and injuring themselves. Some of these measures include the following:

>> Assessing all new clients for their risks of falling

>> Maintaining a patient's toileting schedule throughout the day and night

>> Providing adequate lighting

>> Keeping personal items within reach

>> Explaining the use of the call bell system, keeping it within the patient's reach, and answering it in a timely fashion

>> Alerting all staff on the floor to a patient's risk for falling

>> Assigning a patient to a room near the nurses' station

>> Using any other safety and antifalling devices or systems that the institution may have

The following question is an example of a fall-related NCLEX-RN question:

EXAMPLE

A patient is admitted to the nursing unit from a skilled nursing facility. In the nurse's assessment, she notes that the patient may be at a higher risk for falling than another patient who's in the room directly across from the nurses' station. What would be an appropriate intervention for the nurse to do first?

(1) Put the patient in an available room down the hall.

(2) Put the patient in a chair by the nurses' station while the nurse checks for a room change.

(3) Have the patient transferred to another floor.

(4) Send the patient back to the skilled nursing facility.

Keywords for this question are *admitted, nurse's assessment, higher risk for falling than another,* and *appropriate intervention for the nurse to do first.* Higher risk for falling patients needs to have interventions put into place to protect them from injury. The correct answer is Choice (2). Patient safety is the primary concern, so the first intervention is to put him in a chair while requesting a room change. The other actions listed aren't in the patient's best interest.

Disaster Planning and Emergency Response

Your role in disasters varies dramatically depending on the type of institution you work in as well as the type of unit you work on. You must know the disaster plan of the facility you work in. Disasters come in many different scenarios:

>> **Internal disasters** occur inside the facility and put it and its inhabitants in danger. An example of an internal disaster is a large chemical spill in the laboratory.

>> **External disasters** occur in the community and send victims to a healthcare facility for treatment. An example of an external disaster is a major bus accident.

>> **Man-made disasters** include a structural collapse of something, terrorist attacks, and radiological accidents.

>> **Natural disasters** may be in the form of earthquakes, floods, landslides, forest fires, tornadoes, hurricanes, and so on.

When your healthcare agency is notified of a disaster, follow the guidelines specified in the agency's disaster plan. The nurse's role in disaster planning consists of making his or her own personal and family preparations and being aware of the disaster plans at the place of employment and in the community. If you're present at an internal disaster, your role depends on the directions identified in the disaster plan. In a community setting, nurses are first responders to disasters; you care for victims by attending to those with life-threatening problems first.

Triage in the emergency department is about setting priorities according to patients' needs for care, the types of illnesses they have, and the severity of either the injury or illness. Clients with trauma, chest pain, severe respiratory distress, or cardiac arrest are the number one priorities. Patients with conditions such as simple fractures, lacerations, minor respiratory conditions, fever, abdominal pain, or renal stones are classified as number two priorities. Anything else comes after them.

The following question is an example of disaster- and emergency-related questions on the NCLEX-RN:

EXAMPLE

An emergency department nurse is assigned to triage patients arriving for treatment after an auto accident. The nurse should assign the highest priority to which of the following patients?

(1) The patient with inward movement of an area of his chest when inhaling and outward movement on exhalation

(2) The patient with swelling and bruising to his knee

(3) The patient complaining of muscle aches and a backache

(4) The patient with small lacerations on his head with significant bleeding

This question's keywords are *triage patients, auto accident,* and *highest priority to which of the following patients.* So which patient has the most life-threatening condition or is most unstable? The correct answer is Choice (1). Inward movement of the chest during inhalation describes paradoxical breathing, which indicate respiratory distress. All other options are not life threatening.

Sounding the alarm: When fires break out

Fires aren't uncommon emergencies wherever nurses work, be that at a patient's home, a hospital, or a nursing home. Fires can spread rapidly, so acting quickly can mean the difference between life and death for you and your patients. The following guidelines help you and your patients remain safe in the event of a fire:

>> Keep open spaces free of clutter.

>> Ensure that fire exits are clearly marked.

>> Know the locations of all fire alarms and extinguishers.

>> Know the telephone number for reporting fires.

>> Know the fire drill and evacuation plans of your floor and agency.

>> Never use an elevator during a fire.

>> Turn off oxygen and appliances in the vicinity of the fire.

REMEMBER

Oxygen is frequently in use in hospitals and, if around flames, will increase the fire's ability to spread and grow. When oxygen is in use, no open flames or smoking are permitted in the area. You also need to remove all flammable liquids from the area and post "oxygen in use" signs per institutional policy. Secure oxygen in appropriate places when not in immediate use.

If a fire occurs, you can direct ambulatory patients to walk by themselves to a safe area; in some cases, they may be able to assist in moving clients in wheelchairs or in beds. If a client must be carried from the fire, appropriate transfer techniques should be used, and if fire department personnel are present, they can help evacuate patients.

Most hospitals teach the acronym RACE to make remembering what to do first in case of fire easy:

1. **R**escue: Remove all clients from the vicinity of a fire.

2. **A**larm: Activate the fire alarm. Report the fire before attempting to extinguish it.

3. **C**onfine: Close doors and windows when the fire is detected.

4. **E**xtinguish: Extinguish the fire by using the appropriate fire extinguisher.

You can put out a small fire by smothering it with a blanket, but if you're the one aiming the red can, you must remember that different types of fires need different types of extinguishers. Using the wrong fire extinguisher can make a fire worse! Know these types of fire extinguishers and where to find them in your unit or nursing environment:

>> **Class A:** Wood, cloth, rubbish, paper, and plastic

>> **Class B:** Flammable liquids or gases, grease, and tar

>> **Class C:** Electrical equipment

>> **Class ABC:** Works on Class A, B, and C fires and is the most commonly used extinguisher in hospitals today

Fire extinguishers aren't quite point-and-shoot devices. And when your adrenaline's pumping, you don't want to be fumbling while a fire continues to burn. To use any type of fire extinguisher, remember the acronym PASS, and follow these instructions:

1. **P**ull the pin.

2. **A**im at the base of the fire.

3. **S**queeze the handles.

4. **S**weep the extinguisher from side to side.

Test questions related to fire safety may resemble the following:

EXAMPLE

The nurse enters a patient's room and finds that the wastebasket is on fire. The nurse immediately assists the client out of the room. What is the next nursing action?

(1) Confine the fire by closing the room door.

(2) Activate the fire alarm.

(3) Call for help.

(4) Extinguish the fire.

The correct answer is Choice (2). Keywords for this question are *wastebasket is on fire, immediately assists the client out of the room,* and *next nursing action.* The first priority in the event of a fire is to rescue clients who are in immediate danger, but the nurse in this question has already done that. Use RACE to remember that the next step is activating the alarm. Then you confine the fire by closing all doors and lastly extinguish the fire.

EXAMPLE

A nurse enters a patient's room and discovers that the chair is on fire. She rescues the patient, pulls the alarm, closes the door, and obtains the fire extinguisher to put out the fire. The nurse pulls the pin on the fire extinguisher. The next appropriate action in the use of the fire extinguisher is to

(1) Squeeze a handle on the extinguisher

(2) Sweep the fire from side to side with the extinguisher

(3) Aim at the base of the fire

(4) Sweep the fire from top to bottom with the extinguisher

Keywords for this question are *chair is on fire, rescues the patient, pulls the alarm, closes the door, obtains the fire extinguisher, pulls the pin,* and *next appropriate action in the use of the fire extinguisher.* The correct answer is Choice (3). Remember PASS. The nurse has already pulled the pin, so the next action is to aim at the base of the fire. Then she'll squeeze the handle of the extinguisher and extinguish the fire by sweeping from side to side.

Responding to terrorism or bioterrorism

As the world changes, nurses play more and more of a role in dealing with terrorism and bioterrorism. *Bioterrorism* is warfare with biological or chemical substances that can cause mass destruction and fatalities.

The NCLEX-RN may ask you to identify a biological terror agent or chemical used in this type of terrorism. Some of the agents of terrorism and bioterrorism are

» **Biological:** Smallpox, anthrax, plague, botulism, Ebola hemorrhagic fever, ricin, hantaviruses, and tularemia

» **Chemical:** Nerve agents (sarin), blood agents (cyanide), blister agents (mustard gas), pulmonary or choking agents (phosgene), and other agents such as tear gas and pepper spray

» **Small arms and explosives**

» **Nuclear and radiological weapons**

You need to be aware of your facility's policies concerning terrorism or bioterrorism emergencies; policies for such events are usually similar to disaster plans and may vary greatly depending on where your facility is located. Although it's sad to say, today's world requires preparation for such events.

Keeping Infectious Bugs at Bay

Two of nursing's primary functions are to prevent patients from getting infections and to keep infections from spreading to other patients. An *infection* is an invasion of the body by pathogens that multiply and produce injurious effects. An infectious disease that may be transmitted from one person to another is a *communicable disease. Nosocomial infections*, also referred to as *hospital-acquired infections* or *healthcare-associated infections*, are acquired in a hospital or other healthcare facility and weren't present or incubating at the time the patient was admitted.

Illness impairs the body's normal defense mechanisms, and a hospital environment provides exposure to a variety of organisms that a patient hasn't been exposed to in the past. Therefore, the patient hasn't developed resistance to these organisms. Healthcare personnel who fail to practice proper hand-washing procedures or fail to change gloves between client contacts can transmit infections. Most healthcare agencies have dispensers containing an alcohol-based solution for hand rubs mounted at the entrance to each client's room as well as a stock of gloves usually available outside and inside a patient's room for healthcare workers to use. However, you must remember that different bugs require different sprays — or precautions, rather.

This section has a rundown of all things infection-prevention-and-protection-related and states loud and clear the laundry list of precautions you must take when being near or handling potentially hazardous infections or materials. I even provide a handful of example questions similar to those you're likely to find on the NCLEX-RN.

Maintaining medical and surgical purity

Germs are everywhere. You're covered with them no matter how clean you are! Keeping germs to a minimum in healthcare facilities is important for keeping patients safe from infection, especially in areas such as surgery or with patients who have diseases that lower their resistance to infection.

REMEMBER

Asepsis is the absence of disease-producing organisms. The two types of asepsis are medical and surgical. Medical asepsis is often referred to as a *clean technique.* Surgical asepsis is often referred to as a *sterile technique.*

Medical asepsis is practiced to reduce the number of microorganisms that leave the body or to reduce transmission of microorganisms to other clients. Hand-washing and decontamination are the primary components of medical asepsis, but in general, medical asepsis

>> Uses standard precautions

>> Uses isolation techniques

>> Involves the cleaning and disinfecting of equipment

For the details of these precautions and techniques, see the following section.

Surgical asepsis is the practice of destroying pathological organisms before they enter the body through an open wound. Surgical asepsis

>> Uses physical barriers (masks, gowns, drapes, and protective eyewear)

>> Is practiced during procedures with a high risk for infection, such as

- Catheter insertion of any kind

- Surgical wound dressing changes

- Special medication injections

- Transplantation

- Treatment of burns, especially third-degree and those requiring total removal of the skin

- Treatment of immunosuppressed and immunocompromised patients, such as those receiving chemotherapy and those with AIDS

The *sterile field* is an area in which sterile materials for sterile procedures are placed. A sterile field is usually a table covered with a sterile drape; in an operating room, you find multiple sterile areas covered with sterile drapes. When working with and around sterile fields, remember the following rules; if you don't, someone *will* yell at you, especially in the OR!

>> A dry field is necessary to maintain sterility of the field.

>> Sterile containers are no longer sterile after being opened.

>> Barrier techniques, as discussed in the following section, are required.

>> Keep your hands in front of you and above your waist at all times.

>> Never reach across a sterile field with unsterile items, including ungloved hands.

>> Movement in and around the sterile field must not contaminate the field.

>> A sterile field must remain sterile throughout the entire procedure.

Here are two examples of NCLEX-RN questions related to asepsis:

Which of the following is a proper technique for medical asepsis?

(1) Wearing gloves for all patient contact

(2) Changing the linen weekly

(3) Using your hands to turn off the water after you wash them

(4) Putting on a gown to care for a 1-year-old child with infectious diarrhea

The keywords for this question are *proper technique* and *medical asepsis.* The correct answer is Choice (4). A nurse should wear a gown when infected material is likely to soil his or her clothing. Gloving isn't required for all patient contact, and linen should be changed as necessary. When washing hands, a nurse should use a paper towel to turn off the faucets.

Which of the following procedures requires a nurse to use surgical asepsis?

(1) Changing a central-line dressing

(2) Cleaning around a urinary catheter

(3) Changing linen for a patient in isolation for a drug-resistant infection

(4) Preparing food for a toddler

Keywords for this question are *procedures* and *surgical asepsis.* The correct answer is Choice (1). Surgical asepsis is required for a central-line dressing change. Cleaning around a urinary catheter and changing linen for a patient in isolation both require medical asepsis. Surgical aseptic technique isn't required for food preparation.

Differentiating among the types of infection precautions

Nurses must practice standard precautions with all clients in any setting, regardless of the diagnosis or presumed infectiousness. *Standard precautions* apply to blood, body fluids, secretions, and excretions (except sweat), regardless of whether they contain blood or are on intact skin or mucous membranes. In addition to standard precautions, you also need to know about the different types of infectious precautions to use depending on the type of infection a patient has. In this section, I cover the major types of infection-related equipment and interventions you need to keep in mind as you click away at the NCLEX-RN.

Standard precautions that you absolutely must remember, in practice and in test-taking, are as follows:

>> **Handle all blood and body fluids as if they were contaminated.**

>> **Wash hands** between client contacts; after contact with blood, body fluids, secretions, or excretions and after contact with equipment or articles contaminated by them; and immediately after removing gloves.

>> **Wear gloves** when touching blood, body fluids, secretions, nonintact skin, mucous membranes, or contaminated items. Remember to remove gloves and wash hands between patient contacts.

>> **Wear a mask, eye protection, or face shield** when involved with client-care activities that may generate splashes or sprays of blood or body fluid.

>> **Wear a gown** if soiling of clothing is likely.

>> **Clean and disinfect patient equipment** properly, and discard single-use items.

>> **Place contaminated linen in leak-proof bags** and handle carefully to prevent skin or mucous membrane exposure.

>> **Discard all sharp instruments** and needles in a puncture-resistant container, and dispose of needles uncapped or use a mechanical device for recapping if necessary and available.

>> **Clean spills of blood and body fluids** with a solution of bleach and water or an agency-approved disinfectant while wearing gloves.

REMEMBER

You use standard precautions with HIV patients and any other patient unless the patient has an infectious condition. Unless the HIV patient has another condition that requires a different type of precaution, standard is the only one used.

Transmission-based precautions include airborne, droplet, and contact precautions. Each is handled differently, but you need to know them all!

>> **Airborne precautions** are taken for diseases such as chickenpox (varicella) and tuberculosis. When dealing with these diseases, remember the following:

• Area barrier protection for airborne precautions includes having the patient in a single room under negative pressure with the door closed except when somebody enters or exits the room.

• The nurse should maintain negative airflow pressure in the room with a minimum of 6 to 12 air exchanges per hour, depending on the healthcare agency standard.

• Healthcare providers must use a respirator that is specific to the infectious agent (for example, an N-95 mask to prevent tuberculosis). The client must wear a mask when leaving the room and should leave only when necessary.

>> **Droplet precautions** are taken for diseases such as adenovirus, epiglottitis, influenza, mumps, pertussis, pneumonia, rubella (German measles), and sepsis. When dealing with these diseases, remember the following:

• The patient must have a private room or must be paired with patients with the same infection(s).

• Healthcare providers must wear masks when in the same room as the client.

• The client must wear a mask when leaving the room and should leave only when necessary.

>> **Contact precautions** are taken for diseases or infections with multidrug resistant organisms; enteric infections such as clostridium difficile; respiratory infections; wound infections; skin infections such as cutaneous diphtheria, herpes simplex, impetigo, scabies, herpes zoster (shingles); and eye infections such as conjunctivitis. When dealing with these types of diseases and infections, remember the following:

• You must wear gloves and a gown when in contact with the client.

• The client must have a private room or must room with a patient who has the same infection(s).

TIP

Table 6-1 shows some of the most common infectious conditions with the type of transmission-based precautions used for those conditions. Setting up charts such as this one for studying purposes can be a helpful aid.

TABLE 6-1   **Common Infectious Conditions and Precautions**

Condition	Transmission-based precautions	Infectious Material
Varicella (chickenpox)	Airborne and contact	Airborne droplets; Skin lesions
Clostridium difficile	Contact	Feces
German measles/rubella	Droplet (doesn't require a room with airflow ventilation)	Respiratory secretions
Herpes simplex	Contact	Lesion secretions
Tuberculosis	Airborne	Airborne droplet nuclei
Pertussis	Droplet	Respiratory secretions

Protective precautions are taken for patients who are immunosuppressed and have very low white blood cell counts. The measures are to protect the patient, not the nurse or others. When dealing with these types of patients, remember the following:

> ❯❯ You must wear gloves, a gown, a mask, and goggles when in the room with the patient.

> ❯❯ The client must have a private room.

Here are a few examples of exam questions that deal with infection precautions:

EXAMPLE

A nurse is caring for the following patients who are on different types of infection control precautions. The nurse isn't required to wear a mask when caring for which of these patients?

(1) A 6-year-old with meningitis

(2) A 33-year-old with diphtheria

(3) A 14-year-old post bone marrow transplant patient

(4) A 6-month-old with cholera

Keywords in this question are *different types of infection control precautions, isn't required to wear a mask,* and *which of these patients.* The correct answer is Choice (4). Knowing the transmission-based precautions for each patient helps make this question easy. Cholera is a contact infection and therefore doesn't require the nurse to wear a mask. Meningitis and diphtheria are transmitted by respiratory means, and a bone marrow transplant patient is susceptible to airborne germs.

EXAMPLE

The nurse is caring for a client with a healthcare-associated infection caused by penicillin-resistant staphylococcus aureus. Contact precautions are initiated as the nurse prepares to provide colostomy care to the patient. Which protective equipment is required to perform this procedure?

(1) Gloves, gown, and eye protection

(2) Gloves and eye protection

(3) Gloves, gown, and shoe covers

(4) Gloves and gown

This question's keywords are *healthcare-associated infection, penicillin-resistant staphylococcus aureus, contact precautions, colostomy care,* and *which protective equipment is required to perform this procedure.* The correct answer is Choice (1). Colostomy care can involve splashing and spray, so the infectious item in penicillin-resistant staphylococcus aureus is the feces. Protective eyewear is warranted to protect the mucous membranes of the eyes during interventions that may cause splashes. In addition, contact precautions require the use of gloves and a gown if direct patient contact is anticipated. Shoe protectors aren't necessary and usually aren't required unless the nurse wants to protect his or her shoes from splashes.

EXAMPLE

An adult has been treated for pulmonary tuberculosis (TB) and is being discharged home with his wife and two children. His wife asks how TB is passed from one person to another. To help the wife prevent anyone else from catching it, how should the nurse respond?

(1) "You should wear gloves when handling his linen and bedding because you can get tuberculosis by touching the germs."

(2) "You should keep the windows and doors closed so as not to spread the droplets."

(3) "He must be careful to cough into a handkerchief that's washed in hot water or discarded after use."

(4) "Make sure to boil all milk before drinking or using it."

Keywords for this question are *pulmonary tuberculosis*, *discharged home*, *wife and two children*, *the wife asks how TB is passed*, and *how should the nurse respond*. The correct answer is Choice (3). TB is transmitted by airborne droplets, specifically the airborne droplet nuclei, so the answer you're looking for limits access to these droplets. Tuberculosis may remain in the air for long periods of time. Thus, care should be taken when coughing or sneezing to limit the spread of residue.

Handling hazardous and infectious materials

The handling and disposal of infectious/hazardous waste must adhere to very strict guidelines set by the state and federal governments. If these materials aren't handled appropriately and within all legal rules and regulations, an institution can face serious fines. The following are some general guidelines for handling infectious/hazardous waste:

» Handle all infectious materials as hazardous.

» Dispose of waste in designated areas, using only proper containers and making sure that red bags are used for red bag waste only.

» Don't put any contaminated waste in undesignated bags.

» Ensure that infectious material is labeled properly.

» Needles shouldn't be recapped or broken.

» Dispose of sharps immediately after use in closed, puncture-resistant disposal containers that are leak-proof and labeled or color-coded. Most sharps containers are red or have a red top and are clearly marked as a biohazard and a sharps container.

» Never remove the cover from the sharps container or attempt to retrieve anything from it.

Radiation safety is also a hazard issue in certain areas of the hospital. The following precautions need to be taken to avoid serious radiation exposure:

» Know the protocols, procedures, and guidelines of the healthcare agency in which you work.

» Label all potentially radioactive material.

» Limit the time spent near sources of radiation.

» Distance yourself as much as possible from the radiation source.

» Use a shielding device, such as a lead apron, whenever you must be close to the source of radiation.

» Anyone caring for a patient undergoing radiation treatment should monitor their own radiation exposure with a personal film badge.

>> Place a client with a radiation implant in a private room, and post an appropriate notification that there's a radiation hazard in the room.

>> Never touch dislodged radiation implants.

Exam questions related to radiation and radiation safety may resemble the following:

EXAMPLE

A nurse is caring for a patient with an internal radiation implant. Which of the following is an inappropriate component for the nurse to include in the plan of care?

(1) Place the client in a semiprivate room at the end of the hall.

(2) Wear gloves when emptying the client's bedpan.

(3) Keep all linens in the room until the implant is removed.

(4) Wear a lead apron when providing direct care to the patient.

The keywords for this question are *internal radiation implant, inappropriate component,* and *include in the plan of care.* The correct answer is Choice (1). Think about the appropriate actions to take for a patient with internal radiation implants to help you find the inappropriate choice. You'd wear gloves when emptying the client's bedpan, keep linens in the room until the implant is removed, and wear a lead apron when providing care (to protect yourself). That leaves Choice (1). A private room with a private bath is essential because it prevents accidental exposure of other patients or healthcare workers to the radiation.

Keeping Clients Down in a Way That Lifts Them Up

Restraints are protective devices used to limit the physical activity of the patient or to immobilize the patient (or just an extremity). Documenting the use of restraints is an important nursing requirement. Whereas the use of restraints was once fairly common, regulatory agencies pay very close attention to their use today; therefore, restraint use must be limited and meet rigorous regulatory requirements.

The two types of restraints are

>> **Physical restraints,** which restrict patient movement through the application of some kind of device

>> **Chemical restraints,** which are medications administered to inhibit specific behaviors in patients

You should try everything in your professional arsenal before you resort to restraining a patient. Some alternatives to restraining patients are

>> Explaining everything to the client and family and encouraging family and friends to stay with the patient. If the patient needs supervision, you may suggest that the family arrange for sitters.

>> Assigning confused and disoriented patients to rooms near the nurses' station and orienting the patient and family to their surroundings.

>> Instituting exercise and walking schedules as the client's condition allows while placing familiar items such as family pictures near the client's bedside. These personal items help clients become oriented to their surroundings.

>> Maintaining toileting routines and eliminating treatments that may be unnecessary as soon as possible.

REMEMBER

If the patient does require restraints, you must document the reasons for their use in detail and frequently. Documentation for a patient in restraints needs to include the following information:

>> The reason for the restraint

>> The method of restraint

>> Date and specific time of application

>> Duration that the restraint was applied, or the duration of the use of a chemical restraint

>> The client's response to restraints

>> Record of release from restraints with periodic exercise and circulatory, neurovascular, and skin assessments

>> Assessment of continued need for restraint

>> Evaluation of the client's response to restraints

REMEMBER

If you didn't document it, you didn't do it! Always document the preceding information when using restraints.

As I mention earlier in this section, you can't just slap restraints on a patient who's getting on your nerves — you have to follow some strict protocol, and you have to have valid reasons for suggesting the use of restraints. Some of the legal requirements include the following:

>> If restraints are necessary, a physician's order must state the type of restraint called for, identify the specific behaviors for which the restraints will be used, and limit the time frame for their use.

>> Physicians' orders for restraint should be renewed within the time frame established by agency policy.

>> Restraints can't be ordered "PRN" or "as needed."

>> Permission to use restraints should be granted by the patient and family if restraints are necessary.

>> Restraints can't be secured to the side rails; rather, the nurse should use an easy slipknot to secure the device to the patient's chair or bed frame.

>> Assure enough slack on the straps to allow some movements of the body or body parts that are restrained.

>> Skin integrity and neurovascular and circulatory status must be checked and documented every 30 minutes.

>> The restraint must be removed at least every two hours to permit muscle exercise and promote circulation. This activity must be documented as well.

>> The need for restraints must be continually assessed and documented.

Here are some sample questions related to the proper use of restraints:

EXAMPLE

A nurse is delegating care to unlicensed assistive personnel (UAP) who will be caring for a patient in wrist restraints. The nurse instructs the UAP to document the skin integrity at the restraint site

(1) Every half hour

(2) Every two hours

(3) Every three hours

(4) Every four hours

Keywords for this question are *delegating care, unlicensed assistive personnel (UAP), wrist restraints,* and *document the skin integrity at the restraint site.* Reworded, the question asks how often skin integrity for a restrained extremity must be documented. The correct answer is Choice (1). The nurse must instruct the UAP to check the restraints and skin integrity every half hour. Agency policy should always be followed regarding this aspect of care.

EXAMPLE

You're a nurse in a skilled nursing facility, and you're supervising several unlicensed assistive personnel (UAP). Which UAP best understands the use of restraints?

(1) The UAP who places all clients into bed with the side rails up

(2) The UAP who ties the ends of the restraints to the side rails

(3) The UAP who applies a jacket restraint to the client who pulls out IV lines

(4) The UAP who fastens the restraints with an easy slipknot to an area the client can't reach

This question's keywords are *skilled nursing facility, supervising several unlicensed assistive personnel (UAP),* and *understands the use of restraints.* Which nursing action shows an understanding of restraint use? The correct answer is Choice (4). Fastening the restraints with an easy slipknot to an area the client can't reach allows the UAP to easily remove the restraint if an emergency occurs. However, the client can't reach the knot or untie himself or herself. Choice (2) is wrong because the client can be injured if the side rails are moved. Choice (3) is wrong because a jacket restraint doesn't restrain the client's hands, and Choice (1) is wrong because most patients should be put into bed with the side rails down. With the side rails down, the patient is less likely to fall because he or she doesn't have to climb over the rails.

Accidents Happen: Knowing the Next Steps and Preparing an Incident Report

In my experience, the area of incident or variance reports is one that can get students in trouble on the NCLEX, so here's what you need to know. An incident report should be filled out whenever a negative event occurs or could have happened. For example, you should fill out a report if you find a patient has fallen, medication errors were made, or a visitor is injured while at the facility. This information is used to put procedures into place that help prevent similar incidents from happening in the future. Recording the facts helps determine what procedures need to be implemented. Be sure to know the steps to dealing with and filling out the report.

Briefly, the nursing process (covered in detail in Chapter 4) in the aftermath of an accident is as follows:

1. **Assess.**

2. **Treat any injuries found.**

3. Notify the charge nurse who will get help.

4. Make the client safe until the nurse returns.

5. Notify the doctor.

This step may include getting orders for treatment.

6. Return to reassess the client.

After following orders, you then fill in the incident report. Remember, the incident report includes just the facts, not what you think happened. When the report is complete, you give it to the nursing supervisor. It's confidential, so it cannot be copied or placed in the chart. This report is for the facility quality assurance which puts in place procedures that prevent incidents like this one.

The last step is to chart the incident, again including only facts, such as the following:

» Where did you find the client?

» What did you do for the client?

» When was the doctor notified, and what orders were received?

» What orders were completed, and what's the condition of the client now?

Make sure that, no matter where a test question places you in the process, you're able to state the next step.

Exam questions related to incident reporting may resemble the following:

A nurse walks into the room of a postoperative client to find the client on the floor. The nurse assesses the client for injuries and notifies the charge nurse. The nurse and other staff assist the client back to bed. Which of the following should the nurse do next?

(1) Notify the MD

(2) Fill in the incident report

(3) Chart that the client fell

(4) Make sure the client is safe

Keywords for this question are *find the client on the floor, assesses the client for injuries, notifies the charge nurse, assist the client back to bed,* and *nurse do next.* The correct answer is Choice (4). The safety of the client is the priority. Choices (1) and (2) are things the nurse does do, but not at this time in the process. Choice (3) is incorrect because the nurse doesn't know for a fact that the client fell. The nurse just found the client on the floor. Unless the question specifically says the nurse saw the client fall, always chart how the client was *found.*

Code Pink: Understanding the Protocol for Infant Abduction

Hospitals now initiate a *code pink* when an infant goes missing. At the time of birth, the mother is fingerprinted and baby has footprints taken and they get matching bracelets. The parents receive education about how to identify who can and who can't take the baby from their presence. If a baby comes up missing, the code pink is called and the unit and building go into lockdown mode. Then the staff asks the mother about who took the baby from their room, searches the hospital, and talks to staff and visitors in the area about whether they've seen the baby. Security from the hospital and police are involved in looking for the infant. A nurse is assigned to keep the parents informed as to the investigation and search.

Exam questions related to infant abduction may look like this:

EXAMPLE

A new mother calls the nurse for her baby to be brought back to her room. The nurse finds the baby isn't in the nursery. The nurse checks to ensure the doctor doesn't have the baby in a procedure room. What is the priority action by the nurse?

(1) Question the mother as to who took the baby from the room

(2) Search the whole hospital for the baby

(3) Call a code pink and lockdown the unit

(4) Question the staff and visitors on the floor as to seeing the baby

The keywords for this question are *baby isn't in the nursery, doctor doesn't have the baby in a procedure room,* and *the priority action by the nurse.* The answer is Choice (3). The other answers are things that do happen as part of the process, but calling a code pink and locking down the unit are a priority to stop the baby from being able to leave the unit or the building.

Chapter 7

Health Promotion and Maintenance

Keeping clients healthy is easier — not to mention cheaper — than curing them when they get sick. For this reason, knowing how to promote good health and how to recognize developmental norms are important skills for nurses. The NCLEX-RN includes questions related to maintaining good health. This category of questions isn't the largest on the exam, but it's one that many students find baffling, confusing, and stressful.

In this chapter, I show you how basic knowledge of the different stages of growth and development helps you to plan and implement nursing care. I also review common health and wellness assessment techniques and discuss the importance of family involvement in planning care as well as the importance of teaching patients to care for themselves. I include test questions in each section to illustrate what to expect from this area of the NCLEX-RN.

Surveying the Stages of Growth and Development

The best way to get a handle on the stages of growth and development is to know general milestones. For example, if you know what a 3-month-old can do and you know what a 6-month-old can do, you can figure out what a 5-month-old may be doing. You don't need to memorize all the different growth and development charts for the NCLEX-RN — just know the basics.

REMEMBER

Growth and development are different but interrelated in that they have profound effects on one another. *Growth* is a physiological process that's influenced by nutrition, environment, and development. *Development* is the acquisition of skills that's influenced by nutrition, environment, and physical growth. Keep these definitions in mind when reading questions that ask how you'd provide the most effective care for a patient of a particular age or one who's experiencing a specific developmental process.

Think of developmental milestones as a pass-fail system. To meet a milestone, all your client has to do is pass with a minimum grade. For example, if 74 out of 100 is a failing grade on a test, you pass whether you get a 75 or a 95. As a nurse, you're only concerned if patients don't meet their developmental milestones; you're not concerned with whether they get a 75 or a 95 on the "test." (Note, however, that many parents *are* concerned with their kids' "scores." They really don't want to hear that their child is "meeting his milestones" — they know he's a genius and want you to back them up!)

For children

Both parents and nurses need to give patients who are meeting developmental milestones tasks and experiences (and toys) that help them move forward to the next stage. Here are some basic guidelines on what developmentally appropriate items look like:

>> Babies learn best from adult stimulation and attention. They need things that they can see and hear.

>> Toddlers learn from experimentation with the environment. They need things that they can touch and that respond to them.

>> Preschoolers learn from things that stimulate the imagination. They need things with which they can create and pretend.

>> School-age kids like competition. They need to play games that allow for interaction with others and engage in activities that demonstrate their accomplishments.

>> Adolescents strive for independence and peer acceptance, so they need exposure to experiences that allow them to make decisions and take responsibility.

The following pointers, combined with your working knowledge of the growth-and-development fundamentals, will help you answer development questions:

>> Always choose an answer that relates to the child's developmental age, not his or her chronological age.

>> Patients who don't meet expected developmental milestones need further evaluation.

Questions concerning childhood growth and development may look like the following:

The nurse is choosing an activity for a slightly developmentally delayed 5-year-old whose interests are in line with those of a younger child. Which of the following items would the nurse choose to help the child achieve developmental milestones?

(1) Coloring books and crayons

(2) A 20-piece puzzle

(3) Modeling clay

(4) A video game

The keywords for this question are *slightly developmentally delayed 5-year-old, interests in line with those of a younger child,* and *help the child achieve developmental milestones.* The correct answer is Choice (3). The child in the question is achieving younger children's milestones and is showing interest in their interests, so you need to consider the developmental age of the child, not the chronological age. This 5-year-old is mildly delayed, so he's more likely to be interested in things that a toddler finds stimulating. Coloring is more for school age children. The 20-piece puzzle is appropriate for a preschooler. And playing a video game is an activity more for school age children and adolescents.

EXAMPLE

A 6-month-old is admitted to the hospital with a diagnosis of seizure disorder. He's placed in a crib and has an IV ordered. The nurse enters the room to start the fluid infusion and notes that the mother is sitting in a chair at the bedside, the infant is in the crib, and the side rails are partially raised. The nurse also sees a small stuffed toy and a rattle in the crib. As the nurse makes an assessment, which of the following would be of concern?

(1) The small stuffed animal in the crib within reach of the baby

(2) The rattle in the crib

(3) The partially raised side rails

(4) The child's mother sitting in a chair near the crib

Keywords for this question are *6-month-old, admitted to the hospital, seizure disorder, in a crib, IV ordered, the nurse enters the room, side rails partially raised,* and *a small stuffed toy and a rattle in the crib and most concern.* The correct answer is Choice (3). No matter what else is going on, safety is a priority. This question is an example of a safety question disguised as a growth and development question.

Picture the scene. Partially raised side rails are also partially down (just like the half-full glass is also half empty). Your knowledge of a 6-month-old's development should tell you that the side rails' being down is a safety issue. Any crib with a baby in it must have the side rails pulled all the way up. The other options are appropriate for a 6-month-old: soft toys, stimulating rattles, and, of course, Mom close by. Knowing what's appropriate at what age helps you eliminate things that aren't of concern.

EXAMPLE

A 16-year-old who is recovering from an appendectomy is refusing to allow her friends to visit her in the hospital. She says they really don't like hospitals and she'll see them when she gets discharged. Which of the following interpretations of the patient's statement explain her behavior?

(1) She is experiencing an altered body image.

(2) She is afraid that her friends may think she's contagious.

(3) She doesn't want her friends to feel inconvenienced by visiting her.

(4) She isn't feeling well enough for the company of friends.

This question's keywords are *16-year-old, recovering from an appendectomy, refusing to allow her friends to visit, says they really don't like hospitals and she'll see them when she gets discharged,* and *which of the following interpretations of patient's statement explains behavior.* The correct answer is Choice (1). Adolescents are very concerned about body image issues and how they're accepted by their peers. A 16-year-old would normally want her friends to be around her, but being in the hospital affects her body image and thus her ability to have her friends with her. Refusing to see friends or participate in social activities when they're experiencing health-related issues is typical of this age group.

EXAMPLE

The nurse is caring for a 9-year-old who is admitted to the hospital with an exacerbation of asthma. Which of the following items would the nurse present to the patient?

(1) A coloring book and markers

(2) Checkers

(3) Blowing bubbles

(4) A book about being in the hospital

Keywords for this question are *9-year-old, admitted to the hospital, exacerbation of asthma,* and *which of the following items would the nurse present to the patient.* The correct answer is Choice (2). A 9-year-old is school age, and school-age kids are competitive. Checkers is a game that facilitates competition.

REMEMBER

Don't put anything into the question that isn't already there. Most nursing students would choose coloring books in the preceding example because they read too much into the question and ask who would be available to play checkers with the patient. The NCLEX-RN wants to know whether you know what's developmentally appropriate for children of different ages and conditions. Blowing bubbles is used for respiratory chest expansion or as a distraction intervention. A book about being in the hospital may address some of the child's concerns, but it doesn't help the child meet developmental milestones.

For normal pregnancy and the birth of newborns

The growth and development of the mother and the fetus, the newborn/infant, and the care of that infant are all part of what the NCLEX-RN tests. Pregnancy- and birth-related concepts you need to know for the exam include the following:

» How to calculate the expected due date

» How culture plays into the childbearing and how it affects the care you give

» Prenatal tests and care needed

» Normal ranges for heart rate for during prenatal exams

» Newborn care needed

» Postpartum care and instructions, and education as needed

» How to evaluate the parent's ability to care for their newborn

Questions concerning pregnancy-related issues may look like the following:

EXAMPLE

A mother at 39 weeks gestation has arrived at the clinic for a prenatal check. The fetal heart rate (FHR) is 170 at the beginning of the visit. When the doctor monitors it again 10 minutes later it's 168. Which of the following is a possible cause of this condition?

(1) Maternal fever

(2) Fetal heart failure

(3) Structure defects

(4) A blood sugar reading of 50 for the mom

Keywords for this question are *39 weeks gestation, prenatal check, fetal heart rate is 170, 10 minutes later it's 168,* and *a possible cause of this condition.* FHR greater than 160 is considered tachycardia, so the correct answer is Choice (1). Maternal fever is a cause of tachycardia in the fetus. All the other answers are the causes of FHR bradycardia.

EXAMPLE

A new graduate is caring for a set of four expectant mothers. Which expectant mother would the graduate nurse expect to see a *partera*, or traditional midwife, during labor?

(1) African American mother

(2) Hispanic mother

(3) European mother

(4) Native American mother

The keywords for this question are *new graduate; four expectant mothers; which expectant mother;* and *partera, or traditional midwife.* The correct answer is Choice (2). Of these choices, only Hispanic mothers use midwives called *partera* for labor.

During a patient's first prenatal visit, the new nurse needs to figure the expected due date. Using Naegele's rule, what would the expected due date be for this patient if she states her last period was December 4, 2019?

(1) October 11, 2020

(2) September 11, 2020

(3) November 4, 2020

(4) August 11, 2010

Keywords for this question are *first prenatal visit, figure the expected due date, last period, using Naegele's rule,* and *last period was December 4, 2019.* Using Naegele's rule, first subtract 3 months from December (September), then add one year to 2019 (2020), and add 7 days to 4 (11). So Choice (2) is the correct answer.

For older adults

Older adults have milestones of adjusting to retirement and change in income, role changes in function and social life, and especially the loss of spouses or close friends.

You may see questions like these about older adults' developmental milestones:

The nurse has entered the home of a new client who lost wife three months ago. Which of the following mental health concerns would the nurse be monitoring for? Select all that apply.

(1) Depression

(2) Mania

(3) Schizophrenia

(4) Isolation

(5) Dementia

The keywords for this question are *a new client, lost his wife three months ago, which of the following mental health concerns would the nurse be monitoring for,* and *select all that apply.* The correct answers are Choices (1) and (4). If the client lost his wife three months ago, the nurse's main concerns would be grief, depression, isolation, and suicide. Mania and schizophrenia aren't related to recent spouse loss. Dementia comes on more slowly than the time frame in the question and involves a disorientation not seen in depression.

To Your Clients' Health! Promoting Well-Being

As an RN, you can make a huge difference in patient's lives by encouraging health- and wellness-oriented behaviors over crisis management of illness. Nurses provide information to help patients make healthy lifestyle decisions. Knowing who's at risk and what can be done to prevent disease and injury is a major nursing responsibility.

To keep your patients healthy and well, you need to be able to identify who's at risk for what. The common threads in risk assessments are age, family history, genetics, and lifestyle. For example, age is the number one risk factor for almost all diseases. If you're ever unsure about who's at the greatest risk for a disease, choose the patient with the most advanced age. Knowing to pay particular attention to these elements will help you choose the correct answer when facing a question related to health and wellness, such as the following:

THE IMPORTANCE OF SLEEP TO LONG-TERM MEMORY

Okay, you've all studied the effects of sleep deprivation on patients. But what's it doing to you and your study skills? Research has shown that people who are well rested have stronger memories and longer attention spans than those who are sleep deprived. Alertness, performance, thought, and creativity are all affected by how much you sleep. During a good night's sleep, the information you take in is transferred to your long-term memory. So sleep, already! At least seven to eight hours each night.

EXAMPLE

The nurse would identify which of the following patients as the highest priority in needing a mammogram?

(1) A 35-year-old woman who has never given birth

(2) A 49-year-old woman whose sister was diagnosed with breast cancer

(3) A 50-year-old woman who smokes ten cigarettes a day

(4) A 62-year-old woman who hasn't had a mammogram in five years

This question's keywords are *nurse would identify, which of the following patients, highest priority*, and *needing a mammogram*. The pieces of information you need to answer the question are each patient's risk factors and age. The correct answer is Choice (4). Even though family history and never having given birth are risk factors for breast cancer, the greatest risk factor is age.

EXAMPLE

The nurse is holding a class on child abuse prevention. Which of the following actions would be most likely to prevent child abuse?

(1) Identifying that a father had been abused as a child

(2) Telling parents that child abuse is illegal

(3) Giving parents a child abuse hotline phone number

(4) Teaching parents about discipline

Keywords for this question are *a class on child abuse prevention, following actions*, and *most likely to prevent child abuse*. The first step in any problem with nursing is assessing, so look for the answer that involves assessment. The correct answer is Choice (1). A history of abuse as a child for either parent puts their child at risk. Identifying parents who are at risk for involvement in child abuse allows the nurse to choose an intervention that prevents the occurrence of abuse. The other options aren't correct because simply providing the information is less likely to ensure that child abuse will not occur.

Creating and Implementing Care Plans

You may remember all those care plans you had to create night after night as a nursing student. In the following sections, I review some of the more important things you need to remember regarding assessing a patient and creating a care plan based on what you find. As you move through this chapter (and any other chapters, for that matter), remember the nursing process — in the beginning, assess.

Assessing your patient's physical condition

Assessment is one of the cornerstones of the nursing process. It's the basic premise on which all care and decisions are based. I can't say it enough: You can't treat anything until you know what you're dealing with. You do a physical assessment every time you look at your patient, even if you're just in the room to fill the water pitcher. As a nurse, assessment becomes second nature to you, to the point where you find yourself watching people in restaurants and airports, trying to figure out what's wrong with them!

When conducting a physical assessment, you perform the following techniques in this order — except for abdominal assessments, which require that you do auscultation after inspection.

1. **Inspection:** Paying close attention to observations, looking carefully, and knowing what things are supposed to look like

2. **Percussion:** Tapping the body to determine organ size and placement (only used for abdominal organs)

3. **Light palpation:** Applying pressure with the hands to determine temperature, texture, tenderness, size, and position

4. **Deep palpation:** Applying pressure with the hands to determine masses and tenderness

5. **Auscultation:** Listening to identify breath sounds, cardiac sounds, circulatory sounds, and abdominal sounds

REMEMBER

You don't necessarily use all these techniques for all systems. For example, you don't perform auscultation for urinary retention assessments.

TIP

Any question that asks you to perform an assessment or asks you to make a decision based on an assessment requires you to review the physical assessment steps. Always use an assessment finding to plan your intervention, whether the intervention is giving medication, changing a dressing, changing the patient's position, educating the patient, or notifying the doctor.

When answering questions about assessments (and actually performing them) keep these additional pointers in mind:

>> Always use protective equipment when appropriate.

>> Be sure to explain the procedure to the patient.

>> Always compare one side to the other.

>> Make sure that an abnormal finding isn't the fault of malfunctioning equipment.

Try your hand at the following example NCLEX-RN questions on assessment:

EXAMPLE

The nurse is taking routine vital signs on a 3-year-old. The child is sitting happily playing with a puzzle. Her skin is warm, dry, and intact, and she's looking forward to going to the playroom when it opens. The vital signs are T 104.8 degrees F (orally), P 106, R 22, BP 90/66. Which action should the nurse should take next?

(1) Document the findings.

(2) Call the doctor.

(3) Retake the temperature.

(4) Retake all the vital signs.

Keywords for this question are *routine vital signs; 3-year-old; happily playing with a puzzle; skin is warm, dry, and intact; vital signs are T 104.8 degrees F (orally), P 106, R 22, BP 90/66;* and *which action should the nurse take next.* The correct answer is Choice (3). The temperature of 104.8 degrees Fahrenheit doesn't fit with the other assessment findings, so the most appropriate action is to retake the temperature in case the thermometer is malfunctioning. The other options are all incorrect because documenting findings that aren't accurate and calling the doctor before determining the accuracy of the vital signs aren't appropriate, and retaking all the vital signs isn't necessary and may cause undue concern to the patient and her family.

EXAMPLE

During a morning assessment of an 82-year-old client, the nurse notes that he has 2+ pitting edema on his left lower extremity. Which of the following would be of most concern to the nurse?

(1) The right lower extremity has no edema at all.

(2) The right lower extremity also has 2+ pitting edema.

(3) Both legs feel cool to the touch.

(4) Capillary refill time is three seconds.

Keywords for this question are *82-year-old, 2+ pitting edema, left lower extremity,* and *be of most concern.* Anytime you see "most concern," think "which is most unstable or most life-threatening?" The correct answer is Choice (1). Abnormal findings that are unilateral are more indicative of an acute problem that may be developing, and such findings require immediate intervention. The other options aren't as concerning because Choices (2) and (3) reflect a more chronic or positional problem, and Choice (4) is a normal finding.

Teaching patients from the moment of introduction

Hopefully, you didn't go into nursing to avoid being a teacher, because nurses do a tremendous amount of teaching. One of the underlying themes in nursing is the accountability that nurses have to teach their clients what they need to know about their health, medications, treatments, and care plans. More than that, you have to assess the patient for readiness to learn. This teaching is one of the major components of patient care that you can't delegate to unlicensed assistive personnel (UAP).

Given that patient teaching is so important, you can be sure that you'll encounter questions about it on the licensure exam. Some basic principles to remember about teaching and learning include the following:

>> You *can* teach an old dog new tricks — you just have to find the right motivator.

>> The patient needs to be part of the process; don't forget to include the patient in the teaching plan.

>> Environment affects learning. Does the patient face any barriers to learning what he or she needs to know? If the patient is in pain, tired, worried, or not feeling well, learning can't take place. Address the patient's issues before trying to teach him or her.

>> Learning styles affect outcomes. For effective teaching, you need to know whether you're dealing with a *visual learner* (learns best by seeing), an *auditory learner* (learns best by talking about the subject), or a *kinesthetic learner* (learns best by doing).

Teaching and patient education start the minute you meet your patient. You need to assess knowledge level, be aware of knowledge deficits, and start teaching whatever information the patient is able to take in at the time. Plans for addressing knowledge deficits are an underlying theme in many questions you'll encounter on the NCLEX-RN, such as the following:

TAKING CARE OF YOURSELF

Hydration and nutrition aren't just nursing diagnoses; they also apply to you! Avoid the pitfall of snacking while studying. Not only are you likely to gain weight, but high fat and sugar intake can also make you feel sluggish. If you're a caffeine fiend, know that research has shown that small amounts of caffeine spaced throughout the day are better for maintaining mental alertness than that one extra-large cup. But take care when pouring the java because too much caffeine can make you nervous and jittery, and you're probably already nervous and jittery! Instead of slurping coffee, exercise regularly; you'll feel better and have more energy when you sit down to study.

EXAMPLE

A woman who was admitted in preterm labor is stable and is being discharged home on oral terbutaline (Brethine). Which of the following statements made by the patient indicates that she may require additional teaching about the medication?

(1) "I'm so happy that I won't have to worry about premature labor now that I'm going to be taking medication."

(2) "The medication may make me jittery."

(3) "I'll contact my doctor if I feel fetal movement in a 12-hour period."

(4) "This medication can be taken with or without food."

This question's keywords are *preterm labor, stable, being discharged, oral terbutaline,* and *which of the following statements made by the patient indicates she may require additional teaching about the medication.* In other words, which statement is wrong about the medication terbutaline? The correct answer is Choice (1). Although terbutaline is a smooth muscle relaxant, there are no absolutes to prevent preterm labor. The patient needs reeducation about the medication. Choices (2) and (4) are true statements about the medication, and Choice (3) has nothing to do with the medication.

This next question is an example of one that asks you to identify when and how teaching should take place:

EXAMPLE

A newly diagnosed diabetic is feeling very overwhelmed by the amount of information and skills he needs to learn before being discharged home. He asks the nurse to identify the most important thing he should learn because he can't learn everything so fast. The nurse should address this patient's concern by

(1) Spending a lot of time with the patient to instruct and review all the information with him

(2) Discussing with the doctor the benefit of having this patient receive home care for continuation of the teaching

(3) Giving the patient a lot of literature that he can refer to at home

(4) Telling the patient to focus on the insulin administration because it's the hardest part of managing diabetes

The keywords for this question are *newly diagnosed diabetic, overwhelmed by the amount of information, needs to learn, the most important thing he should learn,* and *the nurse should address his concern by.* The correct answer is Choice (2). The patient is obviously anxious about all the diabetes information and feels that it can't be covered adequately before he's discharged. Continuing the education process by using home care services ensures that the patient has support in meeting his goals of self-care. Choice (1) isn't realistic, Choice (3) doesn't ensure effective learning alone, and Choice (4) assumes that the patient is having difficulty in an area that he may have mastered.

Understanding and explaining screening tests

The NCLEX-RN tests you on tests. As a nurse, you spend a lot of time explaining to your patients what certain tests are and why they're important, so you need to know your tests. In particular, screening tests are diagnostic, not preventative, but early diagnosis leads to early treatment and better outcomes.

Healthcare has a million and one different screening tests, but nobody expects you to know about all of them. (Except your relatives. Nurses are constantly asked by their own family members to interpret test results, so be forewarned and prepared to take your laboratory values book to every family gathering.) But for the exam and nursing practice, the common tests you should be familiar with are glucose testing, cholesterol screening, and mammograms, just to name a few. And Pap smears, tests for sexually transmitted diseases, and tuberculosis tests, just to name a few more.

REMEMBER

Most importantly, know when the tests are done — such as who's more likely to need the testing, what preparation is necessary, and who should be tested — and know what nursing care is required after the test.

Exam questions about screening tests resemble the following:

EXAMPLE

A woman is scheduled to have her first mammogram. She is 40 years old and has never had a mammogram before. What would be the most important information to provide the patient with in preparation for this test?

(1) Ask her why she didn't have a mammogram sooner.

(2) Tell her not to eat or drink after midnight prior to the test day.

(3) Instruct her not to use body lotion or deodorant on the day of the test.

(4) Instruct her not to take any medication the morning of the test.

Keywords for this question are *first mammogram, 40 years old, never had a mammogram before,* and *most important information to provide the patient with in preparation for this test.* The correct answer is Choice (3). Body lotions and deodorants can interfere with test results. None of the other options are relevant. The first screening mammogram is recommended around age 40 to 44 unless the patient has a family history of cancer. Consuming medications, food, and fluids doesn't interfere with the procedure or the results.

EXAMPLE

During a newborn screening test, which of the following tests can't be taken until after a newborn has been fed either formula or breast milk?

(1) PKU (phenylketonuria)

(2) Glucose

(3) Galactosemia

(4) Sickle cell trait

The keywords here are *newborn screening test* and *can't be taken until after a newborn has been fed either formula or breast milk.* The correct answer is Choice (1). PKU is a test that requires the consumption of protein, and formula and breast milk are protein sources. (Phenylalanine hydroxylase is an enzyme that breaks down the amino acid phenylalanine. When phenylalanine hydroxylase is lacking, the phenylalanine doesn't break down but instead accumulates causing the phenylketonuria.) Glucose can be tested at any time (and isn't part of a normal newborn screening); galactosemia is an enzyme deficiency, not a test, and is present with or without food consumption. Sickle cell trait has nothing to do with food intake. Reading the question carefully can help you find the right answer even if you aren't sure what the tests are for.

Handling High-Risk Behavior and Alternate Lifestyle Choices

You don't have to be a nurse for very long before a basic truth really hits home: Not everybody is like you. Nurses treat patients whose lifestyles range from nontraditional to dangerous or socially unacceptable. Nurses encounter all kinds of people who have made all kinds of lifestyle choices, so you always must demonstrate a professional attitude toward your patients regardless of what you think of their lifestyles.

REMEMBER

Remaining therapeutic and nonjudgmental is a fundamental responsibility in nursing, but it isn't always easy. Here are a few do's and don'ts for dealing with patients who engage in high-risk behaviors (think drug abuse, unprotected sex, and the like) and practice lifestyle choices that may not be common or socially acceptable:

>> Do give factual information.

>> Do give the patient correct health information so the patient can make informed choices.

>> Do accept the choices the patient makes.

>> Don't give your opinion.

>> Don't blame the patient for the circumstances of his or her situation.

At the same time, knowledge of the client's lifestyle practices and how they could affect the patient adversely shouldn't impact the way you interact with the client. But you need to try to educate patients about the prevention and treatment of their high-risk behaviors, be they smoking, unsafe sexual practices, repeated use of the same needle for drug use, or whatever.

Exam questions about lifestyle decisions may go a little something like this:

EXAMPLE

A 39-year-old with a history of chemical substance abuse and alcohol use is diagnosed with cirrhosis of the liver. He is feeling very concerned that his wife and three children won't be able to manage without him. He tells the nurse that he feels depressed and is really concerned about his family. The nurse's best response would be to

(1) Offer to talk with him in greater detail about his concerns

(2) Tell him he really should've thought about this issue when he was making his lifestyle choices

(3) Tell him that the doctor will talk to him about his choices

(4) Ask him if he wants to start a 12-step program

Keywords for this question are *39-year-old, history of chemical substance abuse and alcohol use, cirrhosis of the liver, concerned that his wife and three children won't be able to manage without him, depressed, really concerned about his family,* and *nurse's best response.* This question asks for a therapeutic response from the nurse, so look for statements that will make the client talk more about his feelings and concerns. The correct answer is Choice (1). Always offer to be available for patients who want to talk about their concerns. Doing so shows respect and interest in the patient and shows that you're unbiased and nonjudgmental. Choice (2) is judgmental and ineffective, Choice (3) avoids the patient, and Choice (4) doesn't address the patient's immediate concern.

Preparing Patients to Leave Your Care

Nurses sometimes have trouble stepping back after teaching patients to take care of themselves. As people with caretaker-type personalities, nurses may rush in to do things for patients that they should let patients learn to do for themselves. When a patient's involved in his care, he's more likely to comply with medications and treatments. So getting patients involved in their care is another important area of health promotion and maintenance.

Helping patients take care of themselves

Self-care can mean many different things in the world of healthcare:

>> **Self-care can be personal healthcare performed by the client.** For example, a client may be able to change his own colostomy bag.

>> **Self-care can be making decisions to sustain life, health, and well-being.** For example, a client signs a consent form for surgery.

>> **Self-care can be practicing safety in the environment.** For example, a client wears a seat belt when traveling by car.

>> **Self-care can be a caregiver helping the patient meet goals.** For example, a child or spouse may assist in caring for the patient.

Helping patients take care of themselves boils down to education. The process of teaching self-care begins at the nurse's very first encounter with the patient, as the following question shows:

EXAMPLE

A 32-year-old who is six weeks pregnant tells the nurse that she's very excited and wants to learn everything about pregnancy. Which of the following responses by the nurse would be most appropriate?

(1) "Tell me exactly what you want to know."

(2) "Wait until you complete the first trimester."

(3) "The doctor will be giving you information at each visit."

(4) "You should enroll in a prenatal education class."

Keywords for this question are *32-year-old, six weeks pregnant, very excited, wants to learn,* and *which of the following responses, be most appropriate*. The correct answer is Choice (4). This question asks for the therapeutic response, but in this case, you need to provide the patient with the ability to do self-care. Referring the patient to education classes to gain further knowledge and information is an appropriate way of assisting her in meeting the goal of a healthy pregnancy and a healthy baby. It also gives the patient an opportunity to practice self-care and become an active participant in her care.

Choices (1) and (3) don't allow the patient to participate in her care, and Choice (2) is unsafe because the first trimester is the critically important period in the development of the fetus and pregnancy outcomes, and the patient should take certain measures during that time.

Embracing the family system

Whether you like it or not, patients come with families, and these families play a crucial role in the overall well-being of your patients (and your patience)! For example, in the case of children as patients, you often find yourself treating entire families. When answering exam questions that address family matters, focusing on answers that keep the family involved is always a good strategy. After all, family members are the ones who influence a patient's decisions, provide basic needs, and have a vested interest in the patient's outcome. But be careful not to assume that all families look the same or interact in the same way, because they don't. Families can include people who aren't part of the nuclear family or who don't live with the patient but who are involved with the patient's daily routines and activities. A good rule when dealing with families is to never assume!

The following is an example of a question that tests your understanding of family systems:

EXAMPLE

The nurse is discharging a newly diagnosed diabetic patient who will be taking insulin and following a specific diet. Who should the nurse be sure to include in the diet teaching?

(1) The patient only

(2) The patient and his wife

(3) The patient and the person who does the food shopping and food preparation in his home

(4) The patient and anyone who lives in the patient's home

Keywords for this question are *discharging, newly diagnosed diabetic, taking insulin, following a specific diet,* and *who should the nurse include in the diet teaching.* The correct answer is Choice (3). With dietary changes and adherence to specific diet instructions, the nurse must educate anyone who's involved with food preparation in the patient's home. Therefore, the person who handles food shopping and food preparation has to know the diet requirements just as well as the patient does. The other options are all people who can be included in the teaching but who don't play a vital role in ensuring that the patient gets the proper diet.

TIP

If you picked Choice (2) on the theory that the patient's wife and the food shopper/preparer may be the same person, you fell victim to reading information into the question that isn't there. The question doesn't specify that the wife handles the food tasks, so you can't factor that possibility into your answer.

Chapter **8**

Psychosocial Integrity

All nurses are psych nurses. Every area of nursing, from med-surg to maternity, deals with patients with emotional problems and mental illness. Developing therapeutic relationships with your patients is essential to their physical and mental well-beings — and it helps your mental well-being as well because you get the satisfaction of truly contributing not only to your patients' physical health but also to their growth as human beings.

In this chapter, I discuss the roots of different types of behavior and how you can handle behavioral issues. I also look at how cultural standards can affect your patients' care and outline the steps that you need to take to deal with grief and crisis situations, including end of life care and how patients deal with change in independence, such as loss of hearing or sight, or family roles. Lastly, I examine behaviors seen in patients with abuse issues. I include test questions in each section to illustrate what you can expect from this area of the NCLEX-RN.

Looking Beyond the Surface: Factors That Influence Behavior

Why do people do the things they do? Behavior is based on a personal and cultural sense of right and wrong, but also it's influenced by what a person is going through at the time. Crisis or grief, for example, can lead people to do things that they normally wouldn't do. Some people get stuck developmentally at a certain stage and never grow past the behaviors common at that stage. Others suffer from psychological disorders that lead to behaviors that they may not otherwise exhibit.

As a nurse, you're sure to work with patients suffering from any of the following mental disorders at some time or another: conduct disorder, attention deficit and hyperactivity disorder (ADHD), major depression, panic disorder, schizophrenia, personality disorder, and substance abuse disorders. Many of these disorders have physical and psychological components that contribute to the behaviors they elicit. The NCLEX-RN tests you on your knowledge of behavioral development as well as cultural diversity in health matters, so the following sections examine some of the many reasons why people do what they do.

Behavioral basics: Important development theories

Many people have tried to explain human behavior over the years by putting actions in different categories related to the different life stages. Theorists, of course, didn't invent these behavior patterns; they just formalized them. To prepare yourself for exam questions related to behavior patterns, know the basic ideas of the most well-known theorists:

>> **Sigmund Freud:** According to Freud, a person's personality consists of the id, the ego, and the superego. Freud taught that development occurs in five psychosocial stages: oral, anal, phallic, latency, and genital. Psychopathology occurs when a person remains fixed at one stage or has difficulty moving to the next stage. Freud also believed that people use defense mechanisms to protect the self from anxiety and painful feelings.

>> **Harry Sullivan:** Sullivan believed that the purpose of all behavior is to get one's needs met through personal interactions designed to decrease or avoid anxiety.

>> **Erik Erickson:** Erickson described eight psychosocial stages of development; he believed that growth occurs in stages and that each stage is dependent on the completion of the previous stage. The stages are trust versus mistrust, autonomy versus shame and doubt, initiative versus guilt, industry versus inferiority, identity versus role confusion, intimacy versus isolation, generativity versus stagnation, and ego integrity versus despair.

>> **Lawrence Kohlberg:** Kohlberg developed the theory of moral development. He stated that these levels are developed in stages but not necessarily in sequential order. The stages are punishment-obedience, instrumental relativist behavior, good boy/nice girl orientation, law and order orientation, social contract and legalistic orientation, and universal ethical principles orientation.

>> **Abraham Maslow:** Maslow defined the five-stage hierarchy of needs, which starts with the most important and basic needs. It proceeds as follows: physiological needs, safety and security, love and belonging, self-esteem, and self-actualization. Following Maslow's model helps you prioritize nursing actions. For example, you stabilize a patient physically before psychologically; a nurse in the ER should triage a patient who's bleeding before a patient with depressive symptoms — unless the depressive patient has a gun!

>> **Hildegard Peplau:** Peplau was a nursing theorist who developed the concept of the nurse-patient relationship. She defined four phases of the nurse-patient relationship: orientation, identification, exploitation, and resolution. Peplau also defined four levels of anxiety: mild, moderate, severe, and panic.

Questions related to development theories may sound like this:

EXAMPLE

A client has been admitted to the ER. After dealing with the patient, the staff determines the client is fearful of the future. He is suspicious of staff members and their care. His family members say he has been this way all his life. At what stage of Erickson's development is the client?

(1) Trust versus mistrust

(2) Autonomy versus shame and doubt

(3) Initiative versus guilt

(4) Intimacy versus isolation

The keywords for this question are *admitted to the ER, fearful of the future, suspicious of staff members and their care, all of his life,* and *what stage of Erickson's development.* The correct answer is Choice (1). Unsuccessful resolution of the trust versus mistrust stage leads to fear of the future, suspicion of others, and difficulty trusting others.

The spice of life: Cultural and family diversity

It's no surprise that upbringing and cultural background have a huge impact on how people behave. How and where a person was raised influences the way she looks at health and illness and also determines what she expects from the healthcare system. For example, if her early illnesses were treated by certain rituals (most types of behaviors are rituals, including going to the doctor for a shot when ill), she won't feel "healed" without that ritual. Ritualized treatment is one reason so many people think that they need the doctor to give them antibiotics to recover from viruses. Some people don't even fill the prescription — just receiving one is considered a cure.

REMEMBER

Your patient's cultural beliefs may differ greatly from your own. Each culture has different patterns of verbal communication, nonverbal communication (such as eye contact, touch, and personal space), beliefs, values, illness, and health. You must be able to adjust your nursing care to meet the needs of the patient's cultural beliefs, practices, and preferences, regardless of your own beliefs. For example, as a sign of respect, Chinese patients may avoid eye contact when they're speaking with nurses or doctors. To remain sensitive to patients' cultural differences, check out some of the many available reference books concerning cultural practices and inform yourself about the basics of a patient's culture.

The following example questions address cultural diversity:

EXAMPLE

The nurse receives a meal tray for a terminally ill Roman Catholic client. Which of the following actions would be inappropriate behavior for the nurse upon entering the room?

(1) Removing the crucifix from the wall

(2) Giving the patient a meal tray with roast beef during Lent

(3) Allowing the priest to enter to see the patient

(4) Allowing family to stay as long as they want

The keywords for this question are *terminally ill*, *Roman Catholic*, and *inappropriate behavior for the nurse*. The correct answer is Choice (1). A terminally ill Roman Catholic patient doesn't need to follow the religion's dietary restrictions. (Neither do pregnant women or children.) Removing the crucifix from the wall would be an inappropriate action by the nurse.

EXAMPLE

A nurse is taking care of a Hispanic American client. Which of the following should the nurse take into consideration while caring for this client? Select all that apply.

❑ **(1)** Clients from this culture may avoid eye contact with people in authority.

❑ **(2)** Clients from this culture may exhibit dramatic body language such as gestures or facial expressions.

❑ **(3)** Clients from this culture may believe that the future is more important than the present.

❑ **(4)** Clients from this culture may view health as a reward from God or the result of good luck.

❑ **(5)** Clients from this culture may give family needs precedence over their own.

The keywords for this question are *Hispanic American client* and *nurse take into consideration*. The correct answers are Choices (1), (2), (4), and (5). Avoiding eye contact with a person in authority actually conveys respect in the Hispanic community. The present is often seen as more important than the future, so Choice (3) is incorrect.

Culture-bound syndromes are sets of symptoms that are common in one cultural group and not another, such as Wind illness in Asian culture groups. Here's an example of a culture-bound syndrome question:

EXAMPLE

A Hispanic American comes to the clinic with her young daughter. The nurse enters the room to provide care and talks to the mother exclusively while looking at her daughter. Which of the following culture-bound syndromes may the mother be concerned about?

(1) *Mal de ojo*

(2) Falling out

(3) Brain fog syndrome

(4) *Mal de pelea*

Keywords in this question are *Hispanic American, young daughter, talks to the mother exclusively, looking at her daughter,* and *culture-bound syndromes.* The correct answer is Choice (1). *Mal de ojo,* or the evil eye, is a culture-bound syndrome in some populations (including Mexican and Central American communities) where staring at someone who's part of a group considered vulnerable — such as young children — is believed to cause illness. The other three answers don't address the information in the question about staring at a child.

Coping, Counseling, and Crisis Intervention

Everyone experiences crises, and some people experience more than others. A crisis state, which can be mental and not just physical, can cause significant distress in the affected individual and lead to personality disorganization. A little stress and anxiety in new or unusual situations is good; it helps keep you on your toes and alert for danger. But anxiety in excess can be maladaptive and can lead to harmful behaviors.

Keep in mind that most patients you see as a nurse are in some sort of crisis. Part of your job is to help them through the crisis stage. Crises come in many forms; even happy situations such as childbirth can cause crises by upsetting the apple cart, so to speak.

REMEMBER

The three categories of crises are these:

>> **Maturational:** Crises that result from life and are part of the developmental cycle, such as getting married or having a child

>> **Situational:** Crises that are sudden and unpredictable, such as losing one's job or experiencing the death of a family member

>> **Adventitious:** Crises that aren't part of everyday life and that threaten one's integrity, such as experiencing an earthquake or fire

Remember the following facts about crisis intervention:

>> The goal of crisis intervention is to assist the patient to return to his precrisis level of functioning.

>> A crisis is self-limiting and typically lasts four to six weeks.

>> A crisis can promote change and growth in the affected individual.

>> The nurse focuses on the immediate problem, on the here and now.

>> The nurse helps the patient set goals, look for solutions, and find new coping skills.

Having a strong support system can make the difference between recovery and no recovery in times of crisis. Mortality and stress levels decrease when people have good support systems, so involve your patient's supporters in his care, and let them know that they're an important part of the team that cares for the patient. Too often, support people are treated as more of a hindrance than a help (and sometimes they are!), but they can really make a huge difference in your patient's mental attitude. Keep them involved!

EXAMPLE

Which of the following can be defined as a crisis? Select all that apply.

❏ **(1)** A terrorist strapped with a bomb boards a bus full of people and blows it up.

❏ **(2)** A tornado destroys a community and kills thousands.

❏ **(3)** A young girl finds out that she is pregnant.

❏ **(4)** A high school senior shoots his peers in gym class because he feels left out.

Keywords for this question are *defined as a crisis* and *select all that apply.* All the answers should be checked because all represent crises. This item is an example of a multiple multiple question, which is one type of alternative question you may see on the exam. In a multiple multiple, as few as one and as many as all the answers may be correct. You can read more about multiple multiples and other alternative question types in Chapter 3.

Dealing with defense mechanisms

When people face danger or overwhelming anxiety, they may use defense mechanisms to help keep them from falling apart in the crisis. Defense mechanisms are behaviors that give people ways to handle the anxiety by changing their perceptions of the situations. Defense mechanisms can be conscious or subconscious. All the defense mechanisms operate on a subconscious level except for suppression. For the NCLEX-RN, you need to be able to identify the type of defense mechanism a patient is using so that you can better intervene in the patient's care.

Of the many defense mechanisms, here are some to be aware of for the NCLEX-RN:

>> **Compensation:** Overachievement in one area to offset real or perceived deficiencies in another area

>> **Conversion:** Expression of an emotional conflict through the development of a physical problem

>> **Denial:** Failure to acknowledge a condition or situation

>> **Displacement:** Expressing intense feelings toward people who are less threatening than the one who arouses those feelings

>> **Dissociation:** Dealing with emotional conflict through a temporary alteration in consciousness or identity

>> **Fixation:** Immobilization of a portion of the personality resulting from the unsuccessful completion of tasks in a developmental stage

>> **Identification:** Modeling actions and opinions of others while searching for one's own identity

>> **Intellectualization:** Separating the emotions of a painful event or situation from the facts involved

>> **Introjection:** Accepting another person's attitudes, beliefs, and values as one's own

>> **Projection:** Unconsciously blaming unacceptable thoughts on an external object

>> **Rationalization:** Excusing one's own behavior to avoid guilt, responsibility, or anxiety

>> **Reaction formation:** Acting the opposite of what one thinks or feels

>> **Regression:** Moving back to a previous developmental stage to feel safe or have needs met

>> **Repression:** Excluding emotionally painful thoughts and feelings from conscious awareness

>> **Resistance:** Overt or covert antagonism toward remembering or processing anxiety-producing information

>> **Sublimation:** Exhibiting acceptable behavior to make up for unacceptable behavior

>> **Substitution:** Substituting a socially acceptable activity for an impulse that's unacceptable

>> **Suppression:** Replacing the desired gratification with one that's more readily available

>> **Undoing:** Conscious exclusion of unacceptable thought from conscious awareness

The following questions deal with helping patients cope with crisis situations:

EXAMPLE

The nurse is performing an assessment of a patient who is in crisis. The nurse knows that the question that assesses the patient's perception of the event is

(1) "Who will pick you up today after the session?"

(2) "Who do you live with?"

(3) "How has this crisis strengthened your family?"

(4) "What caused you to come in today to see me?"

The keywords for this question are *performing an assessment, patient who is in crisis,* and *question patient's perception of the event.* The correct answer is Choice (4). In crisis intervention, the first step is assessment. The nurse must assess the patient's perception of the event. Clients in crisis need to be able to tell the nurse why they're seeking help or the cause of the crisis. Then the nurse can assess situational supports and personal coping skills.

EXAMPLE

The ER has just received a female patient in crisis from a rape. The nurse enters the cubicle of that patient knowing that the goal of crisis intervention that takes the highest priority is to

(1) Maintain patient safety

(2) Identify coping skills

(3) Identify support systems

(4) Reduce anxiety

Keywords for this question are *patient in crisis from a rape, goal of crisis intervention,* and *highest priority.* The correct answer is Choice (1). Maintaining safety takes priority over anything else. According to Maslow, physiological needs come before psychological needs.

Talking through troubles

Sometimes the therapeutic conversations you have with your patients help them heal as much as the medications you administer do. Often, patients need nothing more than a sympathetic, understanding person to hear what they have to say. Learning therapeutic listening isn't easy; some people are born with a knack for it, and the rest have to pick up the skill as they go along. The easiest way to do so is to always get patients talking about their feelings and concerns. For example, a client who just lost his sight and has withdrawn needs to express his feelings and concerns about the loss of his eyesight.

REMEMBER

Worrying that you may say the wrong thing or ask the wrong question when you're working with a patient is normal. Early in your nursing practice, applying the therapeutic techniques you learned in your psychiatric theory class may make you feel uncomfortable, and you may sound stilted until you find your own way to ask questions. You don't have to sound like a psych textbook to be therapeutic!

The key to therapeutic communication is asking open-ended questions — questions that require more than a "yes" or "no" answer. For example, "Tell me about how your anger has affected your husband" is an open-ended question. In contrast, closed-ended questions ask for specific information, such as "How old are you?" Therapeutic communication also involves restating what a patient says, or *mirroring*. For example, the patient says, "Life sucks!" and you respond, "You feel that life sucks." A patient who's silent following your question may be taking time to collect his thoughts, so give him time to answer before jumping in to fill the silence. Remember that silence can be therapeutic!

Nontherapeutic communication techniques shut down communication and don't encourage the patient to keep talking. "Why" questions (such as "Why did you forget to take your lithium?") often imply criticism and make the patient feel defensive.

REMEMBER

Communication involves more than just words. How you present your questions — through tone, posture, and so on — matters just as much as what you ask.

TIP

The NCLEX-RN is likely to have a few questions about therapeutic communication. If you're having trouble identifying the correct answer, look for the response that's most therapeutic. Eliminate any response that starts with "Why," responses that make false reassurance (such as "Don't worry!"), and any other nontherapeutic technique. False assurances make the patient feel as if you're not taking her issue seriously and make her feel belittled. Other nontherapeutic techniques are asking excessive questions, giving approval or disapproval, and changing the subject.

NCLEX-RN questions related to communication may resemble the following:

EXAMPLE

A patient tells the nurse, "I wish I were dead." The nurse knows that the best therapeutic response is

(1) "We all have days that we wish we were dead."

(2) "Why do you feel that way?"

(3) "Tell me more about how you're feeling right now."

(4) "It's a sunny day today."

Keywords for this question are *patient states, "I wish I were dead"; the nurse;* and *best therapeutic response.* The correct answer is Choice (3). This request for more information encourages the patient to verbalize her feelings. The other responses are nontherapeutic communication techniques.

EXAMPLE

A newly diagnosed breast cancer patient has just gotten her treatment options from the doctor. The nurse stands in the patient's doorway with her arms crossed and asks, "Do you have any concerns you want to talk about?" The patient softly says "no" and begins to cry. Which of the following is the reason for the patient's response?

(1) She has no concerns.

(2) Her husband came into the room as they were talking.

(3) The nurse's nonverbal communication.

(4) What the doctor told her has not really sunk in yet.

The keywords of this question are *newly diagnosed breast cancer patient, just gotten her treatment options from the doctor, nurse stands in the patient's doorway with her arms crossed,* and *reason the patient is not responding.* The correct answer is Choice (3). The nurse's wording may have been therapeutic, but her nonverbal communication — standing at the door, crossed arms — indicated she was in a hurry and didn't really want to hear the patient's input.

Teaching stress management

Life is full of stress. Some stress is actually considered to be good for you, but too much stress, or poor coping skills when faced with stress, can be harmful not only physically but also mentally. Chronic long-term stress can be associated with hypertension, decreased concentration and memory, lowered resistance to infections, depression, anxiety, and infertility, among other things. On the exam, you need to know how the body handles stress and reacts or adapts to it.

As you may remember from psychiatric nursing theory, Hans Selye defined the general adaptation syndrome and the three stages of reactions toward stress:

>> **Alarm stage:** The body mobilizes for a fight through increased hormone levels, weight changes, and other physiological changes.

>> **Resistance stage:** The body prepares for fight or flight by undergoing many more physiological changes, such as taking more air into the lungs.

>> **Exhaustion stage:** The body's reserve is depleted because the person didn't respond positively to the stressor or the stressor didn't resolve.

Another way to measure stress is through the Life Events Scale devised by Holmes and Rahe. Each criteria on the scale has a life-change number. For example, marriage is a 50, and the death of a spouse is a 100. A person with a score over 300 is considered to be at risk for stress affecting their health. (Taking the NCLEX-RN isn't on the scale . . . but perhaps it should be!)

Many patients need help to reduce stress. Some stress reducers are music, exercise, and massage. Relaxation techniques, guided imagery, and meditation are all behavioral approaches to managing stress that you can teach your patients. Cognitive reframing is another technique that helps patients reduce stress by recognizing their negative thoughts and replacing them with positive thoughts. For example, a nursing student says, "I'm not going to pass the NCLEX-RN." In cognitive reframing, the thought becomes "I studied for a long time, and that can only make me more successful on the exam."

Here's an example of a defense mechanism question:

EXAMPLE

A nursing director reprimands the nursing manager for consistently going over budget. The next day, the nursing manager has a staff meeting and accuses the staff of wasting supplies. This behavior is an example of

(1) Denial

(2) Depression

(3) Suppression

(4) Displacement

The keywords in this question are *nursing director, reprimands nursing manager, next day, nursing manager accuses staff of wasting supplies,* and *behavior is an example of.* The correct answer is Choice (4). Displacement is the discharging of pent-up feelings on people less threatening than those who made the emotion surface. The other options are incorrect because denial is blocking out painful events or feelings, repression is unconsciously burying unacceptable feelings, and suppression is consciously keeping those feelings away.

Helping Patients through Grief and Loss

Psychiatrist Dr. Elisabeth Kubler-Ross defined five stages to explain what a dying patient experiences: denial, anger, bargaining, depression, and acceptance. The acute grief reaction generally lasts four to eight weeks.

Grief is normal in crisis situations. Normal grief reactions include the following:

» Insomnia

» Depression

» Poor concentration

» Dreams of the loss

Your interventions should focus on helping family members cope with the loss, listening, and, most important, just being present with the family. Remember, you don't have to say a word to communicate!

Grieving becomes dysfunctional when your patient shows signs of prolonged depression, inability to accept the reality of the loss, and severe mood disturbances.

Patients that are dealing with end of life deserve a different type of care, and the NCLEX-RN expects you to know the core principles of care given to end of life patients (typically palliative care). You must give all care with dignity, especially to the client and the caregiver. For this part of the test, be sure you know the symptom management at the end of life, the physical symptoms of nearing death, the symptoms of imminent death, and then what postmortem care entails. You also need to know the psychological support you need to give these patients at the end of life and, especially if the dying patient is a child, what do you need to do for the family as well.

REMEMBER

You need to be aware of culture-specific rituals that your patient's family may want to conduct during times of grief and loss. For example, Chinese Americans often believe in reading scriptures and burning incense to assist the dying patient's body in the afterlife journey. Many Orthodox Jewish Americans don't believe in autopsies and require that a person who has expired be buried within 24 hours. You can easily put your foot in your mouth, therapeutically speaking, if you ask questions or make suggestions that are offensive to the patient's culture. Obviously, you can't know every cultural or religious group's rituals, so always ask the family what their normal procedures are before making suggestions or arrangements.

Questions for this area of the exam may look like this:

EXAMPLE

A 24-year-old female patient has terminal breast cancer. The nurse goes in for the history and finds out that the client is a Jehovah's Witness. Which of the following would be appropriate end of life care for this patient?

(1) The patient may be cremated.

(2) The patient may not receive an autopsy.

(3) The patient may not receive blood transfusions to save her life.

(4) The patient should never be left alone.

Keywords for this question are *24-year-old female patient has terminal breast cancer, Jehovah's Witness,* and *appropriate end of life care.* The correct answer is Choice (3). Because this patient is terminal, she requires end of life care. Members of Jehovah's Witness don't take blood for any reason (the nurse should still verify that refusing blood transfusions upholds the patient's wishes). The other answers don't relate to this religion's end of life care.

EXAMPLE

A client is admitted to the hospital because he isn't grieving appropriately after the death of his spouse. With treatment, the client does well and is ready for discharge. Which of the following is an appropriate outcome?

(1) The client verbalizes the stages of grief.

(2) The client verbalizes connections between significant loss and low self-esteem.

(3) The client verbalizes decreased desire for self-harm.

(4) The client reports three coping strategies.

The keywords for this question are *isn't grieving appropriately after the death of his spouse, with treatment, does well, ready for discharge,* and *appropriate outcome.* The correct answer is Choice (1). This option is the only one that deals with grief. Choices (2), (3), and (4) are unrelated to this patient's diagnosis.

Caring for Patients with Abuse Issues

Many patients suffer from abuse of one form or another. Some are abusers themselves, like abusers of alcohol or drugs. Others suffer from abuse committed by others; this kind of abuse tends to be sexual, verbal/emotional, or physical. Never assume that your patient isn't experiencing some type of abuse. People become very good at hiding the evidence of abuse in their lives and may deny it when first asked about any type of abuse. In the following sections, I talk about different types of situations in which abuse may occur and how to best intervene to provide the most support for the patient.

Recognizing different types of abuse

REMEMBER

Abuse isn't always obvious in patients. Take the time to listen to what they say for hints of abuse. Many patients throw out comments to see how you react before they're willing to open up to you about what's really bothering them.

You may encounter several types of abuse in patients:

>> **Emotional abuse** occurs when an abuser belittles, criticizes, or puts down the victim.

>> **Sexual abuse** occurs when an abuser has sexual contact with the victim without the victim's consent.

>> **Physical abuse** occurs when an abuser harms the victim bodily.

>> **Chemical or substance abuse** occurs when a patient uses alcohol or other psychoactive substances that change mood, behavior, and perception of events. Abused substances include alcohol, barbiturates, cocaine, marijuana, inhalants, opioids, nicotine, and hallucinogens.

Abuse intervention is primarily therapeutic in nature and can take many directions based on the immediate problem and priority.

A test question on different types of abuse may look like this:

EXAMPLE

The nurse is caring for a child who is suspected of being sexually abused. The nurse knows that which of the following is a warning sign that sexual abuse may have occurred?

(1) Red, swollen genitalia

(2) Multiple bruises on the legs and arms

(3) Skull fracture

(4) Lacerations to both arms

The keywords for this question are *caring for a child, suspected of being sexually abused,* and *which of the following is a warning sign that sexual abuse may have occurred.* The correct answer is Choice (1). Sexual abuse involves unconsented sexual acts. Some examples are rape, incest, and fondling. In suspected sexual abuse, you may see a high occurrence of urinary tract infections, and you may see tears or bruising in the genitalia, rectum, or vagina. Choices (2), (3), and (4) may be signs of physical abuse.

REMEMBER

The NCLEX-RN may ask you what your priority would be for a child being brought in with the possibility of sexual abuse. Just remember safety is your number one priority in this instance.

Identifying stages of substance abuse

Nurses see substance-abusing patients in different stages of abuse. In order to offer the most appropriate and effective treatment, you need to know the differences among intoxication, withdrawal, and detoxification:

» **Intoxication** occurs when a person uses a substance in excessive amounts and the substance produces behavioral or psychological changes in the person.

» **Withdrawal** occurs when a patient stops taking the substance and experiences physical or psychological effects.

» **Detoxification** is the process undertaken on a substance abuse unit to safely withdraw the patient from a substance.

REMEMBER

Keep in mind that substance dependence and substance abuse are two terms that usually confuse the graduate nurse. *Substance dependence* has the following characteristics:

» The patient shows tolerance to or withdrawal from the drug.

» The patient uses larger and larger amounts of substances and can't control his desires.

» The patient continues to use substances despite problems that result.

Substance abuse, on the other hand, is a maladaptive pattern of substance use related to

» Significant impairment and distress, which can cause legal and personal problems

» Engaging in hazardous situations while impaired

» Inability to meet obligations at school, work, and home

The NCLEX- RN may ask substance abuse questions such as the following:

EXAMPLE

The nurse is working in a substance abuse clinic. A patient is experiencing signs of alcohol withdrawal. Which of the following signs would the nurse expect to see?

(1) Lip puckering

(2) Fever and muscle rigidity

(3) Hand tremors, nausea, and elevated blood pressure

(4) Weight loss

The keywords in this question are *substance abuse clinic, experiencing signs of alcohol withdrawal,* and *which the following signs would the nurse expect to see.* The correct answer is Choice (3). Signs of alcohol withdrawal are sweating, tremors, elevated blood pressure, nausea, and vomiting. Choices (1), (2), and (4) aren't signs of alcohol withdrawal.

EXAMPLE

The nurse is working on a substance abuse unit. A patient is being discharged on disulfiram therapy. Which of the following statements by the patient indicates an understanding of his discharge instructions?

(1) "I should avoid foods that contain tyramine."

(2) "I should choose cough medicines that don't contain alcohol."

(3) "I can drink 2 ounces of alcohol daily."

(4) "I can take disulfiram every other day."

Keywords for this question are *substance abuse unit, discharged on disulfiram,* and *which of the following statements by the patient indicates an understanding of his discharge instruction.* The correct answer is Choice (2). The patient must avoid any food, medication, or preparation applied to the skin that contains alcohol. As for the other options, tyramine doesn't interact with disulfiram, disulfiram must be taken every day, and any ingestion of alcohol can trigger an adverse reaction.

» Supplying food and fluids

» Ensuring rest and sleep

» Helping patients with hygiene

» Monitoring bodily waste

» Dealing with irrigations

» Going outside the norm with alternative and complementary therapies

» Treating pain without pills or potions

» Addressing mobility

Chapter 9

Basic Care and Comfort

When you walk into your patient's room for the first time, you may find yourself focusing on the tangled IV tubing, multiple pumps, and monitoring systems and lose sight of your real priority — your patient! Never forget that your first priority as a nurse is to ensure that your patient's basic needs are being met. The foundation of your nursing practice is basic nursing care: ensuring adequate nutrition and hydration, providing personal hygiene, promoting rest and sleep, and making sure that waste products are properly eliminated.

The writers of the NCLEX-RN know the importance of these basics and therefore test your knowledge of these concepts. In addition, the exam covers interventions to assist patients with impaired mobility and promote patient comfort.

In this chapter, I review concepts related to the client-needs subcategory of basic nursing care and comfort. (This category contributes 6 to 12 percent of the questions on the test.) To help you fine-tune your ability to answer these types of questions, I use sample NCLEX-RN questions that address this category.

Giving Patients First What They Need Most

In the mid-20th century, a well-known psychologist named Abraham Maslow invented a pyramid called, sensibly enough, *Maslow's hierarchy of needs.* This pyramid prioritizes the needs of human beings from most to least important. Not surprisingly, the most important human needs are the basics: air, water, food, warmth, and cleanliness. You can see an illustration of Maslow's hierarchy in Chapter 4.

You may be thinking that *your* most important need in the world is to pass the NCLEX-RN. Before reviewing basic care and comfort for patients, you need to satisfy your own basic needs, so go get a sandwich, a glass of water, and your *Fundamentals of Nursing* textbook.

REMEMBER

You need to use your knowledge of pathophysiology (see Chapter 12) to answer questions about providing basic nursing care to patients with a variety of health problems. When answering questions about basic care and comfort, keep these pointers in mind:

>> **Answer the question as if you have all the resources and time in the world.** In other words, it's not the real world; it's the NCLEX-RN! Don't fall into the trap of thinking, "But I wouldn't have the time or equipment available to do all those interventions." Assume you have at your disposal all the time, staff, and equipment you need. (After all, if the real world functioned like the NCLEX-RN scenarios, it wouldn't have a nursing shortage.)

>> **Identify your keywords.** Who is your client? What condition or procedure does the question mention? What labs, medications, and signs and symptoms? What does the question want? (Chapter 4 has more on using keywords.)

>> **When answering questions that require you to prioritize, always put safety and security issues before psychosocial needs.** When prioritizing physiological needs, remember the life-threatening and the most unstable conditions are priority one!

>> **Use the steps of the nursing process.** If it's not a life-threatening emergency, assess the patient before you intervene! If one of the answer options is an assessment, consider it very closely before selecting your final answer. (For more on the nursing process, check out Chapter 2.)

>> **Rephrase the question in your mind to determine the concept or general topic.** Most questions pertaining to basic care and comfort test your knowledge of general principles of care. Sometimes rephrasing the question helps you determine what the question is *really* getting at.

Ensuring Adequate Nutrition and Hydration

Although we human beings *think* we can't live without things like cars, candy bars, or the newest electronic gadget, the truth is that the list of what we really need is somewhat shorter. Two of the things we really need are food and fluid (and they weren't even on Julie Andrews's list of her favorite things). Neither needs to be fancy, just adequate. Without enough fuel and fluid, our bodies can't keep going for any length of time, especially when we're ill and need to heal.

REMEMBER

To answer NCLEX-RN questions related to nutrition and hydration, focus on the components of a healthy diet and therapeutic diets. Make sure you know the following:

>> How to assess and identify nutritional deficits

>> How illness can affect dietary needs

>> How to administer enteral feedings and supplements

Identifying the building blocks of nutrition

With all the talk about nutrition and diet these days, even laypeople know that foods are made up of varying amounts of the basic components of nutrition: carbohydrates, fats, and proteins. You need to know how the body uses each of these nutrients and what foods are good sources for each. Here's a quick rundown:

>> **Carbohydrates:** The primary energy sources of the body, carbs are converted to glucose for use as energy. Foods high in carbohydrates include fruits, vegetables, breads, pasta, milk, and sugars.

>> **Proteins:** Made up of amino acids, proteins are required for tissue growth and repair (think wound healing!). Foods high in protein content include meat, poultry, fish, milk and milk products, eggs, nuts, and dried peas and beans.

>> **Fats:** In addition to providing energy and insulation for the body, fats promote absorption of fat-soluble vitamins. Foods high in fat content include whole milk, oils, butter, salad dressings, mayonnaise, bacon, and nuts.

Food also supplies vitamins and trace minerals. Vitamins are needed in small amounts for body maintenance and are classified as *water-soluble* or *fat-soluble.* Test questions commonly deal with the following vitamins:

>> **Vitamin C:** Needed for wound healing

>> **Vitamin A:** Needed for visual acuity in dim light

>> **Vitamin D:** Needed for bone formation

>> **Vitamin E:** An antioxidant

>> **Vitamin K:** Needed for blood clotting

>> **Folate:** Needed during pregnancy to prevent neural tube defects

Be sure to know what conditions the lack of these vitamins can cause and which foods are high in these vitamins. The questions may not specifically ask which vitamin a patient needs for a given condition but rather what foods the nurse should encourage the client to eat more of.

Modifying your patient's diet

Your patient's diet may need to be modified based on his or her specific disease or injury, so you need to apply your knowledge of basic nutrition when creating a care plan. For example, if the test question asks about diet and heart disease, you should know the proper dietary modifications for heart disease (low fat, low cholesterol) and also which foods are appropriate (or inappropriate) on this diet. Here's an example of this type of question:

EXAMPLE

When teaching a client who has been recently diagnosed with hepatic encephalopathy, the nurse should teach the client to avoid excessive amounts of which foods in her diet?

(1) Toast and cereal

(2) Oat bran and dried peas

(3) Citrus fruits and broccoli

(4) Eggs, steak, and cheese

The keywords for this question are *hepatic encephalopathy* and *avoid excessive amounts of which foods*. The correct answer is Choice (4). *Hepatic encephalopathy* is a disease of the liver. If the patient's liver is sick, it has a buildup of ammonia, which is the by-product of protein breakdown. Therefore, the patient with hepatic encephalopathy must follow a low-protein diet, which means limiting the intake of high-protein foods such as meats, poultry, milk and milk products, eggs, and nuts. Toast and cereal are carbohydrates and therefore are allowed. Citrus fruits and broccoli are high in vitamin C, and oat bran and dried peas are high in fiber, so these items are also allowed.

Other things to consider when modifying the patient's diet are the patient's bowel sounds and ability to swallow or chew. A patient without bowel sounds shouldn't be offered any food. Whereas a patient with hyperactive bowel sounds should be offered more fiber in their diet. If a patient can't swallow, aspiration is a true concern. If a patient is unable to chew, then food such as raw vegetables or steak would be avoided in favor of a more tolerable soft diet.

EXAMPLE

A patient is three days post-op from having abdominal surgery and is ready to have the naso-gastric (NG) tube for suction removed. The doctor orders the patient to have a clear liquid diet *after* the NG is removed. Which intervention is a priority for the nurse *prior* to removing the NG?

(1) Place the client in high Fowler's

(2) Assess bowel sounds

(3) Irrigate the NG to remove secretions

(4) Ask the client to swallow as the tube is being pulled out

The keywords in this question are *three days post-op, abdominal surgery, NG tube for suction removed*, and *which intervention is a priority for the nurse prior to removing the NG*. The correct answer is Choice (2). The bowel sounds must return for the client to be able to take fluids and have the NG removed. The other answers may be done but aren't a priority in this situation.

EXAMPLE

A patient has been on full liquids for 24 hours postoperative, and the doctor has ordered an advance to a soft diet. What assessment is a priority for the nurse at this time?

(1) Bowel sounds

(2) I&O

(3) Ability to swallow

(4) Ability to chew

The keywords for this question are *full liquids, ordered an advance to a soft diet*, and *what assessment is a priority*. The correct answer is Choice (4). The client has to be able to chew to tolerate going from full liquid to a soft diet. The client has already been assessed for bowel sounds and ability to swallow to take a clear liquid diet, so Choices (1) and (3) are incorrect. The I&O (intake and output) plays no part in this question.

Recognizing malnutrition

Good nutrition and hydration are essential to human health and are especially important for people suffering some sort of illness. Hospitalized patients are at risk for protein-calorie malnu-trition for many reasons. As anyone who's stayed overnight in a hospital knows, hospital food isn't always the best. In addition, clients may not be able to eat on their own, or they may be weak and unable to consume enough food to make up for protein loss. Additionally, fish, dairy, meat, and poultry contain proteins but may not be available in quantity or palatability for patients to eat. A malnourished patient may not heal well or quickly.

People are creatures of habit, especially when it comes to food, so recognizing when a client hasn't been eating or getting adequate nutrition is very important. Know the following signs and symptoms of malnutrition:

>> Weight loss

>> Fatigue and lethargy

>> Decrease in muscle mass

>> Dry skin

>> Hair changes

>> Poor dentition

>> Decreased reflexes

>> Edema

Lab tests that can indicate possible malnutrition include the following:

>> Albumin

>> Blood Urea Nitrogen (BUN)

>> Hematocrit

>> Hemoglobin

>> Pre-albumin

>> Serum potassium

>> Transferrin

>> Urinary creatinine

Questions related to malnutrition may resemble the following:

EXAMPLE

A client with a history of alcohol (ETOH) abuse is admitted to the nursing unit. The nurse suspects a nutritional deficit when her assessment reveals

(1) Moist buccal cavity mucous membranes

(2) Smooth, shiny hair and creatinine level of 0.8 mg/dl

(3) Decreased muscle mass, weight loss, and serum albumin level of 2.6 g/dl

(4) Skin breakdown and hematocrit of 41%

The keywords in this question are *alcohol abuse, suspects a nutritional deficit,* and *assessment.* The correct answer is Choice (3). Decreased muscle mass and weight loss are signs of a nutritional deficit, and low serum albumin is an indicator of protein malnutrition. (The normal serum albumin level is 3.3 to 5 g/dl.) Patients with a history of alcoholism are susceptible to malnutrition because of poor nutrient intake, altered nutrient absorption, and possible effects of liver disease. Patients with malnutrition may also exhibit dry buccal mucous membranes and dry, brittle hair. The lab values in the other answer options are considered within normal limits.

Administering tube feedings

Many patients are unable to take adequate nutrition by mouth; they may be comatose, on ventilators, at risk for aspiration, or simply unable to take in as many calories as they need to heal. *Enteral nutrition* (tube feeding) can provide nutrition for such a patient as long as he or she has a functioning GI tract. If the patient's GI tract is non-functioning, then this type of feeding is inappropriate, and you need to consider other types of supplemental nutrition, such as *parenteral,* in which nutrition is given intravenously.

Questions pertaining to enteral nutrition are likely to focus on the following key concepts:

» **Contraindications to enteral nutrition:**

- Severe diarrhea

- Paralytic ileus

- Intestinal obstruction

- Peritonitis

» **Primary risk associated with enteral nutrition:** Aspiration (the feeding goes into the lungs)

» **Interventions to minimize risk for aspiration when administering enteral feeds, including the following:**

- Keeping the head of the bed elevated during feeding

- Checking for gastric residual every four to six hours during a continuous feeding

- Assessing for bowel sounds at least once per shift

- Checking for tube placement by testing gastric pH before administering any feedings or medications through the tube

Check out this example question related to enteral feedings:

EXAMPLE

A client who is receiving enteral feedings via a nasogastric tube suddenly becomes dyspneic and cyanotic. What action should the nurse take first?

(1) Stop the feedings and further elevate the head of the bed.

(2) Notify the physician and prepare the patient for an X-ray.

(3) Check the placement of the tube by testing gastric pH.

(4) Assess the patient's bowel sounds.

The keywords in this question are *enteral feedings, suddenly becomes dyspneic and cyanotic,* and *what action should the nurse take first.* The correct answer is Choice (1). The phrase *suddenly becomes dyspneic and cyanotic* indicates that the patient is exhibiting signs of aspiration, a complication of enteral feeding. The nurse needs to provide safety for the patient, so the first action should be to stop the feeding and elevate the head of the bed. The other options should be performed but aren't immediate priorities.

Hydrating your patient

Patients need food, but they need fluids even more. Humans can live much longer without food than they can without water, so keeping your patient hydrated is an essential part of nursing. Questions on the exam related to hydration require you to know the symptoms of dehydration (also known as *hypovolemia*) and fluid excess (also known as *hypervolemia*). You also need to know how to intervene to correct the patient's fluid volume imbalance.

Exam questions on this topic may resemble the following:

EXAMPLE

A client with a history of congestive heart failure comes to the clinic. He reports a nine-day history of shortness of breath, peripheral edema, and weight gain. Your assessment findings include hypertension, distended neck veins, and an S3 gallop on auscultation of the heart. Based on your assessment, you can anticipate that the physician will order which intervention?

(1) Fluid bolus of 250 ml normal saline (0.9% NaCl) solution over 30 minutes

(2) Three-day calorie count

(3) Oral fluid restriction, low-sodium diet, and diuretic therapy

(4) Immediate hemodialysis

The keywords for this question are *a history of congestive heart failure, a nine-day history of shortness of breath, peripheral edema, weight gain, hypertension, distended neck veins,* and *S3 gallop on auscultation and intervention.* The correct answer is Choice (3). The patient is exhibiting signs and symptoms of fluid overload. Treatment for this condition includes restricting food and fluid intake by mouth (per oral or PO), providing a low-sodium diet, and giving medication (diuretic) to promote fluid loss from the body. In regard to the other options, a fluid bolus is a treatment for dehydration, a calorie count is indicated when a patient has experienced recent weight loss, and hemodialysis isn't indicated unless the patient is in renal failure.

Resting Easy, Sleeping Soundly

Considering the fact that you successfully survived nursing school, I assume that you know how crummy it feels to miss a few nights' sleep. Sleep and rest are essential to good physical and mental health. Questions on the NCLEX-RN related to rest and sleep require you to understand the physiology of sleep and the factors that affect sleep patterns. You also need to know how to intervene to promote sleep. (As an added bonus, your knowledge in this area may help *you* get better sleep, and you'll need to sleep well after you start working as an RN!)

The two major stages of sleep are *nonrapid eye movement* (NREM) and *rapid eye movement* (REM) sleep. Simply put, during NREM sleep, your patient's pulse, BP (blood pressure), temperature, and metabolic rate all decrease. During REM sleep, the opposite occurs: Vital signs increase, and active dreaming occurs. REM sleep is believed to be essential for maintaining mental and emotional equilibrium.

Sleep requirements vary across the human lifespan and from person to person. In general, the following guidelines are accurate:

>> Infants sleep 14 to 20 hours each day.

>> Growing children need from 10 to 14 hours of sleep each day.

>> During adolescence, the time needed for sleeping declines somewhat to 8 to 10 hours per day.

>> The average adult needs 7 to 9 hours of sleep per night, with many variations among individuals.

>> Older adults often need more time to fall asleep, wake more frequently during the night, wake earlier, and may nap during the day.

REMEMBER

Sleep deprivation can result in symptoms of irritability, impaired mental ability, and loss of concentration. Interventions to promote sleep include the following:

» Create a relaxing environment, such as a quiet, darkened room away from a nursing station.

» Schedule nursing care to minimize interruptions to sleep in the hospital setting.

» Offer a patient sleep medication if ordered.

» Avoid exercising right before going to sleep; daytime activity and exercise are beneficial.

» Abstain from caffeine, alcohol, and tobacco use.

» Avoid eating less than three hours before bedtime (although a light snack may be helpful).

» Establish a routine to facilitate relaxation prior to sleep.

Here are two sample questions related to sleep and rest:

EXAMPLE

A nurse is planning care for a 76-year-old client who is experiencing difficulty sleeping. In developing the care plan, the nurse takes into account the understanding that elderly individuals

(1) Are deeper sleepers and are more difficult to rouse than younger people

(2) Have a decline in Stage 4 NREM sleep

(3) Take less time to fall asleep than younger people

(4) Require more sleep than middle-aged adults

The keywords in this question are *76-year-old client, experiencing difficulty sleeping, care plan, the understanding that,* and *elderly individuals.* The correct answer is Choice (2). Stage 4 NREM sleep is a stage of deep sleep, and aging produces a decline in the amounts of Stages 3 and 4 NREM sleep. In regard to the other answer options, in general, elderly individuals take more time to fall asleep and awake more frequently during the night than younger people. Also, they don't require more sleep than middle-aged adults (although they may spend more time in bed).

EXAMPLE

The nurse is teaching a family with a newborn about infant safety during sleep. What information is most important for the family to understand?

(1) The infant should be placed on his back to sleep.

(2) Small pillows should be used to support the infant.

(3) The infant should be covered loosely with a blanket.

(4) A stuffed animal may be placed in the crib for comfort.

The keywords for this question are *family with a newborn, infant safety during sleep,* and *what information is most important.* The correct answer is Choice (1). Research has demonstrated that placing an infant on its back to sleep reduces the incidence of *sudden infant death syndrome* (SIDS). To decrease the risk of suffocation, pillows, stuffed animals, and loose blankets shouldn't be placed in the crib with the infant.

Keeping 'em Clean: Personal Hygiene

What's personal hygiene got to do with staying healthy? A lot! Maintaining clean skin helps keep it from breaking down and helps prevent infection if skin breakdown occurs. Keeping your patient and his environment clean and in order also promotes psychological well-being. Questions on the

NCLEX-RN related to personal hygiene focus on what you can do as a nurse to maintain good personal hygiene in your patient — and keeping your own personal hygiene at a high level is always a good idea as well!

In regard to personal hygiene, you need to have a good understanding of the following concepts:

>> Care of the skin, including cleanliness, moisture, and circulation to pressure points

>> Nail care appropriate to age and disease conditions, especially diabetes

>> Cultural and age-specific considerations related to performing hygienic care

>> Techniques for implementing hygiene measures

>> Care of the client's environment, which is anywhere the client is located — at home, in a hospital room, in a testing area, and so forth

>> Information and supplies, such as shower chairs, grip bars, and so forth, to help client independence in performing hygiene

Questions dealing with personal hygiene may look like the following:

EXAMPLE

When assisting an elderly client with hygienic care, the nurse pays special attention to the client's skin. The nurse's assessment is based on an understanding of which normal age-related skin changes?

(1) As clients age, skin becomes drier and more easily injured, and healing time increases.

(2) Secretions from the sebaceous glands become more prevalent with age.

(3) Bowel and urinary incontinence result in skin breakdown.

(4) Eczema and psoriasis are common skin alterations in the elderly.

Keywords for this question are *elderly client, hygienic care, special attention, client's skin,* and *age-related skin changes.* The correct answer is Choice (1). These age-related skin changes are normal and can make an elderly client more susceptible to skin breakdown. In regard to the other options, sebaceous gland secretions decrease as a person ages, and normal age-related changes don't result from bowel and urinary incontinence or include eczema or psoriasis.

EXAMPLE

What instruction related to foot care should the nurse include in the discharge teaching plan of a client who has diabetes and peripheral vascular disease?

(1) Carefully cut the toenails once a week with nail clippers.

(2) Soak the feet for at least 30 minutes every day.

(3) Using a mirror, inspect the feet for breakdown every day.

(4) Use commercial corn removers if needed.

The keywords in this question are *instruction, foot care, discharge teaching, diabetes,* and *peripheral vascular disease.* The correct answer is Choice (3). Diabetics have trouble feeling due to *peripheral neuropathy* (nerve damage), and peripheral vascular disease can cause additional issues. The combination places the diabetic at increased risk for injury, infection, and amputation of the extremities. Therefore, careful daily inspection is vitally important to detect skin breakdown. You should also teach the patient to immediately report any breakdown or reddened areas to his or her physician. In regard to the other options, the client should file toenails, not cut them; wash and dry the feet, not soak them; and avoid commercial corn removers because they can damage the skin.

EXAMPLE

A homecare nurse is making the first visit to a newly diagnosed stroke client who is experiencing weakness on the right side. Which of the following items would the nurse expect to see in the house to help regain independence performing activities of daily living (ADLs)? Select all that apply.

(1) Grab bar in the shower

(2) A rolling walker

(3) A shower chair

(4) A deep soak tub

(5) Handrails on the stairs on the left side

Keywords for this question are *first visit*, *newly diagnosed stroke*, *weakness on the right side*, *items*, *expect to see*, and *help with independence*. Choices (1), (3), and (5) apply. A grab bar in the shower would help with balance. A shower chair to sit while taking a shower would help with decreasing falls in the shower. Having handrails on the left side of the staircase encourages the client to use her stronger side. A rolling walker requires use of both upper extremities; the weakness on her right side would make this intervention unsafe. A deep soak tub would require the patient be able to stand up using both upper and lower extremities, which she isn't able to do at this time.

Understanding the Process of Elimination

Although it's not discussed much in civilized company, it's a fact of life: Everybody has to "go," society's polite term for elimination of bodily waste. Going too much, too little, too often, or too infrequently can all be signs of serious illness and require prompt intervention from you, the nurse. So paying attention to what comes out of your patient's bodily orifices is an important part of your job — just ask any nurse who spent the last hour of his or her shift tallying I&Os (intake and output).

Measuring your patient's urinary health

When answering questions about nursing care for patients with alterations in urinary elimination, focus on factors affecting urination, common assessment findings, nursing interventions to promote normal urination, urinary diversions, and bladder catheterization.

Many factors affect urination, including what went into your patient's body that day. Two factors, in particular, are important to note:

>> **Aging:** *Nocturia* (urination at night) is common as clients age. Decreased bladder muscle tone may result in frequent urination, urinary retention, and stasis, which can lead to urinary tract infection and incontinence.

>> **Medications:** Some medications (such as narcotics) carry a side effect of urinary retention, and others are *nephrotoxic,* or damaging to the kidneys.

Examining urine

Normal urine output should be approximately equal to intake; in other words, the amount that comes out should be equal to the amount that went in.

REMEMBER

Output less than 30 ml/hour for an adult may indicate decreased blood flow to the kidney and should be reported immediately to the physician.

A routine urinalysis examines the following components and results:

>> **Color:** The normal range is yellow to light orange. The lighter the color, the better hydrated the person is.

>> **Specific gravity:** Specific gravity is an indicator of hydration status: A high value indicates dehydration, and a low value indicates over-hydration. The normal range is 1.005 to 1.030.

>> **pH:** The normal range is 4.6 to 8.0.

>> **Other components:** Glucose, ketone bodies, protein, and blood aren't normally found in urine.

Foley catheter: Handle with care!

REMEMBER

Because of immobilization or inability to void, many patients have indwelling Foley bladder catheters. Foley catheters are a major cause of hospital-acquired infections, so you must use strict aseptic technique when inserting catheters and maintain a closed system. (Head to Chapter 6 for more on aseptic technique.) Catheters should be used only when absolutely necessary and for as short a time as possible because of the incidence of sepsis. Nursing assessment of catheter outputs is important for maintaining patient status.

Here's an example of the type of question you may encounter about urinary catheters:

EXAMPLE

The nurse is aware of the potential complications associated with the use of an indwelling urinary catheter. What is the most important nursing assessment for a patient with a Foley catheter?

(1) Draining the catheter bag once per shift and documenting the task

(2) Assessing the patient for elevated temperature and cloudy urine

(3) Monitoring intake and output every shift

(4) Checking urine for gross hematuria and signs of trauma

Keywords in this question are *potential complications, indwelling urinary catheter, most important nursing assessment,* and *patient with a Foley catheter.* The correct answer is Choice (2). Elevated temperature and cloudy urine are signs of urinary tract infection (UTI). The presence of an indwelling Foley catheter is a major risk factor for *nosocomial* (hospital-acquired) infection. The nurse is aware of this risk and monitors the patient accordingly. The assessments listed in the other options are also performed when a patient has a catheter, but the priority here is recognizing the signs of UTI so the patient can be treated.

Maintaining a healthy urinary tract

Following are the important things nurses must remember to maintain a healthy urinary tract in clients who are under medical care:

>> Maintain the patient's usual voiding schedule as much as possible while hospitalized.

>> Teach the patient Kegel exercises to strengthen pelvic floor muscles and improve control of urination.

>> Assess the patient for urinary retention by palpating the bladder and checking urine output.

>> Discourage the use of alcohol and caffeine.

>> Advise limiting fluid intake at bedtime.

>> Teach bladder retraining, if necessary.

>> Maintain adequate fluid intake of 1,700-2,500 ml/day.

>> Teach proper hygiene (in particular, female clients should wipe the perineal area from front to back after voiding).

Keeping bowels healthy

The stool can be loose or hard and come in a variety of colors. As unpleasant as it may sometimes seem, your patient's stools are your concern. Nobody said that looking at poop was fun, but it can be instructive.

When answering questions about nursing care for patients with alterations in bowel elimination, focus on factors that influence bowel elimination (such as diet, sleep, fluid balance, and certain medications), common bowel problems, and care of patients with bowel diversions.

Treating common bowel problems

You need to know how to deal with several common stool issues, among them

>> **Constipation:** Inability to defecate or passage of dry, hard stools. You need to assess the patient's usual patterns of elimination and laxative use.

REMEMBER

Some patients may say they're constipated if they don't have bowel movements every day; you need to teach these patients that the frequency of bowel movements is less important than the difficulty passing stools. Teach patients to increase fluid intake, activity levels, and the amount of fiber in their diets to correct constipation.

>> **Impaction:** The accumulated mass of feces in the rectum that can't be expelled. Symptoms of impaction include distended abdomen, the absence of bowel movements, decreased bowel sounds, and/or frequent passage of small amounts of liquid stool.

>> **Diarrhea:** Increased frequency of bowel movements as well as the passage of liquid, unformed stools. With diarrhea, identifying and treating the cause — be it impaction, GI tract infection, antibiotic use, or certain foods — is important. If a patient has continued diarrhea, assess him or her for fluid volume deficit, hypokalemia, and metabolic acidosis.

Caring for ostomies

An *ostomy* is a surgically created opening (or *stoma*) in the abdominal wall through which feces pass. An ostomy can be temporary or permanent and is classified by its location in the bowel and the construction of the stoma. As a nurse, you may deal with two types of ostomies:

>> **Ileostomy:** An opening into the distal end of the small intestine (the ileum). Because of its location, an ileostomy drains liquid stool, which contains digestive enzymes that can be irritating to the skin.

>> **Colostomy:** An opening into the colon. The location of this type of ostomy determines whether the stool is liquid in consistency or semi-solid: The more distal the location, the more formed the stool.

REMEMBER

Inspect the stoma regularly; a stoma should be rose to brick red in color and moist. A dark blue or purple stoma indicates compromised circulation, and the physician should be notified immediately.

Follow these tips to maintain an intact, healthy ostomy site:

>> Keep the skin around the stoma clean and dry. Ileostomy drainage, in particular, can be irritating to surrounding skin.

>> Measure intake and output.

>> Encourage the patient to participate in his care and to look at his ostomy. Alteration in body image is a common problem.

Postoperatively, an ostomy begins to drain when peristalsis returns (usually about two to five days). Initially, the patient may be placed on a low-residue diet. Foods that are high in fiber can be introduced gradually, and the patient can eventually resume a normal diet.

On the NCLEX-RN, ostomy-related questions may look like this:

EXAMPLE

A nurse is teaching a client with a newly formed ileostomy. Which statement by the client indicates a need for further teaching?

(1) "I will need to irrigate my ileostomy every day."

(2) "The skin around my ileostomy will need to be protected from prolonged contact with secretions."

(3) "I will need to follow a low-roughage, low-residue diet."

(4) "I should inspect my stoma daily and report any change in color."

The keywords in this question are *newly formed ileostomy, which statement,* and *indicates a need for further teaching.* The correct answer is Choice (1). Irrigation of an ostomy is intended to regulate bowel function and stimulate the bowel to function at a specific time every day, but irrigation isn't possible with an ileostomy because drainage is frequent and loose. The patient's other comments are accurate. Drainage from an ileostomy can irritate the skin because digestive enzymes and gastric secretions are irritating to the skin. Diet with an ileostomy is highly individualized; often, a low-roughage diet is ordered initially, and foods containing fiber are reintroduced gradually. Later, the patient may have no dietary restrictions and should aim to return to a normal, presurgical diet. The stoma should be assessed daily.

Wading through Irrigations

The basic care and comfort section also covers irrigations, including eye, ear, and bladder irrigations; how to do them; and the order in which you perform them.

REMEMBER

Don't forget any conditions that result from irrigations. For example, bladder irrigation places the client at risk for *hypornatremia* (low sodium concentration in the blood).

Here are some other irrigation items to remember:

>> Eyes

- Know the normal saline to use to irrigate the eye for chemical burn.

- Position the client supine with his or her head turned toward the affected eye.

- Check the pH of the eye prior to and after irrigation to ensure it matches the pH of the nonaffected eye. The pH of the affected eye will need to be same of the unaffected eye or the client is at risk for injury from chemical or foreign body.

>> Ears

- Visualize the tympanic membrane prior to irrigation for being intact. Not visualizing puts client at risk for irrigation entering behind tympanic membrane and infection if a tear or hole exists in the membrane.

- Warm the solution to body temperature of 98.6 degrees Fahrenheit. Cool solution puts the client at risk of becoming nauseated and issues with vertigo.

- Aim the solution at the wall of the ear canal rather than the tympanic membrane.

- The ear being irrigated is facing up during the irrigation.

>> Bladder

- Know that performing a bladder irrigation occurs with transurethral resection of the prostate (TURP) with a three-way catheter.

- The solution to be used is ordered by the doctor.

- Bladder irrigations are at risk for TURP or severe hyponatremia-water intoxication. Signs and symptoms of these conditions include change in mental status, confusion, increased blood pressure, and bradycardia.

EXAMPLE

An elderly client needs ear irrigation due to cerumen blocking the ear canal. The nurse prepares to irrigate the ear. Which of the following would the nurse do to prevent a complication from the ear irrigation?

(1) Warm the irrigation solution

(2) Inspect the tympanic membrane

(3) Place the irrigated ear down after the procedure

(4) Have the client move his or her head slowly prior to irrigation

Keywords for this question are *elderly client, ear irrigation, cerumen blocking the ear canal,* and *prevent a complication from the ear irrigation.* The correct answer is Choice (2). The primary complications of ear irrigation are otitis media (infection) and rupturing of the tympanic membrane, and inspecting the membrane ahead of time would prevent fluid from getting behind it and causing an infection. Warming the solution, placing the ear down after irrigation, and moving the head slowly prior to irrigation don't prevent these complications.

EXAMPLE

A postoperative TURP client has become confused, and blood pressure has gone from 90/50 to 140/90 with pulse of 80 to 56. Which of the following should the nurse suspect?

(1) Hemorrhagic Shock

(2) Sepsis

(3) TURP syndrome

(4) Infection

The keywords for the question are *postoperative TURP client, confused, blood pressure has gone from 90/50 to 140/90, pulse of 80 to 56,* and *nurse suspect.* The correct answer is Choice (3). Hemorrhagic shock, sepsis, and infection don't match the symptoms the client is experiencing.

Providing Holistic Care with Alternative and Complementary Medicine

Nursing has always focused on the holistic side of patient care — looking at the whole patient when planning treatment rather than just the disease process. Many patients as well as medical personnel are interested in pursuing alternative treatments, called *CAM* (complementary and alternative modalities), in addition to or in place of traditional medical treatment. Nurses need to be knowledgeable about CAM because they're being incorporated increasingly into patient care. Some examples of CAM modalities are these:

>> Acupuncture

>> Relaxation techniques

>> Imagery

>> Therapeutic touch

>> Music therapy

>> Herbal therapies

REMEMBER

To answer questions about CAM, you need to know that alternative modalities are techniques outside of the scope of conventional medicine, but when they are used in conjunction with conventional medicine to enhance the treatment, they are called complementary. For example, a patient with end-stage cancer is experiencing nausea and vomiting that antiemetic medication doesn't relieve. She visits an acupuncturist for therapy to help relieve her symptoms. As her nurse, you need to know the basics about this therapy to plan her care. In addition, asking about herbal therapies is important when taking a nursing admission history because certain herbal therapies can interact with prescribed medications.

Exam questions on this topic may resemble the following:

A patient who is undergoing abdominal surgery in two weeks asks the nurse about the use of acupuncture as a complementary modality for pain control. Which response from the nurse demonstrates her knowledge of the use of alternative therapies?

(1) "Acupuncture has been studied and found to complement postoperative pain relief and reduce nausea and vomiting."

(2) "No study has shown any difference in the postoperative course after patients have received acupuncture."

(3) "Acupuncture is a relatively new procedure and has shown limited effects."

(4) "Acupuncture works best for smoking cessation and back pain."

This question's keywords are *undergoing abdominal surgery, two weeks, the use of acupuncture,* and *pain control.* The question wants the nurse to show her knowledge of the use of alternative therapies such as acupuncture. The correct answer is Choice (1). Studies have shown a positive effect from acupuncture in relieving post-op pain when used in conjunction with traditional pain relief medications. One of the oldest, most commonly used medical procedures in the world, acupuncture is rapidly gaining acceptance in mainstream medicine in the United States.

Decreasing Pain without Pills

Have a headache? Take a pill. Our society thrives on the notion of a quick fix, but sometimes palliative measures such as distraction or music therapy can be used successfully as adjuncts for pain relief. These techniques are beneficial because they help increase the client's sense of control, are inexpensive, require no special equipment, and are easy to administer.

NCLEX-RN questions pertaining to these topics focus primarily on approaches to relieve pain and promote comfort that are used in conjunction with pain relief medications. These nonpharmacologic techniques include the following:

>> Distraction

>> Music therapy

>> Relaxation

>> Cutaneous stimulation

>> Guided imagery

>> Biofeedback

Massage and heat/cold applications are examples of cutaneous stimulation that nurses use to relieve pain. The success of these techniques is explained by the gate control theory of pain.

Questions dealing with nonpharmacologic techniques may look like the following:

A client is experiencing chronic back pain and receiving analgesics. The nurse first suggests which nonpharmacologic measure to help relieve his pain?

(1) Hypnosis

(2) Herbal therapy

(3) Guided imagery/distraction

(4) Epidural analgesia

Keywords for this question are *chronic back pain, receiving analgesics, nurse suggests,* and *nonpharmacologic measures.* The correct answer is Choice (3). Guided imagery has proven successful for patients with chronic pain. The nurse helps the patient develop a picture in his mind of a favorite place or setting, and the mental images help the patient to relax both mentally and physically. As for the other options, hypnosis is a technique that requires specially trained individuals; though it would be a good option for back pain, the nurse isn't likely to start with that suggestion. Epidural analgesia is a pharmacologic therapy, and herbal therapy is considered an alternative or complementary method (see the preceding section), but is not nonpharmacologic.

Helping Patients Get Around (and What to Do if They Can't)

Moving is good for you; it helps keep all your body systems in shape. However, many clients are unable to get around without assistance, and others are unable to move as much as they should for continued health. For the NCLEX-RN, you need to know about devices patients can use to ambulate as well as the ins and outs of immobility.

Training patients to use crutches, walkers, and canes

If you've ever had to use crutches, canes, a walker, or a wheelchair for any length of time, you know that it's not as easy as it looks! NCLEX-RN questions about *assistive devices* refer to devices used to help patients with limited mobility to ambulate. Many patients leave the hospital dependent on an assistive device to get around, and as a nurse, you're instrumental in teaching them how to navigate without hurting themselves — or anyone else! For the NCLEX-RN, keep in mind the following facts about assistive devices:

>> **Crutches:** Crutches aren't as stable as walkers and canes, and they require upper body strength and balance. Teach patients to support their body weight with their hands and arms and not with the axillary area because the pressure in that area can damage nerves and cut off circulation. Know the different types of gait use with crutches: Two point, three point, four point, swing to and swing through gait. Two-point gait is used for partial weight-bearing restrictions. Three-point gait is used for partial or no weight-bearing restrictions, and four-point and swing-through gaits are used when no weight-bearing restrictions exist. Each gait requires the client to move the crutches and lower extremities in a certain pattern.

>> **Walker:** Walkers provide patients with more support and stability than canes and are useful for clients who have poor balance. Depending on the patient's ability, the walker may be a rolling type, with wheels on the feet, or a pickup type, in which the patient lifts the walker ahead of himself and steps toward it. The nurse must know the amount of weight the patient's allowed to bear. Regardless of the type of walker used, patients should wear nonskid shoes.

>> **Cane:** A cane provides patients with a wider base of support when they're standing and walking. The three basic types of canes are the *quad cane,* which has four feet; the *tripod cane,* which has three feet; and the *straight cane,* which has a single foot. Teach your patient to hold his or her cane on the unaffected (strong) side to give support to the weaker leg, hold the cane close to the body, and advance the weaker foot forward parallel with the cane.

Here's a sample question related to assistive devices:

EXAMPLE

The nurse is teaching a client with right-sided weakness how to ambulate with a cane. The nurse determines that the client knows how to use the cane properly when she observes that

(1) The client holds the cane on the left side.

(2) The client leans into the cane, placing all his weight on the cane.

(3) The client advances the stronger foot forward, parallel with the cane.

(4) The client relies on the cane for total support.

Keywords in this question are *right-sided weakness, ambulate with a cane,* and *knows how to use the cane properly,* and *observes that.* The correct answer is Choice (1). The patient should hold the cane on the unaffected (stronger) side, which in this case is his left side. Proper posture and even weight distribution is important. When walking with a cane, the client should advance the cane between 4 and 12 inches and then advance the weaker foot forward parallel with the cane. Next, the stronger leg should advance ahead of the cane. The client should never rely on the cane for total support.

EXAMPLE

The healthcare provider has ordered that the client be taught a four-point gait for crutches. Which of the following shows the nursing student understands the four-point gait?

(1) The right crutch is moved forward, followed by the left foot, the left crutch, and lastly the right foot.

(2) The crutch on the affected side and unaffected foot are moved forward at the same time. Then the unaffected side crutch and affected foot are moved forward.

(3) Both crutches and the affected foot move forward together, followed by the unaffected foot.

(4) Both crutches are moved forward and then the legs are moved to just next to the crutches.

Keywords for this question are *four-point gait* and *shows the nursing student understands.* The correct answer is Choice (1). Choice (2) describes two-point gait. Choice (3) is three-point gait, and Choice (4) is swing-through gait.

Avoiding complications from immobility

Many patients are unable to move as much as they should and, as a result, are at high risk for many different complications. Exam questions about immobility require you to know the effects of prolonged immobility and the nursing interventions to combat these complications. To make things a bit easier for you, I've broken the effects of immobility on the body down into systems:

» **Neurological/mental status:** Body image issues, poor self-concept and lack of social interaction leading to decreased support systems, powerlessness, sensory deprivation

» **Cardiovascular:** Venous thrombosis, increased cardiac workload, orthostatic hypotension

» **Respiratory:** Atelectasis, pneumonia, pulmonary embolism

» **Musculoskeletal:** Muscle atrophy, fatigue, joint contracture, negative nitrogen balance, calcium loss, bone demineralization

» **Gastrointestinal:** Decreased appetite, constipation

» **Urinary:** Urinary stasis, urinary tract infection, renal stones (calculi)

» **Skin:** Skin breakdown, pressure ulcers

Patients should be mobilized as early as possible and to the extent possible. If they can't be mobilized, then in-bed range-of-motion exercises and other exercises should be performed to the extent possible and within the parameters possible based on the patient's condition.

Immobility-related questions may look something like this:

EXAMPLE

When assessing a female client who is immobilized from a motor vehicle accident last evening, which assessment finding would prompt the nurse to take immediate further action?

(1) Laboratory result called to the unit with a hematocrit of 37%

(2) Client complaining of decreased appetite

(3) Rapid, shallow respirations with an O_2 saturation of 89%

(4) Weight loss of 3 pounds over the past five days

Keywords for this question are *immobilized, motor vehicle accident, last evening,* and *assessment finding would prompt the nurse to take immediate further action.* The correct answer is Choice (3). Rapid, shallow respirations and a drop in O_2 saturation (hypoxemia) can indicate a pulmonary embolism, a complication of immobility. The nurse should immediately notify the physician of these findings. Other assessment findings with a pulmonary embolism can include chest tightness, hemoptysis, and respiratory alkalosis. As for the other options, decreased appetite and weight loss are expected possible results of immobility and shouldn't prompt immediate action, and hematocrit of 37 percent is normal for a female patient (the reference range is 37 to 47 percent).

Chapter **10**

Meditating on Meds: Pharmacological and Parenteral Therapies

Some days, it seems as if a nurse's job consists mostly of handing out pills, giving injections, and hanging intravenous bags. Nursing isn't that robotic, however; ensuring that patients get the proper medications in the proper doses at the proper times is a big part of your nursing responsibility. But trying to remember which medication does what and what interacts with something else, and potential side effects, can cause the mere word *pharmacology* to strike fear in your heart. Trust me — you're not alone!

Questions on the NCLEX-RN related to these tasks and topics focus on how to safely administer medications, and they address basic principles of pharmacology, pain management, dosage calculation, and IV therapy skills (remember, that last one is also called *parenteral therapy*). In this chapter, I review these topics and provide practice questions to help you conquer your fear and decrease your pharmacology phobia!

Remembering the Factors You Must Verify before Giving Meds

Hardly anything is as basic to nursing as the "rights" of medication administration. (Not all text-books include documentation "right," but I put it in this list because it's good to know.) Even though these "rights" undoubtedly were crammed into your head during nursing school, reviewing them here doesn't hurt:

» **Right patient:** When checking the patient's identity prior to med administration, guidelines call for you to identify the patient in two ways, such as checking the patient's armband and asking him to state his name and birth date. Checking the patient's room number isn't an effective way of verifying identity because patients often change rooms.

>> **Right drug:** Drugs have several names. The *generic name* is the common name assigned to the drug when it's first developed. The *trade* or *brand name* is the name that the pharmaceutical company gives the drug to market it. In the past, generic and brand name were both on the NCLEX-RN, but now the generic name is the only name you see. Be sure you know the generic name of the common medications given.

REMEMBER

A drug has only one generic name, but it can have several trade names. For example, ibuprofen is a generic name; common trade names for ibuprofen are Motrin, Advil, and Nuprin.

Questions most often use the most common drugs. You can find a list of these usual suspects in any drug book, typically listed under the 100 most common drugs.

>> **Right dose:** You need to know that the dose to be administered is a safe dose. The current NCLEX-RN expects you to know the common dosage used for the drugs in the question. (Previously, you could consult a drug reference guide or ask the pharmacist.) The dosage of a drug may be stated in either the apothecary, household, or metric system, but regardless, you're responsible for correctly calculating drug dosages (see the section "Calculating dosages" later in this chapter for more on the topic).

>> **Right route:** The route of the medication must be specified in the medication order. You need to know whether a medication is to be given by mouth, by IV, by injection, or in a suppository. If the patient's condition changes and you can't follow the ordered route, you should notify the physician to get a new order written.

>> **Right time:** Nurses need to be aware of the general principles of drug timing, such as which medications should be given with meals or around the clock. Generally, every medication should be given within a half hour of the scheduled time (either before or after).

>> **Right documentation:** Documenting is a critical part of the med administration process, and you need to do it immediately after the med is given. Remember the saying "If it wasn't documented, it wasn't done."

Over time, the list of "rights" has expanded to include the following important reminders:

>> **Right history and assessment:** Check a client's medication history as well as her condition and labs prior to giving medication.

>> **Right to refuse medication:** Remember the client always has the right to refuse prescribed medication, but the nurse needs to make sure the client knows the consequences of not taking the medication.

>> **Right drug-to-drug interaction:** Nurses need to know whether any of the prescribed medications might have adverse effects if taken together as well as what reactions to watch for and when to notify a healthcare provider prior to giving the medication.

>> **Right education:** Nurses help explain what medication the client has been prescribed, why, and any possible side effects.

NCLEX-RN questions about medication may ask you how you'd give medication: an hour before meals or an hour after meals. Or they may ask whether you'd give it through an IV (and how fast), subcutaneously, or by mouth (also referred to as per oral or PO).

TIP

You can eliminate the majority of medication errors by quickly running through this checklist before giving any patient any medication.

Medicating Patients Safely

I want to get something straight: You don't have to be a walking *Nurse's Drug Guide* to pass the NCLEX-RN! Although you aren't expected to memorize long lists of drug names, side effects, interactions, and dosages, understanding certain general guidelines can help you answer questions about medication.

Assessing before medicating

NCLEX-RN questions are designed to find out whether you can think critically before you dispense a medication; therefore, remember to assess the patient before giving any medication. The parameter you assess depends on your knowledge of the medication being given. Specific areas to assess include the following:

>> **Vital signs, if appropriate:** Most cardiac medications and antihypertensives require a pulse and/or blood pressure check.

>> **Allergy history:** Make this assessment before administering any drug.

>> **Harmful drug interactions:** In addition to standard drug interactions, be aware of interactions with herbal supplements.

>> **Medical history and current diagnosis:** Ask yourself whether the client's condition has changed since admission. For example, an elderly patient admitted with pneumonia has recently suffered a stroke while in the hospital. He has an order for a PO medication; however, his level of consciousness has decreased and resulted in impaired swallowing. In this situation, you need to call the prescriber to question the order.

>> **Pertinent lab values:** Review the chart for all values that pertain to the drugs you're administering. For example, check serum digoxin level and serum potassium prior to administering digoxin, and check serum potassium level prior to administering certain diuretics.

>> **Necessary drug-related patient teaching:** Before administering medication to a patient, you need to teach the patient about the drug and any side effects that may occur. For example, when administering insulin in a newly diagnosed diabetic, assess patient's knowledge of diabetes, symptoms of low blood sugar, dietary modifications, and administration techniques.

Here are two questions to show you how to use these assessment concepts:

EXAMPLE

Verapamil has been prescribed for a patient with a supraventricular arrhythmia. Prior to administering this medication, the nurse performs which priority assessment?

(1) Check the patient's heart rate and blood pressure.

(2) Check the patient's serum potassium level.

(3) Hold the drug if the patient is experiencing palpitations.

(4) Monitor liver function studies.

The keywords in this question are *verapamil, supraventricular arrhythmia, prior to administering this medication,* and *which priority assessment.* The correct answer is Choice (1). Knowing the classification for the drugs helps. Verapamil is a calcium channel blocker. Calcium channel blockers affect blood pressure and are indicated for treatment of supraventricular arrythmias, hypertension, and vasospastic angina. Hypotension and bradycardia are side effects; therefore, an important nursing assessment is to check blood pressure and pulse prior to administration. Verapamil moves potassium but does not elevate or lower the level. There is no need to check the patient's potassium level. Palpitations are to be expected in a patient experiencing a supraventricular arrhythmia, and liver function studies should be monitored over the long term but aren't the priority here.

EXAMPLE

A nurse will be administering albuterol to a 65-year-old client with chronic obstructive pulmonary disease (COPD). The nurse will assess which of the following parameters before and during therapy?

(1) Hemoglobin (Hgb) and hematocrit (HCT)

(2) Presence of dyspnea and lung sounds

(3) Diarrhea

(4) Urine output and creatinine

The keywords in this question are *administering albuterol*, *65-year-old client*, *chronic obstructive pulmonary disease*, and *assess which of the following parameters*. The correct answer is Choice (2). Albuterol is a bronchodilator that's being used in this case to treat bronchospasm in a patient with obstructive airway disease. The nurse should check for shortness of breath (dyspnea) and lung sounds in order to assess the effectiveness of the therapy. The other options don't indicate the effectiveness of the therapy.

Calculating dosages

The NCLEX-RN currently tests medication calculation very seldom; students often get only one or two math questions in the entire test. But that doesn't let you off the hook for knowing how to do the calculations.

Although trying to calculate grams (g) versus grains (gr) and milligrams (mg) versus micrograms (mcg) may make your eyes cross, you still need to understand how to calculate medications in order to pass the NCLEX-RN. Yes, most medications now are unit-based and arrive prepackaged by the pharmacist. Most, but not all. On some occasions, you still may need to convert medications from milligrams to grams, for example. You also need to know how to calculate IV rates and mix IV solutions because not all IV medications run on pumps that figure it out for you.

To make things even more confusing, medication therapy uses three different systems of measurement: metric, apothecary, and household. Remember, a drug dosage is usually ordered by weight (mcg, mg, or g), but it may be administered by volume (ml or L). Fortunately, the medication calculation questions you find on the NCLEX-RN are fairly straightforward. To answer the questions, make sure that you memorize the following metric conversions for weight:

1,000 micrograms (mcg)	=	1 milligram (mg)
1,000 mg	=	1 gram (g)
1,000 g	=	1 kilogram (kg)

You also need to store the metric conversions for volume in your noggin:

1 cubic centimeter (cc)	=	1 milliliter (ml)
1,000 ml	=	l liter (L)

Sometimes you need to convert from one system to another, so I've summarized some of the most important equivalents of measurement, converted from metric to household, in the following list:

1 L	=	1 quart (qt)
30 ml	=	1 ounce (oz)
240 ml	=	8 ounces (oz)
5 ml	=	1 teaspoon (tsp)
60 mg	=	1 grain
1 kg	=	2.2 pounds (lbs)

REMEMBER

When performing mathematical calculations to convert dosages, follow this three-step process and you'll be good to go:

1. **Ask yourself whether a conversion is necessary, and if so, convert the measurements to the same system.**

   A conversion is necessary if the measurements are in different systems (apothecary, metric, or household) or different size units (mg and g, or ml and L). If the measurements are in the same system, no conversion is necessary.

2. **Calculate the answer by using the following formula:**

   (Dose ordered ÷ Dose on hand) × Amount on hand = Amount to administer

   The difference between dose on hand and amount on hand is an important one: The *dose* is the weight or volume of medication available, and the *amount* is the basic unit or quantity of medication that contains the dose on hand (supplied by pharmacy). For example, for liquid medications, the amount on hand may be one or more ml or L; for solid medications, the dose on hand may be one capsule or tablet.

3. **Ask yourself whether your answer makes sense.**

   Use estimation to come up with what you think is a reasonable answer. If your calculation doesn't agree with your estimation, check your math.

Practicing the math for tablet meds

REMEMBER

A general rule of thumb is to always question any situation in which you're administering more than three tablets. When administering ½ tablet, be sure it's a tablet that can be cut in half. If the tablet's enteric coated or gelation or sustained release in any form, the drug isn't evenly distributed, and when you break the enteric coating or otherwise alter the tablet, the drug doesn't work as manufactured.

NCLEX-RN questions about calculating numbers of tablets, capsules, or ml may look like this:

EXAMPLE

A physician has prescribed levothyroxine, 150 mcg PO daily. The medication label reads Synthroid, 0.1 mg per tablet. The nurse should administer how many tablet(s) to the client?

(1) 2 tablets

(2) 2.5 tablets

(3) 1.5 tablets

(4) 1 tablet

Keywords in this question are *levothyroxine, 150 mcg PO*, and *label reads Synthroid, 0.1 mg per tablet.* How many tablets should the nurse administer? The correct answer is Choice (3). To work through this calculation, follow the three-step method:

1. **Ask yourself whether a conversion is necessary.**

In this case, yes, so first convert 150 mcg to mg by moving the decimal three places to the left: 150 mcg = 0.15 mg.

2. **Calculate the answer as follows:**

(Dose ordered ÷ Dose on hand) × Amount on hand = Amount to administer

(0.15 mg ÷ 0.1 mg) × 1 tablet = 1.5 tablets

3. **Ask yourself whether your answer makes sense.**

For this question, your calculation is right on the money. If each tablet contains 0.1 mg and you need to give 0.15 mg, your answer makes sense.

Crunching numbers for oral and subcutaneous, intradermal, and intermuscular medications

Here's a sample question for liquid medication calculation:

EXAMPLE

Digoxin elixir is available with 0.05 mg of the drug in 1 ml of solution. How much of the elixir should the nurse administer if the physician's order is for Lanoxin 0.125 mg PO bid?

(1) 2.25 ml

(2) 2.5 ml

(3) 2 ml

(4) 2.75 ml

The keywords in this question are *digoxin elixir, 0.05 mg of the drug in 1 ml of solution*, and *how much of the elixir should the nurse administer if the physician's order is for Lanoxin 0.125 mg PO bid.* The correct answer is Choice (2). To work through this calculation, follow the three-step method:

1. **Ask yourself whether a conversion is necessary.**

In this case, conversion isn't necessary because the drug measurements are in the same system (metric) and units (mg).

2. **Calculate the answer as follows:**

(Dose ordered ÷ Dose on hand) × Amount on hand = Amount to administer

(0.125 mg ÷ 0.05 mg) × 1 ml = 2.5 ml

3. **Ask yourself whether your answer makes sense.**

Yep, it sure does. You can estimate that 0.125 mg is approximately 2.5 times the dose on hand per tablet.

Counting fingers, toes, and everything in between for IV dosages

A question about parenteral dosages may go like this:

EXAMPLE

A prescriber has ordered heparin 1,000 units intravenously every hour as a continuous IV infusion for deep vein thrombosis prophylaxis. The pharmacy has supplied a vial containing 10,000 units/500 ml. How many ml/hour of heparin should the nurse administer?

The correct answer is 50 ml/hour, which you determine through the following steps:

1. Ask yourself whether a conversion is necessary.

In this situation, no, you don't need to make a conversion because the drug units ordered are in the same system and size (measurement units) as the supply.

2. Calculate the answer like so:

(Amount of medication in solution ÷ Total diluent = Amount of medication per ml)

(10,000 units ÷ 500 ml = 20 units/ml)

Then calculate milliliters per hour:

(Desired dose per hour ÷ Concentration per milliliter = Infusion rate or ml per hour)

(1,000 units ÷ 20 units/ml = 50 ml/hour)

3. Ask yourself whether your answer makes sense.

Yes! Your answer makes sense in that 20 units/ml would take a lot to get to 1,000 units/hour!

Recognizing the effects of meds

You always have a reason for giving a medication. Keeping that fact in mind helps you assess, post-administration, whether you're helping the patient by giving the med. To gauge whether a medication is effective, consider the following:

» **Therapeutic effect:** The desired or expected response to the drug. For example, the therapeutic response to nitroglycerin is to reduce cardiac workload and increase myocardial oxygen supply.

» **Side effect:** An unintended, secondary effect of the drug. For example, a side effect of morphine is constipation.

» **Toxicity:** The severe or even lethal effects of excess amounts of the drug in the bloodstream. For example, vancomycin toxicity can result in kidney damage, also known as nephrotoxicity.

For example, when you're giving furosemide, check for the desired effect (diuresis) and any side effects (hypotension, hypokalemia, and so on).

REMEMBER

You also need to know what to do when you see such effects in your patient, both on the test and in real life. Know when to call the doctor for side effects and for when the patient is showing signs of toxicity.

The following are examples of questions related to the therapeutic effects, side effects, and toxicity of drugs:

EXAMPLE

The nurse understands that neomycin is being given to a patient before ileostomy surgery primarily to

(1) Decrease the incidence of postoperative infection by suppressing intestinal bacteria

(2) Increase the body's immune response to the surgery

(3) Reduce the possibility of infectious diarrhea post-op

(4) Decrease production of ammonia in the intestine

The keywords for this question are *neomycin, given to a patient before ileostomy surgery*, and *primarily to*. The correct answer is Choice (1). The therapeutic effect of neomycin given preoperatively is to decrease the number of intestinal organisms that may result in a postoperative infection. Administering neomycin doesn't boost the body's immune response or decrease the production of ammonia in the intestine. The medication does reduce the possibility of infectious diarrhea post-op, but that isn't the primary reason neomycin is administered and therefore isn't the best answer.

EXAMPLE

The nurse is teaching a patient with chronic pulmonary disease about the side effects of long-term corticosteroid therapy. The nurse realizes that the patient will need further teaching when he states

(1) "I may experience some facial swelling."

(2) "I will need to take the drug every day in order to avoid serious side effects."

(3) "My doctor will be checking my blood sugar levels regularly."

(4) "I will heal faster if I get injured."

The keywords for this question are *chronic pulmonary disease, side effects of long-term corticosteroid therapy*, and *realizes that the patient will need further teaching when he states*. The correct answer is Choice (4). This question is checking to see whether you know the side effects of the stated drug. Patients taking long-term steroids have impaired wound healing, so this patient needs further teaching if he indicates he thinks injuries will heal more quickly.

For this type of NCLEX-RN question, rephrasing the question in your mind is helpful. This question is really asking you to identify what side effects you expect to see in a patient with chronic pulmonary disease who's receiving long-term corticosteroid therapy. Any that aren't expected effects are the correct choice. Facial swelling and high blood glucose are both side effects, so Choices (1) and (3) are accurate statements. Choice (2) is also a correct statement; patients shouldn't abruptly discontinue steroids, because doing so may result in adrenal suppression.

EXAMPLE

A patient with a history of atrial fibrillation is currently receiving digoxin 0.25 mg PO daily. Prior to administering the medication, the nurse will assess the patient carefully for which condition and what other condition that may precipitate?

(1) Hypokalemia, digitalis toxicity

(2) Hypocalcemia, hyperkalemia

(3) Hyperthyroidism, hypocalcemia

(4) Hypotension, heart failure

The keywords for this question are *history of atrial fibrillation, digoxin, prior to administering the medication*, and *assess the patient carefully*. The correct answer is Choice (1). Knowing that toxicity happens with low potassium leads you to the correct answer. Hypokalemia (decreased serum potassium) may precipitate digitalis toxicity, and the nurse should check the patient's potassium level prior to administering the drug. Hypocalcemia does not cause hyperkalemia with the use of digoxin. Hyperthyroidism does not cause hypocalcium with the use of digoxin. Hypotension does not cause heart failure with use of digoxin. Digoxin is used for heart failure.

REMEMBER

NCLEX questions may also test you on unusual side-effects, such as coloring all body secretions orange-red — the drug Streptomycin has this effect. Make sure you know these abnormal effects and the medications that cause them.

Answering questions about unfamiliar meds

You're in the middle of the test and you see a question with the name of a drug you've never heard of. Take some deep breaths and follow these steps:

1. Consider the patient.

If the question asks you about an unfamiliar drug, you may be able to figure out the general classification of a drug by looking at the patient it has been prescribed for. For example, if the question starts out "A nurse prepares an IV nitroprusside drip for a patient admitted in a hypertensive crisis . . .," you can deduce that nitroprusside is an antihypertensive drug.

2. Break down the name of the drug.

With a generic name, usually the ending is consistent within a drug classification. Table 10-1 shows some examples of common medication endings and how they may help you classify drugs. Brand names or trade names aren't on the test, though I've listed some in the table for reference.

TABLE 10-1   Endings Common to Drug Classifications

Class of Drug	Common Ending	Examples
Angiotension-converting	-pril	captopril (Capoten), enalapril (Vasotec), enzyme inhibitors
Anticoagulants	-arin	warfarin (Coumadin), heparin, enoxaparin (Lovenox)
Anticholinergics	-ine	atropine
Antilipemics	-statin	pravastatin (Pravachol), simvastatin (Zocor)
Antivirals	-vir	acyclovir (Zovirax), ganciclovir (Cytovene)
Beta blockers	-lol	metoprolol (Lopressor), propranolol (Inderal)
Calcium channel blockers	-pine	amlodipine (Norvasc)
Corticosteroids	-sone	prednisone (Deltasone), methylprednisolone (Medrol)
Proton pump inhibitors	-zole	lansoprazole (Prevacid)
Thrombolytics	-ase	alteplase (Activase)

Try these questions for practice identifying unknown drugs:

EXAMPLE

The nurse notes that a patient with a history of an anterior wall myocardial infarction (MI) is currently taking simvastatin. The nurse would suspect the client has which disorder?

(1) Myalgia

(2) Hyperlipidemia

(3) Arrhythmia

(4) Gastric reflux

The keywords for this question are *history of anterior wall myocardial infarction, simvastatin,* and *suspect the client has which disorder.* The correct answer is Choice (2). Simvastatin is a lipid-lowering agent. If you aren't familiar with this drug, first consider the patient. This patient has a history of myocardial infarction. What concurrent disorder is a patient with an MI likely to have? Of the options listed, possibly hyperlipidemia (high blood lipids) or arrhythmia (irregular heartbeat). You can eliminate myalgia and gastric reflux because these conditions are unlikely with this diagnosis. Next, look at the drug's name: Because it ends in -statin, you deduce that this drug is used as an antilipemic. Well done, Sherlock!

EXAMPLE

The nurse is monitoring a patient with a pulmonary embolism who is receiving a continuous intravenous heparin infusion. Which lab finding would indicate an adverse effect of the medication and the need to notify the physician?

(1) Platelet count of 80,000/mm³

(2) Prothrombin time (PT) 12.0 sec

(3) Hematocrit (HCT) 42%

(4) Blood urea nitrogen (BUN) 28 mg/dl

The keywords for this question are *pulmonary embolism, continuous intravenous heparin infusion, lab finding, indicate an adverse effect of the medication,* and *need to notify physician.* The correct answer is Choice (1). Heparin-induced thrombocytopenia (low platelet count) is an adverse effect of heparin, an anticoagulant. The normal range for a platelet count is 150,000 to 400,000/mm³. Thrombocytopenia caused by heparin may be linked to a type of arterial or venous thrombosis known as white clot syndrome. The medication may have to be discontinued, so a call to the physician is necessary.

If you aren't familiar with heparin (or its adverse effects), use the following strategy to answer the question "Who is the patient?" The patient has a pulmonary embolism, which you know is a blood clot; therefore, you deduce that the patient needs an anticoagulant. You can also use the -arin ending of heparin to figure out the classification (anticoagulant; see Table 10-1). Then examine your answer options: The patient's PT and HCT are within normal limits, and the BUN is abnormal (normal BUN is 5 to 20 mg/dl) but isn't an adverse effect of heparin therapy.

Using Medicine to Manage Pain

Many, if not most, patients in the hospital experience some pain, which is referred to as the "fifth vital sign." You should be assessing your patients for pain every time you take their vital signs. In order to answer exam questions about pain management, you need to remember the following key points:

>> **Believe the patient.** As a subjective sensation, pain is whatever the patient says it is. This concept is the foundation for your care of patients in pain.

>> **Assessment is important.** Use a pain rating scale to determine the intensity of the pain. One example is a numerical rating scale. Ask the patient to rate his pain on scale of 1 to 10. Pediatric clients can use a visual scale with faces drawn to represent expressions ranging from happy and smiling to sad and tearful. When patients have an altered level of consciousness, be aware of nonverbal indicators of pain, such as moaning, grimacing, or guarding. Reassess pain after administration of medication in order to determine its effectiveness.

REMEMBER

Cultural norms can play a role in how patients respond to pain. For example, in Filipino culture, it's considered rude to accept something on the first offer, so the nurse may need to offer pain medication more than once.

>> **Use a combination of drug and nondrug therapies.** Complementary therapies (such as massage, relaxation techniques, and acupuncture) are beneficial when incorporated into pain management. See Chapter 9 for a discussion of complementary therapies.

>> **Don't wait until the patient is in severe pain to administer the drug.** Medications work best when given around the clock or by continuous IV infusion (if controlled by patient, then it is called *patient-controlled analgesia*), or by pump. You should administer the drug before the pain gets too bad because waiting too long results in inadequate pain control. The goal is a constant serum level of pain medication at a therapeutic dose.

>> **Be alert to the side effects and symptoms of overdosage.** Many medications used for pain (such as opiates) have serious side effects ranging from excessive sedation to respiratory depression and arrest. As the nurse, you assess for these side effects before administering the drug; if any exist, you shouldn't administer the drug.

>> **Patient teaching is necessary.** The client receiving medication for pain should be taught about the side effects of the drug and how to manage them, the need to report pain levels, the need to take the drug before pain becomes severe, and signs of toxicity.

REMEMBER

When it comes to pain medication, you need to know the differences among addiction, tolerance, and physical dependence.

>> **Addiction** is characterized by the need to obtain and take substances for other than the prescribed therapeutic value. The risk of addiction to pain medication in acute-care patients with no history of substance abuse is very low.

>> **Tolerance** is characterized by the body's need for an increased dose of the drug in order to maintain the same level of analgesia. Thus, patients experiencing chronic pain (cancer patients, for example) may require large doses of the drug to achieve relief of their pain.

>> **Physical dependence** is a physiologic response that results in symptoms of withdrawal when a drug is discontinued or the dose is decreased. Drugs such as opiates should be tapered gradually when a patient has used them for a long period of time.

NCLEX-RN questions may ask about specific drugs prescribed for different levels of pain. Here's a quick summary:

>> **Mild pain:** When pain is mild, nonopioid analgesics should be used initially for pain control. These drugs don't produce tolerance or physical dependence, and some are available without a prescription. Examples of drugs in this category include

- Acetaminophen (Tylenol)
- Aspirin
- NSAIDs (nonsteroidal anti-inflammatory drugs) such as ibuprofen
- Ketorolac (Toradol)
- COX-2 inhibitors such as celecoxib (Celebrex)

>> **Moderate pain:** Drugs commonly used for moderate pain are more potent than nonopioid analgesics and have side effects that include sedation, bradycardia, nausea, constipation, and urinary retention. Examples include

- Opioids such as codeine
- Hydrocodone (Vicodin) and tramadol (Ultram)

>> **Severe pain:** Drugs used for moderate to severe pain are potent. Common side effects — including constipation, nausea and vomiting, urinary retention, and dizziness — usually can be managed by administering other medications. Respiratory depression and excessive sedation are two adverse effects of drugs of this kind. Elderly patients and patients with lung disease

are particularly at risk for these effects; therefore, you must assess level of consciousness and respiratory rate prior to administering these drugs. Examples include

- Morphine
- Fentanyl (Duragesic)
- Hydromorphone (Dilaudid)
- Oxycodone with Acetaminophen (Percocet)

REMEMBER

With the opioid crisis happening in the United States, be aware that a question may ask for the antidote (naloxone) and its usage in the community. Naloxone is given either by autoinjector into the outer thigh or by nasal spray. Administering this antidote requires training before a person in the community can use it.

You also need to remember the common routes and delivery systems for administering pain medication:

>> **Oral:** Route of choice for a patient with a functioning GI system.

>> **Transdermal:** Useful for patients who can't tolerate oral analgesics. An example of this kind of medication is the fentanyl transdermal patch.

>> **Intramuscular:** Quicker relief of pain than oral or transdermal because the medication is absorbed directly into the tissue and into the bloodstream.

>> **Intravenous:** Used most often in hospitals. Almost immediately relieves pain. Used postoperatively and in the emergency room for people suffering from trauma and heart attacks.

>> **Intraspinal (epidural):** Involves inserting a catheter into the subarachnoid or epidural space and injecting an analgesic. Morphine is an example of a drug that can be administered by this route. Complications of this route are infection and catheter displacement.

>> **Patient-controlled analgesia (PCA):** Involves a pump, which administers a dose of opioid when the patient decides a dose is needed and pushes a button to receive a bolus of the drug. PCA pumps are commonly used for postoperative and cancer pain, and patient teaching is important with a PCA pump. The nurse must assess for level of sedation and respiratory depression.

On the NCLEX-RN, pain management questions may look like this:

EXAMPLE

A client with metastatic breast cancer and bone metastasis has continuous, poorly localized pain. The nurse teaches the patient to use pain medications

(1) As often as necessary to keep the pain controlled

(2) On an around-the-clock schedule

(3) By alternating two different types of drugs to prevent addiction

(4) When the pain cannot be controlled with complementary therapies

The keywords for this question are *metastatic breast cancer and bone metastasis, poorly localized pain,* and *how to use pain medications.* The correct answer is Choice (2). The best control of chronic pain can be achieved by taking pain medication around the clock to obtain a constant serum drug level. The client should take the medication as per the scheduled time and not exceed the recommended dosage. Alternating two drugs doesn't achieve a therapeutic level of either drug. Complementary therapies should be used in conjunction with medication for this patient.

Here's an alternative question format for this topic (refer to Chapter 3 for details on question formats):

EXAMPLE

A postoperative patient is receiving IV morphine via a PCA pump for severe incisional pain. Nursing assessment will include what parameters? Select all that apply.

❑ **(1)** Respiratory rate and depth

❑ **(2)** Level of sedation

❑ **(3)** Pain level and quality

❑ **(4)** Frequency of bowel movements

❑ **(5)** Urine output

❑ **(6)** Serum glucose level

Keywords for this question are *postoperative patient, receiving IV morphine, PCA pump, severe incisional pain,* and *assessment will include what parameters.* The correct answers are Choices (1), (2), (3), (4), and (5). IV morphine administered via a PCA pump carries the side effects of respiratory depression, excessive sedation, constipation, and urinary retention. In addition, the nurse must always perform a pain assessment when a client is receiving pain medication. Choice (6) is incorrect because serum glucose level shouldn't be affected by a morphine infusion.

Giving Meds and More with a Stick and a Poke: Parenteral Therapy

Parenteral medications are any medications given through a route other than through the digestive system; in other words, they're medications given through an intravenous infusion or by injection. In this section, I talk about intravenous administration of various fluids and the different types of access for intravenous medications. I don't cover how to start IVs because ... well ... that's one hands-on skill that the NCLEX-RN can't test!

REMEMBER

However, you still need to know which veins are appropriate for various therapies. The exam may give you a specific type antibiotic like vancomycin and ask what kind of vein you'd use to administer it.

Solving the puzzle of solutions

You know that IV therapy provides your patient with life-sustaining fluids, electrolytes, and medications. Different patients and situations call for different types of solutions. For the exam, you need to know which solution is which and why you give different fluids for different outcomes.

Separating the parts from the whole

In order to safely administer IV fluids, you need to know about the types of solutions and the effects they have on the body's fluid balance. Remember that giving an IV fluid may cause fluids to shift from one body compartment to another. Here's a summary of what you need to know:

>> **Isotonic solutions** have a concentration (or osmolality) equal to that of the body's intracellular fluid. They're used when expanding the intravascular volume is necessary, as in shock or fluid volume depletion.

>> **Hypertonic solutions** have a concentration greater than that of intracellular fluid, so they're used to draw water out of the cells into the vascular space and cause the cells to shrink. They're commonly used with postoperative patients. Fluid overload is one complication when giving hypertonic solutions, so you must monitor levels closely.

>> **Hypotonic solutions** have a concentration less than that of intracellular fluid, so they're used to hydrate the cells. Water is pulled out of the intravascular space and into the cells. You must use hypotonic solutions with caution because they can result in increased intracranial pressure due to fluid shifts into brain cells, and they can cause intravascular fluid depletion.

For specific examples of these types of solutions, see Table 10-2.

TABLE 10-2 **Solutions and Their Applications**

Solution	Type of Solution	Used For
0.9% sodium chloride	Isotonic	Shock, fluid challenges, blood transfusion (normal saline)
Lactated Ringer's solution	Isotonic	Dehydration, burns, hypovolemia
5% dextrose in water (D5W)	Isotonic but turns hypotonic when glucose is metabolized	Total body water replacement
5% dextrose in 0.45% NS	Hypertonic	Diabetic ketoacidosis after treatment with normal saline
10% dextrose in water	Hypertonic	Water replacement, low serum glucose
0.45% sodium chloride	Hypotonic	Hypertonic dehydration, water replacement, sodium and chloride depletion

Here's an example of an NCLEX-RN question related to IV solutions:

EXAMPLE

The nurse is caring for a 90-year-old client with a history of heart failure. When making rounds, the nurse notes that an IV of 0.9% normal saline solution was mistakenly hung for the patient an hour before and has since infused 600 ml. The nurse should observe this patient for which of the following symptoms?

(1) Crackles upon auscultation of lungs, dyspnea, and neck vein distention

(2) Decreased skin turgor, dry mucous membranes, and concentrated urine

(3) Confusion, muscle cramping and twitching, and paresthesias of toes

(4) Diaphoresis, increased respiratory rate, and hyperreflexia

The keywords for this question are *90-year-old client, history of heart failure, normal saline solution mistakenly hung, infused 600 ml,* and *observe this patient for which of the following symptoms.* The correct answer is Choice (1). These symptoms are signs of fluid overload and congestive heart failure. The patient has three risk factors for fluid overload: He is elderly, has a history of heart failure, and has received a large amount of an isotonic solution (normal saline) very quickly. Choice (2) contains the symptoms of dehydration, Choice (3) contains the symptoms of hypocalcemia, and Choice (4) contains the symptoms of respiratory alkalosis.

TIP

The NCLEX-RN is likely to ask you to calculate IV drip rates. To refresh your memory, an *IV drip rate* refers to the number of drops of solution to be infused over one minute. The IV drip rate formula to calculate drops (gtts) per minute is

(Total number of ml ÷ Total number of minutes) × drop factor = gtts/minute

In order to do the math, you need to know the drop factor on the IV tubing. Questions on the NCLEX-RN provide you with the drop factor as part of the question. Here's an example question:

EXAMPLE

Clindamycin 0.3 g in 100 ml normal saline is to be administered over 60 minutes. The drop factor on the IV tubing is 10 gtts/ml. The nurse sets the flow rate at how many drops per minute? (Round answer to the nearest whole number.)

The correct answer is 17 gtts/min. With this type question, be sure you get only the things you need to know — the keywords — and ignore any distracters. The keywords for this question are *100 ml, administered over 60 minutes, drop factor on the IV tubing is 10 gtts/ml,* and *how many drops per minute.* The dose in the 100 ml of normal saline isn't a keyword; it's a distracter.

This is an intermittent infusion calculation:

(100 ml ÷ 60 minutes) × 10 gtts/ml = 16.6 gtts/min (round to 17 gtts/min)

This type of question can also be written as

EXAMPLE

A physician orders 500 ml of 5% dextrose in water to infuse IV in 5 hours. Calculate the flow rate in drops per minute if the drop factor is 15 gtts/ml.

The correct answer is 25 gtts/min. The keywords here are *500 ml, in 5 hours, calculate the flow rate in drops per minute,* and *drip factor is 15 gtts/ml.* The 5% dextrose in water bit is a distracter. Use the IV drip rate formula to figure out the answer. Remember that because the medication is ordered in hours, you need to multiply that number by 60 to get the number of minutes:

(500 ml ÷ [5 hours × 60 minutes]) × 15 gtts/ml = 25 gtts/min

Administering a mighty solution that's chock-full of nutrition

Total parenteral nutrition (TPN) is a type of IV solution that's highly concentrated and hypertonic. It provides nutrition to patients with nonfunctioning gastrointestinal (GI) tracts in that it provides calories and replaces essential fluids, vitamins, electrolytes, and trace elements. TPN helps with wound healing and can be used to reduce activity in the GI tract to give the bowel a chance to heal. The TPN formula is tailored to the patient's individual nutritional needs. Because it's so highly concentrated, TPN is always infused into a central vein. The complications of TPN therapy include the following:

>> Hyperglycemia

>> Infection

>> Electrolyte imbalance

>> Heart failure

Important points to remember about TPN are

>> Always use an infusion pump for rate control.

>> The IV line shouldn't be used for anything except TPN.

>> A single bag of solution shouldn't hang for more than 24 hours.

>> Inspect the solution for particles prior to hanging.

» Check the patient's serum glucose as per policy.

» Watch for signs of infection.

» Don't discontinue TPN abruptly.

Here's a sample question related to TPN:

EXAMPLE

A patient with Crohn's disease is receiving total parenteral nutrition (TPN) via a subclavian triple lumen catheter. The nurse recognizes that a priority is to

(1) Assess the insertion site for signs of infection

(2) Complete the administration of the feeding within 8 hours

(3) Discontinue the infusion if the patient experiences hyperglycemia

(4) Change the IV tubing and dressing every 72 hours

Keywords for this question are *Crohn's disease, total parental nutrition, subclavian triple lumen catheter,* and *priority*. The correct answer is Choice (1). When the question asks for a priority, look for the choice that is life threatening. Infection is a complication of TPN therapy, and the insertion site should be assessed every nursing shift. With regard to the other options, the feeding usually is administered via continuous drip. The infusion should never be abruptly discontinued, because doing so may result in hypoglycemia. The IV tubing should be changed every time a new bag is hung, and the dressing should be changed according to hospital policy.

Providing med therapy all in vein

As a nurse, you care for many patients who require intravenous (IV) therapy. IV therapy is accomplished in one of two ways: via a peripheral IV catheter placed in the patient's arm or via a central venous access device placed in one of the major veins of the neck, chest, or groin. In this section, I highlight the essential facts you need to know about central venous access devices in order to answer NCLEX-RN questions. (Although you'll see some questions about peripheral lines, central catheters are more complicated to understand and manage.)

Start with the basics of central venous access devices:

» The distal tip of a central venous catheter lies in a central vein, usually the superior vena cava (SVC). The large size of the SVC is ideal for administering IV fluids, antibiotics, chemotherapy, blood products, and total parenteral nutrition.

» Blood samples and hemodynamic monitoring measurements are fairly easy to obtain from a central venous catheter (CVC).

» Several different types of CVCs exist:

● A **multilumen catheter** is commonly used in the inpatient setting for short-term use. Most commonly, it has three lumens (called a "triple lumen") and can be inserted at the bedside by the physician and other healthcare workers. The disadvantages of this type of catheter are the high risk for infection and insertion complications, such as pneumothorax. For this reason, strict asepsis is required when inserting and caring for the line, and a chest X-ray is required after insertion. (You can read about asepsis in Chapter 6.)

● A **tunneled catheter** is used for patients requiring longer-term therapy, such as cancer patients needing chemotherapy. The Hickman or Broviac catheters are examples of tunneled catheters. The catheter is placed in a central vein, tunneled several centimeters under the skin, and then brought out through the skin. The major advantage of a tunneled catheter is a lower risk of infection.

- An **implanted port** (such as a Mediport or Portacath) is indicated for long-term use. The port is inserted in the operating room under the subcutaneous tissue and attached to a catheter, which is threaded into the SVC. The port must be accessed with a needle puncture through the skin.

- A **peripherally inserted central catheter (PICC)** is used in the inpatient, outpatient, or home healthcare setting when therapy is expected to last for weeks. A specially trained nurse generally inserts the catheter via the basilic or cephalic vein.

You also need to know the complications of central venous catheters. Here's the rundown:

>> Risks of insertion that include bleeding, pneumothorax, nerve injury, and dysrhythmia

>> Infection that may be local or systemic

>> Air embolism

>> Phlebitis

>> Circulatory overload

>> Occlusion, catheter damage, and migration

Exam questions can be related to minimizing the risks of these complications by using strict sterile technique and maintaining a closed system with careful assessment of the insertion site to detect any changes. The lines must be flushed periodically with normal saline solution to keep them patent and functioning. Be sure to have an idea of how to flush each type of catheter.

Port placement must be checked by aspirating blood return prior to giving medications. Dressing changes involve inspection of the exit site, cleansing of the skin, and covering with a sterile dressing.

A question pertaining to central lines may go something like this:

EXAMPLE

A 26-year-old client had a triple lumen central venous catheter inserted into his subclavian vein 30 minutes ago. The physician prescribes chemotherapy to begin as soon as possible. Before beginning chemotherapy, what must be done first?

(1) The dressing must be changed using strict sterile technique.

(2) The site must be cleaned with alcohol.

(3) A blood return from the port must be aspirated to confirm catheter placement.

(4) The patient must undergo a chest X-ray showing placement and lung expansion.

The keywords for this question are *26-year-old client, triple lumen central venous catheter, 30 minutes ago, prescribes chemotherapy to begin as soon as possible,* and *what must be done first.* The correct answer is Choice (4). Because the patient had the central venous catheter placed 30 minutes ago, the nurse needs to check to see whether any complications have arisen from that placement. When administering any medication into a central line, the nurse first must check for placement of the catheter. A chest X-ray confirms its placement in the superior vena cava. Blood return would only show patency of the tube, not placement. The dressing doesn't need to be changed before administering medication, and the other two actions are also incorrect.

Hanging blood and blood products

Administering a blood transfusion can help restore your patient's blood volume and temporarily correct coagulation deficits. But hanging blood takes special care because the blood must be crossmatched correctly, hung within the proper time frame, and closely watched because of the risk of transfusion reaction. To answer questions related to blood transfusions on the NCLEX-RN, you need to retrieve some key facts about blood products from your RN studies:

» To correct blood losses or anemia, you give packed red blood cells (PRBCs) or whole blood.

» Fresh frozen plasma (FFP) is the plasma portion of the blood and contains plasma proteins, water, fibrinogen (needed for blood clotting), and other clotting factors. Your patient may need a transfusion of FFP if he has a coagulation deficiency or if the doctor wants to treat hypovolemia (fresh frozen plasma is a volume expander).

» Patients who have thrombocytopenia (low platelet count) get platelets.

Transfusions aren't without risk. Transfusion reactions can (and do) occur, and as the nurse, you have to recognize a reaction and respond appropriately. In short, here are a few key points to remember as you study for and take the NCLEX-RN:

» An **allergic reaction** to a blood product is usually caused by the recipient's sensitivity to plasma proteins of the donor's blood. Symptoms of an allergic reaction range from chills, pruritis (itching), and urticaria to a more severe anaphylactic reaction with laryngeal edema, facial swelling, and wheezing.

» A **febrile reaction** is caused by leukocyte incompatibility. These reactions may be prevented by using additional filters in the blood administration tubing. A febrile reaction may result in chest tightness, chills, facial flushing, fever up to 104 degrees Fahrenheit, tachycardia, and headache.

» A **hemolytic reaction** results from transfusion of ABO incompatible blood and may be the result of mislabeling a blood specimen. Luckily, these reactions are rare. Symptoms develop rapidly (usually in the first 15 minutes of the transfusion) and include hypotension, chest pain, chills, dyspnea, and shock.

NCLEX-RN questions related to administration of blood require you to know the following:

» Proper identification of the patient is vitally important, with two nurses required to verify the information.

» Assess your patient to establish a baseline prior to beginning the transfusion.

» Use a large-bore IV to administer the transfusion (at least 18-gauge is best), and administer the transfusion over two to four hours.

» Time is limited after you pick up the blood before you have to start the blood transfusion. If the test asks you to prioritize the order of action in a transfusion (for example, in a drag-and-drop question), start the IV and then go get the blood from the lab. You don't know how long gaining access for an IV time may take. Chapter 3 has more on drag-and-drop questions.

» Transfuse blood through Y-type tubing, and use only normal saline solution to flush the tubing (other solutions hemolyze the RBCs).

» Remain with the patient and monitor him or her closely during the first 15 minutes of the transfusion.

» If the patient experiences a reaction of any kind, immediately stop the transfusion and maintain patent venous access in case medications are ordered. Monitor vital signs and notify the physician immediately.

» Don't forget to document everything you do!

Questions related to blood transfusion may resemble the following:

EXAMPLE

About ten minutes after the nurse begins an infusion of packed RBCs, the patient complains of chills, chest and back pain, and nausea. His face is flushed, and he's anxious. Which is the priority nursing action?

(1) Administering antihistamines STAT for an allergic reaction

(2) Notifying the physician of a possible transfusion reaction

(3) Obtaining a urine and serum specimen to send to the lab immediately

(4) Stopping the transfusion and maintaining a patent IV catheter

Keywords for this question are *about ten minutes; infusion of packed RBCs; complains of chills, chest pain and back pain, and nausea; face is flushed, and he's anxious;* and *priority nursing action.* The correct answer is Choice (4). The patient is experiencing a transfusion reaction. The immediate nursing action is to stop the transfusion and maintain a patent IV line. The other options may be indicated but aren't the priority in this case.

EXAMPLE

The nurse is preparing to administer a blood transfusion of PRBCs. The correct solution to use to flush the tubing when administering a blood transfusion is

(1) 5% dextrose in water (D5W)

(2) Lactated Ringer's solution (LR)

(3) 0.9% NaCl (normal saline) solution

(4) Plasmalyte–A

Keywords for this question are *preparing to administer a blood transfusion, correct solution to use to flush,* and *blood transfusion.* The correct answer is Choice (3). Normal saline solution is the only solution used to flush the tubing during a blood transfusion. The other solutions listed aren't indicated and may hemolyze the RBCs.

Chapter **11**

Reduction of Risk

Interpreting test results and assisting with procedures are big parts of being an RN. They're also areas of the profession that carry some of the greatest risks. This area is one many students struggle with when they appear in my office. Misinterpreting lab results or not knowing complications of some procedures can lead to real harm. The NCLEX-RN checks to make sure you know these complications for the labs and the diagnostic tests. No, you don't have to memorize your entire lab values book, but you do need to know the general parameters for the most common blood and urine tests and also know what deviations from the norm may indicate. Knowing how to assist with common procedures, including conscious sedation, is also important. In this chapter, I go over the most common lab values and their significance and explain how to assist safely and effectively during procedures.

REMEMBER

Nothing in nursing or medicine is purely black-and-white. Everything is a shade of gray because no patient or diagnosis is exactly the same every time. The nurse's duty is to think through the symptoms and test results he or she sees to make appropriate treatment plans. So analyze all your information to come up with appropriate answers, not only on the test but also in real-life patient care.

Interpreting Lab Results without a Hitch

In nursing school, you probably memorized lab values related to whatever body system you were studying at the time and then promptly forgot them as soon as your tests were over. During clinical rotations, the emphasis is on interpreting what the values mean in order to treat the patient appropriately. As an RN, this area is where your focus lies. Memorization of numbers is fine but usually unnecessary in the hospital today because most laboratory reports print the normal values right on the report. However, the NCLEX-RN isn't the real world, so questions on the exam don't provide you with a list of the normal lab values. You're on the hook to know normal lab test results and normal lab values, at least for the most common tests.

When you're familiar with normal lab values, you're able to determine whether an abnormality exists. Then you can think about the value in terms of taking care of the patient.

TIP

When you see a question regarding a specific laboratory value, make a mental note of the illness or disorder presented in the question and the associated body organs and systems that this disorder affects. Thinking through the pathophysiology, the laboratory result, and the system affected gives you great insight into how to answer the question correctly.

For example, if you encounter a question about a patient who comes into the hospital with complaints of fever, vomiting, and diarrhea, you should focus on the urine specific gravity and the hematocrit. Why? Because when the patient loses fluid volume, both the specific gravity of urine and the hematocrit become elevated. In order to answer this question correctly, you need to know the physiological response to a fluid volume deficit. The treatment for this patient involves replacing the fluid volume and correcting the cause of the fever, vomiting, and diarrhea.

Lab values are one of those things you just have to know; take a look at the list in Table 11-1, Table 11-2, and Table 11-3, and memorize the normal values. You'll be able to answer questions that concern the results of laboratory tests more easily if you know them well.

Separating the oozing red stuff

As an RN, you absolutely need to know normal lab values and what diagnosis an abnormal lab test may indicate. Also make sure you know whether the patient needs to do any preparation, such as fasting, for the test. In Table 11-1, I present the main tests in alphabetical order, detail normal values, and explain what problems may exist with a patient who has values outside the normal range.

REMEMBER

The lab values of the cardiac markers — creatine kinase, CK-MB, LDH, and troponin — help diagnose cardiac infarction.

REMEMBER

Depending on the laboratory references used, the values in Table 11-1 may differ slightly. No list of lab values that you've seen is guaranteed to be the values the NCLEX-RN uses. Use your judgment and the question information to determine whether the lab is abnormal.

TABLE 11-1 **Normal Blood Values**

Lab Test	Normal Value	Significance
Activated partial thromboplastin time (APTT)	20–36 seconds depending on the type of activator used	This test evaluates how well the clotting sequences function. It's most commonly used to monitor heparin therapy and screen for coagulation disorders.
Albumin	3.4–5.0 g/dl	Albumin is a mean plasma protein of the blood and maintains osmotic pressure, transports of bilirubin, fatty acids, medications, hormones, and other substances that are insoluble in water.
Alkaline phosphatase	4.5–13.0 King-Armstrong units/dl	Alkaline phosphatase is an enzyme normally found in bone, liver, intestine, and placenta. The level rises during periods of bone growth, liver disease, and bile duct obstruction.
Ammonia	35–65 mcg/dl	Ammonia is metabolized by the liver and excreted by the kidneys as urea. It's a waste product from nitrogen breakdown during protein metabolism, and elevated levels resulting from hepatic dysfunction may lead to encephalopathy.

Lab Test	Normal Value	Significance
Amylase	25–151 units/L	Amylase is an enzyme produced by the pancreas and salivary glands; it assists in the digestion of complex carbohydrates and is excreted by the kidneys. In acute pancreatitis, the amylase level is greatly increased and is a good diagnostic tool for this disease.
Bicarbonate	22–29 mEq/L	Bicarbonate assists in acid-base balance.
Bilirubin	Direct: 0–0.3 mg/dl; Indirect: 0.1–1.0 mg/dl; Total: less than 1.5 mg/dl	Bilirubin is produced by the liver, spleen, and bone marrow and is also a by-product of hemoglobin breakdown. Total bilirubin levels rise with any type of jaundice, whereas direct and indirect levels rise depending on the cause of jaundice.
Blood urea nitrogen (BUN)	8–25 mg/dl	BUN is a nitrogen protein of urea, a substance formed in the liver through an enzymatic protein breakdown process.
Calcium	8.4–10.2 mg/dl	Calcium aids in blood clotting by converting prothrombin to thrombin. Calcium is the cation that's absorbed into the bloodstream from dietary sources and functions in bone formation, nerve impulse transmission, and contraction of myocardial and skeletal muscles.
Chloride	98–107 mEq/L	Chloride is a hydrochloric acid salt that's most abundant in the extracellular fluid. Chloride functions to counterbalance cations such as sodium and acts as a buffer during oxygen and carbon exchange in red blood cells.
CK-MB	0–5% of total	CK-MB is an isoenzyme found mainly in cardiac muscle.
Clotting time	8–15 minutes	This factor is the time required for the interaction of all factors involved in the clotting process.
Creatine kinase (CK)	26–174 units/L	Creatine kinase is an enzyme found in muscle and brain tissue that reflects tissue catabolism resulting from cell trauma. This test is performed to detect myocardial or skeletal muscle damage.
Erythrocyte sedimentation rate (ESR)	0–30 mm/hour depending on the age of the patient	ESR is the rate at which erythrocytes settle out of anticoagulant blood in one hour. It isn't diagnostic of any particular disease but is indicative that a disease process is ongoing.
Fasting blood glucose	70–110 mg/dl	Glucose is the monosaccharide found in fruits; it's formed from the digestion of carbohydrates in the conversion of glycogen by the liver. Fasting blood glucose levels are used to help diagnose diabetes mellitus and hypoglycemia.
Glucose tolerance tests	Varies based on glucose intake	This test aids in the diagnosis of diabetes mellitus. If the glucose levels peak at higher than normal at one and two hours after injection or ingestion of glucose and are slower than normal to return to fasting levels, then diabetes mellitus is confirmed.
Glycosylated hemoglobin	4–6%	Glycosylated hemoglobin is the blood glucose bound to hemoglobin. Hemoglobin A_{1C} is a reflection of how well blood glucose levels have been controlled for up to the prior four months. Be sure to know the ranges for good, fair, and poor control.
Hemoglobin and hematocrit (H&H)	Hemoglobin: adult male: 14.0–16.5 g/dl; adult female: 12–15 g/dl; Hematocrit: adult male: 42–52%; adult female: 35–47%	Hemoglobin is the main component of erythrocytes and is the main vehicle for transportation of oxygen and carbon dioxide. Hemoglobin is important in identifying anemia. Hematocrit is the red blood cell mass and is an important measurement in the identification of anemia or polycythemia.

(continued)

TABLE 11-1 *(continued)*

Lab Test	Normal Value	Significance
International Normalized Ratio (INR)	2.0–3.0 for standard warfarin therapy; 3.0–4.5 for high-dose warfarin therapy	The INR measures the effects of oral anticoagulants.
Lactate dehydrogenase	140–280 units/L; LDH_1 14–26%, LDH_2 29–39%	LDH is an isoenzyme that's particularly affected with acute myocardial infarction (MI). LDH level (LDH) begins to rise about 24 hours after MI, peaks in 48 to 72 hours, and then returns to normal.
Lipids	Cholesterol: 140–199 mg/dl; Low-density lipoproteins (LDL): less than 130 mg/dl; High-density lipoproteins (HDL): 30–70 mg/dl; Triglycerides: less than 200 mg/dl	Lipid assessment includes total cholesterol, low-density lipoprotein, high-density lipoprotein, and triglycerides. Blood lipids consist primarily of cholesterol, triglycerides, and phospholipids.
Magnesium	1.3–2.1 mEq/L	Magnesium is used as an index to determine metabolic activity in renal function. It's needed in the blood-clotting mechanism, and it regulates neuromuscular activity, acts as a cofactor that modifies the activity of many enzymes, and affects the metabolism of calcium.
Platelet count	150,000–400,000 cells/μL	Platelets, which are produced in bone marrow, function in hemostatic plug formation, clot retraction, and coagulation factor activation.
Potassium	3.5–5.1 mEq/L	Potassium regulates cellular water balance, electrical conduction in the muscle cells, and acid-base balance. The body obtains potassium through dietary ingestion, and kidneys preserve or excrete potassium depending on cellular needs. Potassium also plays a huge role in repolarization in heart cells. You can use this information to assist in understanding the ECG reading.
Protein	6–8 g/dl	Protein reflects the total amount of albumin in globulins in the serum. Protein regulates osmotic pressure and comprises coagulation factors for hemostasis, enzymes, hormones, tissue growth and repair, and pH buffers. The loss of protein causes the fluid to shift from the vascular area to the tissues. This shift could cause edema and fluid buildup in the lungs that causes crackles.
Prothrombin time (PT)	Adult male: 9.6–11.8 seconds; Adult female: 9.5–11.3 seconds	Prothrombin is a vitamin K-dependent glycoprotein produced by the liver; it's necessary for firm fibrin clot formation. Each lab establishes a normal value based on the method used to perform the tests. The PT time measures the amount of time it takes for clot formation and is used to monitor response to Coumadin therapy or to screen for a dysfunction of the liver, vitamin K deficiency, or disseminated intravascular coagulation. A value within two seconds plus or minus the control is considered normal.
Red blood cells (RBCs)	Adult male: 4.7–6.1 million/mm3; Adult female: 4.2–5.4 million/mm3	RBCs show how many red blood cells are in the body. A decreased number could indicate blood loss or that the body is anemic.
Serum creatinine	0.6–1.3 mg/dl	An increased level of creatinine indicates a slowing of the glomerular filtration rate and is a specific indicator of renal function.
Serum iron	Adult male: 65–175 mcg/dl; Adult female: 50–170 mcg/dl	Iron is mostly found in hemoglobin. It acts as a carrier of oxygen from the lungs to the tissues and acts indirectly in the return of carbon dioxide to the lungs. Iron aids in diagnosing anemia and hemolytic disorders.

Lab Test	Normal Value	Significance
Serum sodium	135–145 mEq/L	Sodium maintains osmotic pressures and acid-base balance and assists in the transmission of nerve impulses.
Thyroid stimulating hormone	0.2–5.4 μU/ml	Thyroid studies are performed if a thyroid disorder is suspected; they're helpful to differentiate primary thyroid disease from secondary causes and from abnormalities in thyroxine-binding.
Troponin	Usually less than 0.6 mg/ml	Increased amounts of troponin are released into the bloodstream when an infarction causes damage to the myocardium. Greater than 1.5 mg/ml is indicative of possible MI.
Uric acid	Adult male: 4.5–8.0 mg/dl; Adult female 2.5–6.2 mg/dl	Uric acid is formed as purines, adenine, and guanine. It's metabolized continuously during the formation and degradation of DNA and RNA and from the metabolism of dietary periods. Elevated amounts of uric acid deposits in joints and soft tissue can cause gout, and elevated amounts of urinary uric acid precipitate into urate stones in the kidneys.
White blood cells (WBCs)	5,000–10,000 cells/mcL	WBCs show how many white blood cells are in the body. An increase shows an infection. A decrease indicates the body is at increased risk of infection.

Following are some examples of the types of questions you're likely to see on the NCLEX-RN in regard to normal blood values:

EXAMPLE

A cardiac patient is receiving maintenance therapy of warfarin sodium and has a prothrombin time (PT) of 30 seconds. As the nurse caring for this patient, what would be your next anticipated order?

(1) Holding the next dose

(2) Administering the next dose

(3) Increasing the next dose

(4) Adding a dose

The keywords for this question are *cardiac patient, maintenance therapy of warfarin sodium, PT of 30 seconds,* and *anticipated order.* The correct answer is Choice (1). As Table 11-1 notes, the normal prothrombin time is 9.6 to 11.8 seconds for an adult male or 9.5 to 11.3 seconds for an adult female. A therapeutic level is 1.5 to 2 times greater than the client's normal time. Because this patient's value of 30 seconds is high and perhaps near the critical range, you anticipate that the client shouldn't receive any further doses at this time.

EXAMPLE

The patient comes into the emergency department complaining of vomiting blood. Blood tests are done, and it's noted that the patient has a platelet count of 300,000 cells/μL. What is the most appropriate action for the nurse to take after seeing this report?

(1) Report that the platelet count is abnormally low.

(2) Report that the platelet count is abnormally high.

(3) Control the patient's internal bleeding immediately.

(4) Place the report in the patient's chart.

Keywords for this question are *emergency department, vomiting blood, platelet count of 300,000,* and *most appropriate action for the nurse to take after seeing this report.* The correct answer is Choice (4). The platelet count norm is 150,000 to 400,000, so 300,000 cells/μL is a normal platelet count. Choice 3 is incorrect because a patient can still bleed with a normal platelet count.

EXAMPLE

An adult patient arrives at the emergency department complaining of acute epigastric pain. The patient has a history of alcohol abuse. A nurse would interpret that the client may have a diagnosis of acute pancreatitis if the serum amylase level is

(1) 20 units/L

(2) 100 units/L

(3) 142 units/L

(4) 290 units/L

Keywords for this question are *adult patient, emergency department, acute epigastric pain, history of alcohol abuse, a nurse would interpret, pancreatitis,* and *serum amylase level.* The correct answer is Choice (4). A patient with a serum amylase above 151 units/L may have acute pancreatitis. Patients who have an excessive intake of alcohol are prone to this disease. The other options are either within or below normal limits.

EXAMPLE

The nurse reviews the new labs of a patient who is 24 hours post-renal transplant. Which of the following labs indicates the new kidney is functioning?

(1) Creatinine of 1.7 decreased from 2

(2) BUN of 19 decreased from 29

(3) Urine output 15 mls for the last hour

(4) WBCs decreased from 24,000 to 20,000

Keywords for this question are *new labs, 24 hours post-renal transplant,* and *indicates the new kidney is functioning.* The correct answer is Choice (2). The BUN shows the function of the kidney, and this BUN is within the normal range. The creatinine and urine output answers don't show the kidney as functioning properly. The WBC answer shows that an infection still exists, which doesn't relate to kidney function.

Looking closely at immunity defenders

White blood cells function in the immune defense system of the body. The white blood cell count with differentials assesses each leukocyte distribution and is important in looking at infection. The level of each differential is important in discovering more about the type of infection a patient may have. See Table 11-2 for normal values.

TABLE 11-2 ## White Blood Cell Values

Blood Cell or Leukocyte	Normal Value
Bands	3% or 0–700 cells/µL
Basophils	0.3% or 0–200 cells/µL
Eosinophils	2.7% or 0–450 cells/µL
Lymphocytes	34% or 1,000–4,800 cells/µL
Monocytes	4% or 0–800 cells/µL
Neutrophils	56% or 1,800–7,600 cells/µL
White blood cells	4,500–11,000 cells/µL

REMEMBER

The "shift to the left" means that an increased number of immature neutrophils are in the peripheral blood. The shift to the left indicates an infection the body is struggling to fight off. The body has increased the production of WBCs, thus increasing the number of bands or immature WBCs in the system. Unfortunately, bands are weak and can't fight the infection like the mature WBCs. The "shift to the right" indicates the absence of young white blood cells in a differential count; this condition is found in conditions such as liver disease, Down syndrome, or megaloblastic and pernicious anemia.

NCLEX-RN questions relating to white blood cell values may look like the following:

EXAMPLE

A nurse is caring for an immunosuppressed patient. The nurse should consider implementing neutropenic precautions if the client's white blood cell count is

(1) 2,200 cells/μL

(2) 6,100 cells/μL

(3) 9,900 cells/μL

(4) 11,000 cells/μL

Keywords for this question are *immunosuppressed patient, consider implementing neutropenic precautions,* and *white blood cell count.* The correct answer is Choice (1). A normal white blood cell count ranges from 4,500 to 11,000 cells/μL. An immunosuppressed patient has a decreasing number of circulating white blood cells, so the nurse should implement neutropenic precautions when the client's values fall sufficiently below the normal level.

Examining pee (ha-ha)

Normal urine values are important to know so that you can recognize abnormalities. Most of these values, shown in Table 11-3, show up in a urinalysis, which is a common test for most patients.

TABLE 11-3 **Normal Urine Values**

Lab Test	Normal Value
Bacteria	None or < 1000/ml
Bilirubin	Negative
Casts	Negative
Chloride	110–250 mEq/24 hr
Glucose	Negative
Ketones	Negative
Magnesium	7.3–12.2 mg/dl per day
Nitrates	Negative
Osmolality	300–1300 mOsm/kg
pH	4.5–7.8
Potassium	25–125 mEq/24 hr
Protein	40–150 mg/24 hr
Red blood cells	4 RBC/HPF
Sodium	40–220 mEq/24 hr

(continued)

TABLE 11-3 *(continued)*

Lab Test	Normal Value
Specific gravity	1.005–1.030 kg/meters cubed
Uric acid	250–750 mg/24 hr
White blood cells	0-4

EXAMPLE

A client is admitted for acute renal failure. The nurse must continually assess for

(1) Alkalosis

(2) Decreased BUN and creatinine

(3) Hyponatremia and hyperkalemia

(4) Hypercalcemia

Keywords in this question are *acute renal failure* and *continually assess for*. The correct answer is Choice (3). The most common findings in acute renal failure include elevations in BUN and creatinine, hyponatremia, and hyperkalemia. When the kidneys aren't functioning properly, potassium isn't excreted, and sodium decreases due to increase in fluid volume.

Recognizing the Main Diagnostic Assessments

When you're working on a hospital floor, getting your patients ready for diagnostic tests may seem like all you do some days. Diagnostic tests are usually ordered, naturally enough, to help diagnose the patient's condition. Many different diagnostic tests are available, with multiple systems a test could be used for. For example, diagnostic tests for the neurological system include lumbar puncture, cerebral angiography, and MRIs. (Chapter 12 covers MRI information.) In this section, I review some of the most important diagnostic tests. In order to be successful on the NCLEX-RN, you need to know these diagnostic test basics.

The daily routine: Checking vital signs

Maybe you don't think of vital signs as a diagnostic test, but of course, that's exactly what they are — they're a measurement of the patient's vital signs against normal vital signs. In order to make a comparison, you need to know the norms (which are definitely on the NCLEX-RN). For normal adult vital sign values, review Table 11-4.

TABLE 11-4 **Normal Values for Adult Vital Signs**

Vital Sign	Normal Value Range
Blood Pressure	120–130/80–90
Pulse	80–100 beats per minute (bpm)
Respirations	16–20 per minute
Temperature	97.5–99.5°F or 36.4–37.5°C

Not all patients are adults, so in addition to normal adult vital signs, you need to know the normal vital sign values for newborns (see Table 11-5) and toddlers (see Table 11-6). Any vital signs outside these ranges are considered abnormal, so make note of them when answering any questions that contain vital signs.

TABLE 11-5 ## Normal Values for Newborn Vital Signs

Vital Sign	Normal Value Range
Blood Pressure	120/80
Pulse	120–160 bpm
Respirations	25–60 per minute
Temperature	97–99°F or 36.4–37°C axillary

TABLE 11-6 ## Normal Values for Toddler Vital Signs

Vital Sign	Normal Range
Apical heart rate	80–120 bpm
Blood Pressure	92/55 mm Hg
Respirations	20–30 per minute
Temperature	97.5–98.6°F or 36.4–37°C

As a child ages, vital signs get closer and closer to adult ranges. Refer to your textbooks for other age groups up to adult.

The following question gives you an idea of what to expect of vital sign-related questions:

EXAMPLE

An 8-hour-old infant is in his mother's room. Which finding by the nurse indicates that the newborn needs his environment altered to promote adjustment to extrauterine life?

(1) The baby just vomited up his formula.

(2) His axillary temperature is 96.8 degrees F.

(3) His hands and feet are slightly blue.

(4) Petechiae are present on his head.

Keywords for this question are *8-hour-old infant, finding, indicates that the newborn needs his environment altered,* and *promote adjustment to extrauterine life.* The correct answer is Choice (2). His axillary temperature is below the normal range of 97 to 99 degrees F. Infants commonly vomit formula if they ingest too much air while feeding. Petechiae (small spots on the skin) result from pressure on the presenting part at delivery, and slightly blue hands and feet are normal in newborns.

Respiratory tests

The respiratory system is of prime importance because if you can't breathe, you can't live for very long! As you should remember from your ABCs of evaluation (airway, breathing, circulation — in that order), the airway always comes first!

TIP

When studying up on the respiratory system, turn to Chapter 12 to review arterial blood gases and acid-base comparisons for these systems.

The following tests are commonly performed to evaluate the respiratory system:

>> **Pulmonary function test:** This test helps determine whether a patient has any pulmonary dysfunction caused by obstruction, restrictions, or both. The pulmonary function test measures the following:

- **Residual volume (RV):** The amount of air left in the lungs after a maximal expiration
- **Vital capacity (VC):** The amount of air that can be expired following a maximal inspiration
- **Tidal volume (TV):** The amount of air exchanged with a normal respiration
- **Minute volume (MV):** The amount of air expired per minute
- **Functional residual capacity (FRC):** The amount of air left in the lungs after exhaling normally
- **Total lung capacity:** The total volume of the lungs when filled with as much air as possible
- **Forced vital capacity (FVC):** The amount of air expired forcefully and quickly after maximal inspiration
- **Forced expiratory volume (FEV):** The amount of air expired during the first, second, and third seconds of the FVC test
- **Forced expiratory flow (FEF):** The average rate of flow during the middle half of the FVC test
- **Peak expiratory flow rate (PEFR):** The fastest rate that you can force air out of your lungs

Forced vital capacity and forced expiratory volume are the two most common evaluations that healthcare professionals use to help their patients.

>> **Chest X-ray:** This radiologic test is used for screening, diagnosis, and evaluation of respiratory abnormalities such as tuberculosis, foreign objects, pneumonia, rib fractures, or other chest-related problems.

>> **Thoracentesis:** This test is performed to obtain pleural fluid, remove pleural fluid, or instill medication.

>> **Bronchoscopy:** This test involves the use of a flexible tube to directly visualize the inner airway — the larynx, trachea, bronchi, and bronchioles.

The following example question tests your knowledge of bronchoscopy:

EXAMPLE

A patient has just had a bronchoscopy. After the bronchoscopy, the patient develops wheezing, stridor, and cyanosis. What is the highest-priority nursing action at this time?

(1) Encouraging the patient to cough and deep breathe

(2) Calling the patient's physician about the problem

(3) Maintaining an open airway and assessing breath sounds

(4) Checking the patient's gag reflex to make sure that the anesthetic hasn't worn off

This question's keywords are *bronchoscopy; develops wheezing, stridor, and cyanosis;* and *highest-priority nursing action.* The correct answer is Choice (3). If you know that the bronchoscopy deals with the airway, you know you're looking for an answer that deals with maintaining the airway. The airway is always the nurse's first priority. Stridor and wheezing indicate the need to maintain an airway; wheezing also indicates constriction of the bronchioles. Cyanosis shows that oxygen isn't getting into the body. In this case, the nurse should address the airway and then encourage the patient to cough and deep breathe. The last action to take is to notify the patient's physician. Checking the patient's gag reflex isn't appropriate in this situation.

Cardiovascular tests

In assessing the cardiovascular system, you need to know the details about a few major tests. In this section, I cover the descriptions and highlights of the most important ones.

An *electrocardiogram*, often abbreviated as ECG or EKG, is a chart or graph of the electrical forces produced by the heart. The ECG is affected by calcium, magnesium, and potassium levels. If any of these levels are low or high, the heart's rhythm could be affected. It's also the best diagnostic tool for evaluating the effects of medications and fluids on the heart. Most electrocardiograms are taken with 12 leads that produce a three-dimensional graphic representation of different portions of the heart. Lead II is the most commonly used view to do rhythm strips and a quick analysis of the electrical conduction of the heart. Doctors and nurses analyze each portion of the electrocardiogram to identify any abnormalities in the conduction system.

For the NCLEX-RN, you need to know the following components of a normal EKG:

>> P wave < 0.11 second

>> QRS complex: Normal = 0.06–0.10 second

>> T wave

>> P-R Interval: Normal = 0.12–0.20

Abnormalities commonly noted during an EKG include the following:

>> Dysrhythmias: Know some of the common dysrhythmias — atrial fibrillation, atrial flutter, ventricular fibrillation, and ventricular tachycardia — and their most common treatments. They're almost sure to be on the test.

>> Ischemia.

>> Myocardial infarction.

>> Electrolyte disturbances: The main electrolytes that affect the EKG are potassium, calcium, and magnesium.

The following tests are often done in addition to an EKG to assess cardiac function:

>> **Treadmill stress testing:** This test measures the efficiency of the heart during exercise stress. Its value is in diagnosing ischemic heart disease and investigating cardiac signs or symptoms such as arrhythmias and angina. Treadmill testing is also done to measure functional capacities for work, sports, or participation in rehabilitation programs.

>> **Holter monitoring:** This test involves continuously monitoring patients for a period of 24 hours or beyond using a portable EKG recorder.

>> **Echocardiogram:** This noninvasive test uses ultrasound to gather information about position, size, and movements of the heart valves and chambers of the heart. This test may be used to diagnose cardiomyopathies and congenital heart disease issues. An echocardiogram is a definitive test for diagnosing valve problems such as mitral stenosis, mitral valve disorders, and atrial tumors.

The following is a typical question related to EKG testing:

EXAMPLE

During a treadmill stress test, a middle-aged patient becomes short of breath and diaphoretic and complains of chest pain. The EKG shows an elevated ST segment. What is the first nursing action taken?

(1) Offer the patient some fluids.

(2) Have the client take a break and give him some nitroglycerin.

(3) Continue the test.

(4) Stop the test, have the client lie down, and assess vital signs.

Keywords for this question are *stress test, middle-aged patient, short of breath, diaphoretic, complains of chest pain, EKG shows an elevated ST segment,* and *first nursing action taken.* The correct answer is Choice (4). The patient is obviously having some trouble, and an elevated ST segment is a sign of cardiac ischemia. The nurse needs to stop the test immediately. The client may take a break and/or take nitroglycerin, but only after the test is stopped and the nurse assesses the vital signs. Choices (1) and (3) aren't appropriate because they may exacerbate the patient's problem.

Gastrointestinal tests

The gastrointestinal, or GI, system is often evaluated for problems related to digestion and elimination. Know the following tests for evaluating GI function:

>> **Gastroscopy:** Direct visualization of the stomach through a flexible scope to detect inflammatory processors, tumors, hemorrhages, ulcerations, or cancers

>> **Sigmoidoscopy:** Direct visualization of the rectum and sigmoid colon through the sigmoidoscope to detect polyps or tumors or other conditions, such as diverticulitis

>> **Colonoscopy:** Direct visualization of the mucosa of the entire colon

>> **Stool tests:** Lab tests to evaluate for occult blood ova, parasites, and fat in the stools

Musculoskeletal tests

Musculoskeletal testing includes one of the most common tests, the *X-ray.* X-rays are radiological studies that determine changes in bone relationships, density, texture, and erosion. X-rays of the joints show changes in joint structure, narrowing of the joint, spur formation, irregularities, or the presence of fluid.

Another musculoskeletal test is the MRI, but I cover that topic in Chapter 12, where I explain safety issues, because there are so many precautions that must be taken for this exam.

Neurological tests

Diagnostic testing on the brain can be very frightening to patients, so you should always explain these procedures thoroughly to reduce patient fear. Some diagnoses, such as meningitis, can only be definitively confirmed with a lumbar puncture, so I cover common neurological tests, which include these:

>> **Lumbar puncture:** This diagnostic test is given to patients with abnormal neurological signs and symptoms. Its primary use is determining the presence of meningitis or detecting any abnormalities in cerebrospinal fluid (CSF), including the presence of blood or leukemia cells.

During a lumbar puncture, the pressure of the CSF is measured and a small amount of fluid removed for examination. Lumbar punctures aren't performed when there's evidence of greatly increased intracranial pressure because herniation of the brain stem can occur.

Normal CSF is clear; if the procedure has been traumatic, the CSF may have some blood in it. But bloody or cloudy CSF is an abnormal result of a lumbar puncture. Blood in the CSF may indicate an intracerebral bleed, whereas cloudy CSF may indicate meningitis. The abnormal CSF is sent to the laboratory for further evaluations to detect whether it contains any white blood cells or bacteria.

>> **Cerebral angiography:** This test assists in diagnosing vascular disease, aneurysms, and arteriovenous malformations. The study is usually performed by threading a catheter through the femoral artery to the desired level, injecting contrast media into a selected artery, and performing an X-ray study of cerebral circulation.

>> **Computerized tomographic (CT) scan:** A body scanner is used to give a clear, computerized image of any part of the body, including chest, abdomen, and pelvis. The CT scan is an important tool in diagnosing and identifying neoplastic and inflammatory diseases.

The following question relates to neurological testing:

EXAMPLE

An adolescent child is scheduled for a lumbar puncture. His friends told him that his brain is going to sink after the removal of the cerebrospinal fluid. What is the most appropriate response by the nurse?

(1) "Removing CSF has no effect on the brain."

(2) "The amount of CSF removed will be rapidly replaced by the body."

(3) "The body has more fluid than necessary, and the amount removed is insignificant."

(4) "The physician doing the test will monitor the CSF pressure closely during the procedure to minimize any extenuating circumstances or danger."

The keywords for this question are *adolescent child, lumbar puncture, friends told him that his brain is going to sink after the removal of the cerebrospinal fluid,* and *most appropriate response.* The correct answer is Choice (3). Knowing the amount of cerebrospinal fluid being removed helps you answer this question. The body has the necessary fluid to maintain homeostasis. Choice (1) is incorrect because the loss of some fluid may have some effect on the brain in the form of a headache. Choice (2) is incorrect because the fluid is gradually, not rapidly, replaced over time. Choice (4) has to do with the physician, and you can't guarantee what he or she will do.

Being Ready for the Bumps: Complications with Testing and Treating

When you think about complications, you may think of surgical complications or those things that go wrong after surgery. But in reality, complications can arise with any patient at just about any time. Every diagnostic test, procedure, or treatment you do on a patient has the potential for complications. And of course, things go wrong when you least expect it. One of your responsibilities as a nurse is to try to prevent some of those complications from occurring. In this section, I take a look at some of the common complications related to diagnostic tests, procedures, and treatments and what you can do to minimize the damage.

Taking stock of diagnostic risks

Patient safety is the nurse's concern; you need to be sure that your patients are being cared for even when not in your direct care. Sometimes patients have test complications, and you need to know those complications so you can recognize a problem and intervene appropriately.

The following list of diagnostic tests and some of their more common complications isn't inclusive. Please make sure you check out other diagnostic tests for complications that can arise from them.

REMEMBER

>> **Lumbar puncture:** Neck stiffness, irritability, decreasing level of consciousness, altered vital signs

A post-lumbar puncture headache may occur a few hours to several days after the procedure and is caused by leakage of CSF. Bed rest in a quiet, darkened room and analgesics can alleviate the headache. A blood patch is another option the doctor could offer the client.

>> **Cerebral angiography:** Alterations in the level of consciousness, weakness on one side of the body, motor or sensory deficits, speech disturbances.

>> **Cardiac treadmill stress test:** Chest pain.

>> **Cardiac catheterization:** Dysrhythmia, bleeding at the insertion site.

>> **Bronchoscopy:** Bright red sputum, difficulty breathing.

>> **Thoracentesis:** Pneumothorax, shock, subcutaneous emphysema, pyrogenic infection.

>> **Paracentesis:** Hypovolemia, electrolyte imbalances.

Preventing postsurgical complications

Surgery disrupts the homeostasis of every organ and body system. The potential for complications following surgery always exists, and you should always be on watch for signs of complications so they can be treated as quickly as possible.

Carrying out competent post-op care

Before I get into complications from surgical procedures, I need to address postoperative nursing care of the surgical patient and what you should do to prevent complications. This stuff is very likely to be on the exam.

After a patient comes out of the operating room, you should address the following issues in the recovery room or postanesthesia care unit (PACU) in this order:

1. **Ensure that the patient has a clear and patent airway.**
2. **Support respirations by positioning the patient on his or her side with the head of the bed elevated.**
3. **Assess the rate, depth, and quality of respirations.**
4. **Ensure that circulatory status is sufficient by checking vital signs at least every 15 minutes.**
5. **Be alert for signs of shock.**
6. **Check the surgical site for bleeding, hemorrhage, and intact dressings.**
7. **Continually assess the patient's level of consciousness.**

8. Treat the patient for pain and discomfort.

9. Monitor IV infusions, specifically the condition of IV sites, the amount of fluid being infused, and the flow rate.

10. Assess the color and temperature of the skin and the color of nail beds and lips.

11. Check all drainage tubes, and connect them to suction or gravity drainage as ordered; document color, amount, and odor of drainage, if any.

12. Encourage the client to cough and breathe deeply after the airway is removed.

After the patient moves to the surgical floor, the following nursing care should be initiated:

» Monitor respiratory status and promote optimal functioning, encouraging coughing and deep breathing every one to two hours. Encourage the client to splint the incision while coughing, if necessary.

» Monitor cardiovascular status and avoid postoperative complications by encouraging leg exercises every two hours while the patient's in bed. Encourage early ambulation, and apply anti-embolism stockings as ordered.

» Promote adequate fluid electrolyte balance by monitoring IVs and ensuring adequate intake. Measure intake and output, and irrigate the nasogastric (NG) tube properly using normal saline solution.

» Promote optimum nutrition by maintaining an IV infusion and assessing for return of peristalsis. Give diet as ordered, and note the patient's tolerance to food.

» Monitor and promote the return of urinary function, and promote bowel elimination.

» Administer pain medication as ordered, and provide additional comfort measures.

» Encourage optimal activity in the patient by turning every two hours. Promote early ambulation if permitted, and have a client dangle her legs before getting out of bed.

» Provide adequate psychological support and appropriate discharge teaching when the time comes.

The following questions address postsurgical complications:

EXAMPLE

An adult who has had general anesthesia for a major surgical procedure is discharged to the PACU. One of the signs that indicate that his artificial airway should be removed is

(1) Gagging

(2) Increasing pain

(3) Clear lung sounds

(4) Restlessness

Keywords for this question are *adult patient, general anesthesia, discharged to the PACU,* and *signs that indicate his artificial airway should be removed.* The correct answer is Choice (1). The patient's gag reflex usually indicates that he's able to manage his own secretions and maintain a patent airway. Clear lung sounds and increasing pain really have nothing to do with the gag reflex, and restlessness is normal coming out of surgery.

EXAMPLE

A patient has been brought to the recovery room after surgery. When the nurse approaches the patient, he notes that the patient is restless and has a rapid, thready pulse and rapid, noisy respirations. Which term best describes the potential diagnosis of the patient?

(1) Shock

(2) Hemorrhage

(3) Respiratory obstructions

(4) Pain

This question's keywords are *recovery room after surgery*; *patient is restless*; *rapid, thready pulse and rapid, noisy respirations*; and *potential diagnosis*. The correct answer is Choice (1). The pulse, respirations, and restlessness are indicative of shock, which must be treated immediately. Hemorrhage may be a precipitating condition for shock, but it isn't what the nurse sees initially. Respiratory obstruction isn't an appropriate answer because the patient has rapid respirations. Although the patient may be in pain, that problem is secondary to shock.

EXAMPLE

A postoperative GI client has returned to the unit with IV infusing, nasogastric suction, and Foley catheter. The nurse is doing her second post-op check of the client. Which of the following observations would be of most concern to the nurse?

(1) Blood pressure 98/70

(2) Complaints of pain level 4 out of 10

(3) Urine output of 20 ml over an hour

(4) NG suction container with red-tinged drainage

Keywords in this question are *postoperative GI client, IV, nasogastric suction, Foley catheter, second post-op check*, and *most concern to the nurse*. The correct answer is Choice (3). The blood pressure reading, complaints of pain, and red-tinged drainage are all normal after GI surgery. Urine output of 30 milliliters per hour (not 20) is what is normal.

Looking for postoperative complications

Postoperative complications can affect any body system. Watch for the following complications in the following body systems:

>> **Respiratory system:**

- Atelectasis.

- Pneumonia.

>> **Cardiovascular system:**

- Deep vein thrombosis: Predisposing factors include lower abdominal surgery, septic diseases, vein injury caused by tight leg straps during surgery, previous history of venous problems, and increased blood coagulation due to dehydration and fluid loss.

- Shock: The most common causes of shock during post-op are hemorrhage, sepsis, myocardial infarction and cardiac arrest, drug and transfusion reactions, pulmonary embolism, and adrenal failure.

- Pulmonary embolism.

>> **Genitourinary system:**

- Urinary retention: Predisposing factors include anxiety, pain, lack of privacy, narcotics, and certain anesthetics that diminish the patient's sense of a full bladder.

- Urinary tract infection: Most commonly caused by catheterization.

>> **Gastrointestinal system:**

- Paralytic ileus: Predisposing factors are anesthesia and manipulation of the bowel during abdominal surgery. Other possible complications include electrolyte imbalance, wound infections, and pneumonia. Assessment findings are absent bowel sounds, no passage of flatus, and abdominal distention.

>> **Wound complications:**

- Wound infection: Predisposing factors include obesity, diabetes mellitus, malnutrition, advanced age, use of steroids and immunosuppressive agents, and lowered resistance to infection as found in clients with cancer. Assessment findings include redness, tenderness, drainage, and warmth to the touch in the wound area. Fever usually occurs three to five days after surgery.

- Wound dehiscence and evisceration: *Dehiscence* is the opening of wound edge, and *evisceration* is the profusion of bowel or other organs through an incision. Both of these are usually accompanied by sudden escape of profuse pink serous drainage. Predisposing factors to wound dehiscence and evisceration are wound infections, faulty wound closures, and severe abdominal stretching.

NCLEX-RN questions dealing with post-op complications may look like the following:

EXAMPLE

An adult patient is on the surgical floor six days post-abdominal surgery. Which sign would indicate to the nurse that the patient has a wound dehiscence?

(1) Acute bleeding from the incision

(2) A gush of pink serous drainage

(3) Purple drainage

(4) Severe abdominal pain

Keywords for this question are *adult patient, six days, post-abdominal, sign,* and *indicate to the nurse that the patient has a wound dehiscence.* The correct answer is Choice (2). A sudden gush of serous drainage that looks like pink, frothy fluid is usually the major symptom of wound dehiscence. Acute bleeding can be caused by other complications, severe abdominal pain can be caused by other complications, and I've never seen purple drainage before.

EXAMPLE

The patient has just arrived on the general surgical floor from the PACU. Which of the following needs to be the nurse's initial intervention?

(1) Assess the surgical site, noting the amount and character of drainage, if any.

(2) Assess for the amount of urinary output and the presence of any distention.

(3) Allow the family to visit with the client to decrease the client's anxiety.

(4) Take vital signs, assess for a patent airway, and monitor the quality of respirations

The keywords in this question are *arrived on the general surgery floor, from the PACU,* and *nurse's initial intervention.* The correct answer is Choice (4). An initial assessment is the evaluation of a patent airway and respiratory and circulation adequacy. The other options are all secondary to the priority areas.

EXAMPLE

A postoperative adolescent has returned to the unit to a semiprivate room and adolescent roommate. After two hours, the nurse checks on the adolescent patient to see whether he needs to use the restroom. The patient is weak, so the nurse places him on a bedside commode and pulls the curtain. Which of the following would be the most likely cause of urinary retention for this patient?

(1) Being afraid to use the bedside commode with the roommate in the room

(2) Use of antibiotics during surgery and after surgery

(3) Having a urinary tract infection

(4) Not having received enough IV fluids

Keywords for this question are *postoperative adolescent, semiprivate room and adolescent roommate, bedside commode, pulls the curtain,* and *most likely cause of urinary retention.* The correct answer is Choice (1). Adolescents need their privacy. Using a bedside commode with another adolescent in the room may well inhibit this patient from voiding. The use of antibiotics, urinary tract infection, and lack of IV fluids aren't reasons for urinary retention. Also, note that the question doesn't state that the patient hasn't received enough IV fluids.

Taking a Load Off: Therapeutic Procedures and Diagnostic Tests

Regardless of how you may feel at times, your patient is the one who needs therapy, and when you're on duty, it's your job to be sure he gets it. Patients undergo many therapeutic tests and procedures of all types, such as physical, psychological, and so forth. In this section, I review a few of the more important ones that you're likely to see on the exam.

Be sure you know the prep for, care during, and care after receiving therapy. For example, for anticoagulant therapy, you want to know the following:

>> **Prep:** Prothrombin Time (PT) International Normalized Ratio (INR) prior to starting therapy, teaching about diet to avoid vitamin K rich foods

>> **During:** Getting labs of PT INR as ordered, continuing to monitor diet, teaching about possible therapy complications such as bleeding

>> **After:** Applying prolonged pressure to the venipuncture site to stop bleeding

Some of the systems and therapeutic procedures you may be called upon to monitor, perform, or assist with as necessary (this list isn't comprehensive), organized by body system, are

>> **Cardiovascular:**

- Anticoagulants
- Anti-embolism stockings
- Cardiac catheterization
- Cardiac markers: Labs
- Cardiac monitoring
- Echocardiography

- Exercise electrocardiography or stress test
- Holter monitoring
- Monitoring cardiac output
- Myocardial nuclear perfusion imaging

>> **Gastrointestinal:**

- Endoscopic retrograde cholangiopancreatography (ERCP)
- Fiberoptic colonoscopy
- Gastric analysis
- Liver biopsy
- Placement of a Sengstaken-Blakemore tube for bleeding esophageal varices
- Placement of an NG tube
- Stool specimens
- Upper GI
- Upper GI endoscopy

>> **Genitourinary:**

- Bladder ultrasonography (bladder ultrasound)
- Cystoscopy and biopsy
- Hemodialysis: Removes blood from the body and circulates it through a semi-permeable membrane
- Intravenous urography
- Kidneys, ureters, and bladder X-ray (KUB)
- Lithotripsy for renal calculi: Uses large ultrasonic waves to break up stones
- Peritoneal dialysis: Continuous ambulatory peritoneal dialysis (CAPD) or continuous cycled peritoneal dialysis (CCPD)
- Renal biopsy
- Renography: Kidney scan

>> **Musculoskeletal:**

- Arthrocentesis
- Care of an arthroscopy
- Bone mineral density
- Bone scan
- Bone or muscle biopsy
- Buck's traction or an abduction pillow for immobilizing hips
- Electromyography
- Crutch walking
- Skeletal traction: Care of pin sites and monitoring for infection

» Neurological:

- Assessment of different reflexes: Babinski, corneal, and gag
- Assessment of meningeal irritation: Brudzinski and Kernig's sign
- Cerebral angiography
- CT scan/MRI: Show the area of bleed or infarct in a stroke
- Electroencephalography
- Glasgow Coma Scale: Measures the level of coma in patients
- Lumbar puncture

» Respiratory:

- Artificial airways, such as endotracheal tubes
- Blood gases and analysis
- Chest tubes
- Intubation and ventilation
- Laryngoscopy and bronchoscopy
- Lung biopsy
- Mechanical ventilation
- Pulmonary angiography
- Pulmonary function tests
- Oxygen therapy
- Sputum specimen
- Thoracentesis
- Tracheostomy
- Ventilation: Perfusion lung scan or V/Q scan

The following questions review therapies common to nursing care:

EXAMPLE

The nurse is caring for a client who is connected to a volume-cycled positive pressure ventilator when the low volume alarm sounds. What initial assessment should be made by the nurse?

(1) Is the tubing caught in the bed rails?

(2) Is there a leak in the client's ET tube cuff?

(3) Is there a buildup of fluid in the ventilator tubes?

(4) Are the client's lungs becoming noncompliant?

The keywords for this question are *volume-cycled positive pressure ventilator, low volume alarm sounds,* and *initial assessment should be made by the nurse.* The correct answer is Choice (2). A low volume alarm means that not enough air is being cycled to the patient. A leak in the cuff causes much of the volume to leak out. Tubing caught in the bed rails and buildup of fluid in the ventilator tubes trigger a high pressure alarm because of the obstructions in the tubes carrying the air from the ventilator. The client's lungs may be becoming noncompliant, but that change doesn't trigger a volume alarm.

The unlicensed assistive personnel is assigned to care for an 80-year-old patient in Buck's traction. Which statement by the UAP would indicate that the RN needs to clarify the instructions?

(1) "I need to monitor the client's intake and output."

(2) "I will encourage the client to cough and deep breathe."

(3) "I will remove the traction during meals."

(4) "If the client has a productive cough, I need to note the color of the sputum."

Keywords for this question are *unlicensed assistive personnel, 80-year-old, Buck's traction,* and *clarify instructions.* The correct answer is Choice (3). Buck's traction can't be removed at any time unless ordered by the physician. Choices (1), (2), and (4) are all correct statements that describe what the UAP should be doing. An 80-year-old is more susceptible to immobility complications. The answers left are interventions to help prevent those complications.

Administering Conscious Sedation Safely

Many surgical and diagnostic procedures use intravenous conscious sedation, which is extremely safe when given and monitored properly. Sedative and analgesic medications are used to achieve an altered state of consciousness with minimal risk. Patients are able to respond to requests but are free from pain, have reduced anxiety, and experience amnesia for the duration of the procedure. Conscious sedation provides a safe and effective option for clients undergoing minor surgical and diagnostic procedures such as endoscopic procedures, breast biopsy, dental surgery, and plastic surgery.

The following agents are used during conscious sedation:

» Benzodiazepines such as midazolam (Versed) and diazepam (Valium)

» Opiates/narcotics such as fentanyl and morphine

Certified registered nurse anesthetists, anesthesiologists, dentists, oral surgeons, and other physicians are qualified providers of conscious sedation. Specially trained registered nurses may assist in the administration of conscious sedation. Patients can follow simple commands during the procedure, which provides reassurance to a cooperative client and helps monitor neurological status.

The provider who monitors the client receiving conscious sedation should have no other responsibilities during the procedure and should never abandon a client for any reason. Respiratory problems are the most common complication of conscious sedation; because patients aren't intubated, their airways must be constantly evaluated.

A number of tasks must be completed before conscious sedation begins, and many of them fall to the nurse. **Before the procedure,** you should

>> Take a complete health history including medication allergies, a list of current medications, and diagnostic test results.

>> Obtain baseline vital signs, level of consciousness, oxygen saturation, and other vital signs pertinent to the procedure.

>> Make sure that emergency resuscitation equipment is close by.

>> Educate the client and family regarding the effects of conscious sedation.

>> Prepare appropriate antagonists for the medication given as per physician order.

>> Initiate an IV line.

During the procedure, you should

>> Administer any medications ordered by the physician.

>> Maintain the IV line.

>> Continuously monitor the client's physical status; vital signs, LOC, cardiac status, and oxygen saturation.

>> Monitor the patient for signs of adverse medication effects.

>> Document any events and client responses to treatment.

>> Be prepared to administer appropriate antagonists for the sedation given, as per physician order.

After the procedure, you should

>> Continue monitoring the client's physical status.

>> Discharge or transfer the patient with written instructions, as per physician and agency protocol.

>> Verify that the patient has someone to drive him to and from his destination.

NCLEX-RN questions about conscious sedation may go something like this:

EXAMPLE

During a plastic surgery procedure in which a patient is under conscious sedation, the nurse who is administering/monitoring the conscious sedation gets called into another room for an emergency. What is the nurse's first course of action?

(1) Leave the patient and go into the other room.

(2) Explain that he can't leave the patient and get someone else to go.

(3) Tell the physician to stop the procedure and leave.

(4) Do nothing.

Keywords for this question are *under conscious sedation, nurse on hand gets called into another room for an emergency,* and *nurse's first course of action.* The correct answer is Choice (2). After conscious sedation has begun, the nurse can't leave the patient under any circumstances because the patient may have a reaction or some other complication that requires immediate intervention. Leaving the patient and doing nothing are inappropriate and unprofessional, and telling the physician to stop the procedure before leaving the room is unethical, unrealistic, and dangerous for the patient being treated.

Chapter **12**

Physiological Adaptation

Your client's health hangs on balance — the balance of fluid and electrolytes and functioning of the body systems. As an RN, you're the front line of defense for your client's homeostasis, so an understanding of the external or internal forces that tip the body's balance from good health into sudden illness is essential.

In this chapter, I review the flow of fluids and chemicals that keep every system in the body functioning properly. Then I look at the results of imbalance — the pathophysiology of the major body systems. I also cover how patients adapt to illness and the nurse's assessment of their adaptation. Lastly, I explain some of the tests and treatments for fixing problems that occur and some of the side effects and issues related to these tests and treatments. In every section, I include typical NCLEX-RN questions with answers and rationale.

TIP

The people who write the NCLEX-RN questions, smart beings that they are, recognize the importance of understanding physiological adaptation, so 11 to 17 percent of the questions on the NCLEX-RN cover these subjects. These questions are very factual, requiring you to know basics about fluid and electrolyte balance, illness, and disease processes. You also find prioritization questions on these topics. (Prioritization questions set up a situation in which you need to know which actions you should take *first* in a given situation.) The test looks at your clinical judgment closely to make sure your practice as a new RN will be safe in any situation.

Understanding What's Normal So You Know What Isn't

A well-known story — who knows whether it's true — describes the way Canadian Mounties are taught to recognize counterfeit money. They never look at a counterfeit bill; they simply study genuine money in minute detail. The theory is that when you know what's genuine, you're never fooled by counterfeit.

This theory applies to the care of clients as well. If you don't know what's normal, physiologically speaking, you have a hard time recognizing pathophysiology, or what's abnormal, at least in time to keep your client from getting sicker. So in this section, I run through the basics of what's normal and what's not so that you can recognize problems early on.

The water of life: Accounting for fluid

Water is the true fluid of life. It makes up most of the human body, so maintaining appropriate fluid balance and homeostasis is the first priority in treatment situations.

Water, water everywhere

Quick, what makes up over 50 percent of your body weight and is the single largest component of, well, you? Water, you say? You pass! And so does water. Water in the body passes through cells, tissues, and plasma. You can find water in the following places:

>> Inside the cells (intracellular)

>> Outside the cells (extracellular)

Extracellular water is subdivided into two categories:

>> Fluid in the tissues (interstitial)

>> Fluid in the circulatory system (intravascular)

Chemicals in the body fluids

Water in the body contains more than plain liquid. Water contains electrolytes, which are salts or minerals that move between extracellular and intracellular body fluids. Positively charged electrolytes are called *cations*, and negatively charged electrolytes are known as *anions*. Knowing the normal values of electrolytes as well as other common values mentioned throughout the book will assist you in answering test questions.

Some of the most common and important serum electrolyte values are

>> **Sodium (Na):** 135 to 145 mEq/L

>> **Potassium (K):** 3.5 to 5 mEq/L

>> **Calcium (Ca):** 9 to 10.5 mEq/L

>> **Magnesium (Mg):** 1.3 to 2.1 mEq/L

>> **Chloride (Cl):** 98 to 106 mEq/L

TIP

Any word preceded by *hypo* means "low," and any word preceded by *hyper* means "high." Examples are *hypokalemia*, meaning low potassium, and *hypernatremia*, meaning high levels of sodium.

Maintaining balance among fluids and electrolytes

Fluid and electrolyte imbalances are an important thing to monitor when managing your patient because tiny shifts can cause major problems in every body system. Fluid and electrolytes tend to go out of balance when the body is stressed, as it is with surgery, illness, and injury. I tell my students that looking at what each of the electrolytes does for the body makes knowing what happens if a given electrolyte is low or high easier. Most electrolytes have a sedation effect or an excitement effect if the level is abnormal.

Fluids and electrolytes need to move freely between body spaces to maintain homeostasis, and they do so in three different ways:

>> **Diffusion:** The movement of particles from an area of greater concentration to an area of lesser concentration (driven by the gradient of the concentration).

>> **Active transport:** The movement of particles across cell membranes; requires cellular energy. The movement is from a region of lower concentration to a region of higher concentration.

>> **Osmosis:** The movement of solvent particles through a semipermeable membrane from an area of less concentration to an area of higher concentration.

Questions dealing with fluids and balance may look like these:

EXAMPLE

A client with heart failure receives an injection of IV furosemide. Within one hour, a short run of ventricular tachycardia appears on the cardiac monitor. Which of the following electrolyte imbalances should the nurse suspect?

(1) Hypokalemia

(2) Hypocalcemia

(3) Hypernatremia

(4) Hyperkalemia

Keywords for this question are *a client with heart failure; an injection of IV furosemide; within one hour, a short run of ventricular tachycardia;* and *which of the following electrolyte imbalances.* The correct answer is Choice (1). Furosemide is a potassium-depleting diuretic that can cause hypokalemia. When a body is low in potassium, the heart is stimulated, leading to ventricular tachycardia. Calcium helps with muscle contraction; if the calcium is low, the heart rate slows. Hypocalcemia causes brady arrhythmias and AV block by slowing conduction through the AV node. Potassium affects repolarization in the heart cells; too much potassium slows the rate and makes it very thready. Hypernatremia may cause sinus tachycardia as a result of fluid and water loss.

EXAMPLE

A victim of a major fire arrives at the emergency department. He has sustained a major burn injury. Which of the following metabolic alterations is expected during the initial period post-burn?

(1) Hyponatremia and hypokalemia

(2) Hyponatremia and hyperkalemia

(3) Hypernatremia and hypokalemia

(4) Hypernatremia and hyperkalemia

Keywords in this question are *a victim of a major fire, sustained a major burn injury,* and *which of the following metabolic alterations is expected during the initial period post-burn.* The correct answer is Choice (2). When the cell membrane has burned, the contents of the cell spill out into the serum. Potassium is the major electrolyte in a cell, so in this situation potassium floods the serum. With the loss of fluid after a burn, sodium is lost.

EXAMPLE

An admit has had thiazide diuretics and has been diagnosed with hyperthyroidism. The client is complaining of profound muscle weakness and increased blood pressure. Which of the following would the nurse expect to see as the doctor's orders for this client? Select all that apply.

❏ **(1)** Discontinue meds containing vitamin D.

❏ **(2)** Discontinue thiazide diuretics.

❏ **(3)** Order for the medication calcitonin.

❏ **(4)** Monitor for abdominal or flank pain.

❏ **(5)** Instruct the client to increase food containing calcium.

The keywords in this question are *admit, thiazide diuretics, hyperthyroidism, complaining of profound muscle weakness, increased blood pressure,* and *expect to see as the doctor's orders.* The correct answers are Choices (1), (2), (3), and (4). The client is experiencing hypercalcemia as a likely result of thiazide diuretics and hyperthyroidism. The complaints of profound muscle weakness and increased blood pressure are symptoms of hypercalcemia. Discontinuing the meds containing vitamin D decreases the absorption of calcium. Vitamin D helps absorb calcium into the body. Discontinuing thiazide diuretics increases the excretion of calcium. Calcitonin helps the body decrease calcium levels. Abdominal or flank pain is a sign of kidney stones from the hypercalcemia and should be monitored. Choice (5) encourages the client to take in more calcium, which is contraindicated in this situation.

EXAMPLE

A client with heart failure is receiving D5 0.45NaCL at 50 ml per hour. The nurse comes back an hour after starting the IV and finds the client with distended neck veins and an altered level of consciousness. Which of the following conditions has the patient developed?

(1) Pneumonia

(2) Water intoxication

(3) Fluid volume deficit

(4) Cardiovascular collapse

The keywords for this question are *heart failure, D5W and .45% NS at 50 ml per hour, distended neck veins, altered level of consciousness,* and *which of the following conditions has the patient developed.* The correct answer is Choice (2). A patient who has heart failure is prone to develop water intoxication, and D5 0.45NaCL is hypotonic. The symptoms of distended neck veins and altered level of consciousness are from water intoxication.

Getting the right pH: The key to acid-base balance

Acid-base balance sounds more complicated than it is. You need to understand the difference between acidosis and alkalosis as well as the difference between respiratory and metabolic imbalance. Because you *will* see acid-base questions on the NCLEX-RN, and because this can be one of the most confusing and hard to master subjects, I break it down for you.

The acidity or alkalinity of a solution is described by a scale from 0 to 14: A rating of 7 is neutral; anything below 7 is acidic; and anything over 7 is alkaline. The normal human serum pH is 7.35 to 7.45, or slightly alkaline. Anything below this level is considered acidotic in the human body, and anything above is considered alkalotic.

The kidneys and lungs help maintain normal pH. The kidneys excrete acids and reabsorb bicarbonate, and the respiratory system gives off carbon dioxide when the body's in an acidic state. In alkalotic states, the kidneys excrete bicarbonate, and the respiratory system retains carbonic acid.

The four states of acid–base imbalance are

» **Metabolic acidosis:** Decreased pH, pCO_2, and decreased bicarbonate

» **Metabolic alkalosis:** Elevated pH, pCO_2, and bicarbonate

» **Respiratory acidosis:** Decreased pH and elevated pCO_2 and bicarbonate

» **Respiratory alkalosis:** Elevated pH and decreased pCO_2 and bicarbonate

It may seem overly simplistic, but respiratory acidosis and alkalosis are a result of respiratory problems, and metabolic imbalances are caused primarily by renal or gastrointestinal dysfunctions. By looking at the three serum levels — pH, CO_2, and bicarbonate (HCO3) — you can tell whether the problem is being caused by a respiratory problem or by a metabolic problem. Follow these steps:

1. **Look at the pH.**

   Acidosis is always a low pH, and alkalosis is a high pH.

2. **Look at the pCO_2 levels.**

   In respiratory disorders, the pH and pCO_2 change in opposite directions; in metabolic disorders the pH and pCO_2 change in the same direction. By looking at the pCO_2 levels, you can tell exactly what kind of acid-base imbalance you're dealing with.

3. **Determine where to look for the source of the problem.**

   If the pH and pCO_2 levels are both low (or both high), the source is in the metabolic (renal or GI) system. If the pH and pCO_2 levels are opposite, the source is in the respiratory systems.

So if your patient has a pH of 6.9, a pCO_2 of 38, and HCO3 of 21, what's wrong with him? He's below 7.4 on the pH scale, so he's in acidosis, and he has a low pCO_2. That's metabolic acidosis. You need to look for a metabolic, not respiratory, cause for the imbalance. This is a simple method that assumes compensation has not taken place.

TIP

My students also use the ABG tic–tac–toe method. It shows exactly what imbalance the client is in and also tells you whether he or she is compensated, partially compensated, or not compensated. Do a quick YouTube search to find out more about this helpful method.

Keeping an eye on respiratory health — the sum of water and pH

When you're setting priorities, think of the airway first (remember your ABCs). You need a functioning respiratory system to provide oxygen for metabolism in the tissues and to expel carbon dioxide, the waste product of metabolism. The respiratory system also facilitates sense of smell, produces speech, maintains acid-base balance, maintains heat balance, and maintains body water levels.

Illness, disease, and injury to the respiratory system can take many forms; review them all! You should know normal blood gas values and the fraction of inspired oxygen by various delivery devices as well as ventilator settings and the causes of alarms. Suctioning and sampling usually appear as priority-setting questions.

The following are examples of NCLEX-RN questions related to respiratory health and treatment:

EXAMPLE

A nurse is suctioning fluids from a client through an endotracheal tube. During the suctioning procedure, the nurse notes on the cardiac monitor that the heart rate has decreased. Which of the following is the most appropriate nursing intervention?

(1) Continue to suction.

(2) Limit the suctioning to 15 seconds.

(3) Stop the procedure and reoxygenate the client.

(4) Notify the physician immediately.

Keywords for this question are *suctioning fluids, through an endotracheal tube, cardiac monitor that the heart rate has decreased*, and *most appropriate nursing intervention.* The correct answer is Choice (3). Suctioning can cause cardiac irregularities. During suctioning, the nurse should monitor the client closely for side effects, including hypoxemia and cardiac irregularities such as a decrease in heart rate resulting from vagal nerve stimulation, mucosal trauma, hypotension, and paroxysmal coughing. If side effects develop, especially cardiac irregularities, the procedure is stopped and the client is reoxygenated.

EXAMPLE

A client with a chest injury has suffered flail chest. A nurse assesses the client for which most distinctive sign of flail chest?

(1) Cyanosis

(2) Hypotension

(3) Dyspnea, especially on exhalation

(4) Paradoxical chest movement

The keywords for this question are *chest injury, suffered flail chest,* and *most distinctive sign of flail chest.* The correct answer is Choice (4). Flail chest results from a fracture of two or more ribs in at least two places each. The fractures result in a floating section of ribs because the section is unattached from the rest of the ribs. This fractured segment has paradoxical movements, which means that the force of inspiration pulls the fractured segment inward while the rest of the chest expands. In exhalation, the segment balloons out while the rest of the chest moves in. Cyanosis and hypotension occur with many different disorders, and dyspnea can occur with many respiratory disorders.

EXAMPLE

A client with no history of respiratory disease is admitted to the emergency department with respiratory failure. A nurse assesses the arterial blood gas report. Which of the following results are consistent with this disorder?

(1) PaO_2 49 mm Hg, $PaCO_2$ 52 mm Hg

(2) PaO_2 60 mm Hg, $PaCO_2$ 45 mm Hg

(3) PaO_2 59 mm Hg, $PaCO_2$ 32 mm Hg

(4) PaO_2 73 mm Hg, $PaCO_2$ 62 mm Hg

The keywords for this question are *no history of respiratory disease, admitted to the emergency department with respiratory failure, arterial blood gas report,* and *which of the following results are consistent with this disorder.* The correct answer is Choice (1). Respiratory failure is described as PaO_2 of 50 mm Hg or less and $PaCO_2$ of 50 mm Hg or greater in a client with no history of respiratory problems. In a client with a history of respiratory disease and hypercapnia, an increase of 5 mm Hg or more ($PaCO_2$) from the client's baseline is considered diagnostic.

Monitoring hemodynamics

For nurses, *hemodynamics* — a branch of physiology that deals with the circulation of the blood (hemo) — is primarily concerned with the monitoring of cardiovascular function. This monitoring can be done in several ways; one of the simplest and most common is by using a cardiac monitor, which tracks the electrical impulse of the heart (not circulation of the blood). The cardiac monitor provides continuous monitoring of cardiac rhythm and rate and electrical conduction. Knowing what those dips and peaks represent is essential for treating cardiac arrhythmias.

REMEMBER

Be sure you know and can identify the basic cardiac strips: atrial fibrillation, atrial flutter, ventricular fibrillation, ventricular tachycardia, sinus bradycardia, and premature ventricular contractions. You should know the treatment for the most life-threatening of these cardiac strips. For example, you should recognize a cardiac strip showing ventricular fibrillation and know that condition should be treated with defibrillation.

Pulmonary artery catheters provide more detailed and sophisticated cardiac monitoring. A *catheter* is a balloon-tip device that's advanced through the superior vena cava into the right atrium, right ventricle, and pulmonary artery. The balloon is inflated until it's wedged in the distal branch of the pulmonary artery; in this position, it provides accurate measurements of pressure within the heart. Central venous pressure is obtained by generally inserting a catheter into the internal jugular, veins in the arm, or femoral vein and threading it into the vena cava. Clients can also have central venous catheters placed in the subclavian vein to aid in fluid resuscitation or to help maintain fluid balance.

REMEMBER

You need to know the interventions for abnormal monitoring results. You should be able to maintain and manage an arterial line and care for a patient who has a pacemaker.

Here are a few sample questions related to hemodynamics:

EXAMPLE

A client in the ICU has a blood pressure of 88/50; the last hour's urine output was 28 ml, and his skin is cold and clammy. The nurse suspects shock. Which of the following is used as a diagnostic and monitoring tool for determining the severity of a shock state?

(1) Arterial line

(2) Indwelling urinary catheter

(3) Intra-aortic balloon pump (IABP)

(4) Pulmonary artery catheter

The keywords in this question are *blood pressure of 88/50, last hour's urine output was 28 ml, skin is cold and clammy, shock,* and *used as diagnostic and monitoring tool for determining the severity of a shock state.* The correct answer is Choice (4). A pulmonary artery catheter gives an accurate reading of the pressure within the heart, which helps determine a course of treatment. An arterial line is used to continuously measure blood pressure through arterial access. A urinary catheter is used to drain urine from the bladder, and an IABP is a heart-assist device that works with the heart muscle and assists so the heart can rest.

EXAMPLE

A client is about to have a central IV catheter placed. The healthcare provider places the catheter in the subclavian vein. Shortly afterward, the client develops shortness of breath and appears very restless. Which of the following would the nurse do first?

(1) Administer sedatives.

(2) Advise the client to calm down because it's just her nerves.

(3) Listen to breath sounds.

(4) Check to see whether the client can have any medications.

The keywords in this question are *central IV catheter placed, subclavian vein, shortness of breath, appears very restless,* and *which of the following would the nurse do first.* The correct answer is Choice (3). This is an acute episode; the nurse must listen to the client's lungs to assess for shortness of breath and any changes in her condition. Because sedatives may suppress respiration, they aren't appropriate for a client who's short of breath. The nurse may also give emotional support, contact the physician who started the IV, and prepare to give oxygen if appropriate and ordered.

EXAMPLE

A client has been diagnosed with atrial fibrillation. Which of the following will be used to convert the client back to a normal sinus rhythm?

(1) Valsalva maneuver

(2) Cardioversion

(3) Automatic external defibrillator (AED)

(4) Defibrillation

Keywords in this question are *diagnosed with atrial fibrillation* and *used to convert back to normal sinus rhythm.* The correct answer is Choice (2). You treat atrial fib with cardioversion. Valsalva maneuver, defibrillation, and AED aren't treatments for atrial fib patients.

Anticipating the Results of Imbalance

Everyone needs to live in balance, but the body especially does because minor shifts in any system can cause major problems. You need to know the body's requirements for proper vitamins and proper treatment of disease in addition to the signs and symptoms of major diseases. In this section, I dive into the issue of imbalance and look at the kinds of questions you may see on the NCLEX-RN.

Knowing what to do when the body systems are out of whack

Any body system can be altered for better or worse, so this section is a very broad topic. Remember that the main body systems include cardiac, respiratory, endocrine, neurologic, musculoskeletal, immune, genitourinary, gastrointestinal, reproductive, and integumentary. When prioritizing care for alterations in any body system, always remember to *put physiological needs first.*

Test questions on body system alterations include questions on adults and children. Here are some examples:

EXAMPLE

A client comes into the emergency room with complaints of dizziness, nausea, and vomiting. The doctor suspects Ménière's disease. What is the nurse's priority action?

(1) Give an antiemetic

(2) Initiate a sodium-restricted diet

(3) Give an antihistamine

(4) Initiate safety measures

The keywords in this question are *emergency room; dizziness, nausea, and vomiting; Ménière's disease;* and *nurse's priority action.* The correct answer is Choice (4). A Ménière's patient is at high risk for falls; therefore, safety measures need to be put in place. The other answers are interventions for this condition but aren't a priority at this time.

EXAMPLE

A 21-year-old client has just been diagnosed with having a hydatidiform mole. Which of the following is considered a risk factor in developing this mole?

(1) Age in 20 to 40 range

(2) Primigravida

(3) Prior molar gestation

(4) High socioeconomic status

The keywords for this question are *21-year-old client*, *hydatidiform mole*, and *risk factor in developing this mole*. The correct answer is Choice (3). Prior molar gestation increases a woman's risk for developing another molar gestation. Adolescents and women 40 and older are also at increased risk for molar pregnancies. Multigravidas, especially women with prior loss of pregnancies and women from lower socioeconomic classes, are at an increased risk.

EXAMPLE

When performing a neurologic assessment on a neonate, which sign is considered a normal finding?

(1) A positive Babinski's sign

(2) "Sunset" eyes

(3) Closed fontanels

(4) Pupils unreactive to light

Keywords for this question are *performing a neurologic assessment*, *neonate*, and *normal finding*. The correct answer is Choice (1). A positive Babinski's sign is normal in infants up to one year of age but is abnormal in adults. Sunset eyes, where the sclera is visible above the iris, is a result of cranial nerve palsy and may indicate increased intracranial pressure. Fontanels do not completely close till 18 months. An infant's pupils react to light in the same way that an adult's pupils do.

EXAMPLE

Crohn's disease is a chronic relapsing disease. Which area of the GI tract is involved with this disease?

(1) The entire length of the large intestine

(2) The small intestine and colon, the entire thickness of the bowel

(3) The small intestine, mucosa only

(4) The sigmoid area only

The keywords for this question are *Crohn's disease*, *chronic relapsing disease*, and *which area of the GI tract is involved*. The correct answer is Choice (2). Crohn's disease may involve the large intestine, the small intestine, or both, and it affects the entire thickness of the bowel regardless. Choices (1) and (3) probably describe ulcerative colitis, and Choice (4) is too specific and a small part of the bowel; therefore, it isn't a likely answer. In any body system alteration, when an answer involves a very specific part of the body, it's probably an incorrect choice.

EXAMPLE

When assessing a client with a history of genital herpes, which of the following symptoms would indicate that an outbreak of lesions is imminent?

(1) Headache and fever

(2) Vaginal and urethral discharge

(3) Dysuria and lymphadenopathy

(4) Genital pruritis and paresthesia

The keywords for this question are *assessing a client*, *history of genital herpes*, and *following symptoms would indicate that an outbreak of lesions is imminent*. The correct answer is Choice (4). Pruritis and paresthesia, as well as redness of the genital area, are symptoms of recurrent herpes infection. These symptoms appear anywhere from immediately before lesions appear to 48 hours prior. Headache and fever are symptoms of primary infection. Dysuria and lymphadenopathy are local symptoms of primary infection that may occur with recurrent infection, but don't occur prior to the outbreak of lesions.

Looking down the road to infection

Infection is an invasion of the body by pathogenic organisms that multiply and produce injurious effects. A communicable disease is an infectious disease that may be transmitted from one person to another. To prevent the spread of infection, you need to break the chain of events that leads to infection by doing the following:

>> Maintain a clean, dry, well-ventilated environment.

>> Wash your hands — yes, between *every* client!

>> Disinfect, maintain isolation when necessary, and use aseptic techniques.

>> Use universal precautions — on everyone! (That's why they're called "universal.")

You also need to remember treatment protocols, antibiotics and other drug therapy and contra-indications, and how to prevent the continued spread of disease.

Everything that happens, whether it's related to nursing or not, starts with a chain of events. See Figure 12-1 for a visual example.

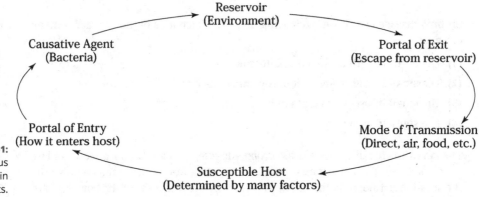

FIGURE 12-1: An infectious illness chain of events.

The following are typical questions related to infectious disease:

EXAMPLE

Which of the following types of cases of pneumonia is most common in children ages 5 to 12?

(1) Enteric bacilli

(2) Mycoplasma pneumonia

(3) Staphylococcal pneumonia

(4) Streptococcal pneumonia

Keywords for this question are *types of cases of pneumonia* and *most common in children ages 5 to 12.* The correct answer is Choice (2). Mycoplasma pneumonia is typically seen in older children. The other three are typically seen in children from 3 months to 5 years old.

EXAMPLE

Pneumococcal vaccine polyvalent and flu vaccination are highly recommended for clients with asthma, chronic bronchitis, and emphysema for which of the following reasons?

(1) These vaccines prevent the patient from getting pneumonia or other serious respiratory infections.

(2) These vaccines help reduce the fast respiratory rates that these clients experience.

(3) These vaccines help reduce the need for maintenance medications for these conditions.

(4) All clients should have these vaccines.

The keywords for this question are *pneumococcal and flu vaccination; recommended for clients with asthma, chronic bronchitis, and emphysema*; and *for which of the following reasons*. The correct answer is Choice (1). Receiving vaccines to protect against respiratory infection is highly recommended for clients with respiratory disorders. Infections can cause these clients to need intubation and mechanical ventilation. Weaning may be difficult or impossible because the client's respiratory system becomes dependent on the assistance provided by the ventilator. The vaccines have no effect on bronchodilation or respiratory rate.

EXAMPLE

An adult client has received an injection of immunoglobulin. The nurse knows that the client will develop which of the following types of immunity?

(1) Active natural immunity

(2) Active artificial immunity

(3) Passive natural immunity

(4) Passive artificial immunity

Keywords for this question are *adult client, injection of immunoglobin,* and *develop which of the following types of immunity*. The correct answer is Choice (4). Passive artificial immunity occurs when antibodies are produced by another person or animal and injected into the recipient.

EXAMPLE

A patient is being admitted to the unit with a diagnosis of chickenpox, or varicella. The nurse needs to set up which transmission-based precautions for this patient?

(1) Droplet

(2) Contact

(3) Airborne and contact

(4) Standard

This question's keywords are a diagnosis of *chickenpox, or varicella; needs to set up*; and *which transmission-based precautions*. The correct answer is Choice (3). Chickenpox is transmitted by touching the rash or contaminated objects and by droplets.

Pathophysiology: Recognizing and Managing Illness and Disease

If you know that *physiology* is the normal functioning of the human body (and you should know that — it's a pretty basic term), you can deduce that *pathophysiology* describes abnormal responses to disease or injury; these can be functional or structural responses and can be positive or negative. The difference between health and disease depends on the body's response and adaptation to stressors. You can expect to see lots of pathophysiology questions covering any system of the body on the NCLEX-RN.

Houston, we have a problem: Focusing on microsystems

Pathophysiologic processes occur when an injury or disease triggers such a rapid response that the body's compensatory mechanisms can't make changes fast enough to remain healthy. As an RN, your observations and knowledge of physiologic and pathophysiologic processes help you determine whether a problem exists and guide you in taking an appropriate course of action — that is, they inform your clinical judgment.

Your study focus in this area should be on specific details of physiologic functioning *microsystems*, which are systems within the system, rather than on the large systems such as renal, cardiac, and so on. You'll then be able to tell how the abnormal condition has affected the microsystem; for example, hypothyroidism affects the hormones the thyroid produces. Examples of these questions follow with explanations:

EXAMPLE

The thyroid gland produces which group of hormones?

(1) Amylase, lipase, and trypsin

(2) Triiodothyronine (T3), thyroxine (T4), and calcitonin

(3) Glucocorticoids, mineralocorticoids, and androgens

(4) Vasopressin, oxytocin, and thyroid-stimulating hormone (TSH)

The keywords in this question are *thyroid* and *which group of hormones*. The correct answer is Choice (2). T3, T4, and calcitonin are all secreted by the thyroid gland. The pancreas secretes the enzymes amylase, lipase, and trypsin, which aid in digestion. The adrenal gland produces glucocorticoids, mineralocorticoids, and androgens, and the pituitary secretes vasopressin, oxytocin, and TSH.

EXAMPLE

The hypothalamus responds to a decrease in blood pressure by secreting which substance?

(1) Angiotensin

(2) Epinephrine

(3) Renin

(4) Antidiuretic hormone (ADH)

The keywords for this question are *the hypothalamus, a decrease in blood pressure*, and *secreting which substance*. The correct answer is Choice (4). ADH works on the renal tubules to promote water retention, which leads to an increase in blood pressure. The other substances listed help increase blood pressure but aren't secreted by the hypothalamus. Epinephrine is in the adrenal medulla. Renin is an enzyme that converts angiotensin, an inactive substance formed by the liver, into angiotensin I. Renin is released by the kidneys in response to decreased renal perfusion. Angiotensin-converting enzyme (ACE) converts angiotensin I to angiotensin II. Angiotensin II, because it's vasoconstrictive, increases arterial perfusion pressure, and increases thirst.

TIP

Take special note of the preceding explanation and rationale; the correct answer requires you to think through systems and the detailed pathophysiology related to them.

EXAMPLE

Stimulation of the sympathetic nervous system produces which of the following responses?

(1) Tachycardia

(2) Bradycardia

(3) Hypotension

(4) Decreased myocardial contractility

This question's keywords are *stimulation of the sympathetic nervous system* and *which of the following responses*. The correct answer is Choice (1). Stimulation of the sympathetic nervous system causes tachycardia and increased contractility. It also causes increased blood pressure as well as dilated pupils. The other listed symptoms are related to the parasympathetic nervous system, which is responsible for slowing heart rate and decreased contractility as well as pupil constriction, and decreased respiratory rate.

EXAMPLE

A client with chronic renal failure is admitted to the unit with pulmonary edema. The client was scheduled for dialysis yesterday but missed her appointment. After blood chemistry is performed, what are the expected results?

(1) Alkalemia

(2) Hyperkalemia

(3) Hypernatremia

(4) Hypokalemia

The keywords in this question are *chronic renal failure, pulmonary edema, scheduled for dialysis yesterday, missed appointment, blood chemistry,* and *expected results*. The correct answer is Choice (2). The kidneys are responsible for excreting potassium. When a patient is in renal failure, the kidneys can no longer perform that function, resulting in hyperkalemia. Hypokalemia is seen in patients undergoing diuresis. The kidneys are responsible for regulating the acid-base balance. Hyponatremia typically appears when patients are retaining water.

EXAMPLE

After an infarct of the brain stem, the nurse would be alert to which of the following conditions?

(1) Aphasia

(2) Bradypnea

(3) Contralateral hemiplegia

(4) Numbness and tingling of the face

Keywords for this question are *infarct of the brainstem* and *alert to which of the following conditions*. The correct answer is Choice (2). The brain stem contains the medulla and the centers that control respiratory, cardiac, and vasomotor functions. An infarct to the brain stem causes changes to vital signs, such as slow respirations (bradypnea). The other options are symptoms of a stroke.

EXAMPLE

A client who had a stroke two months ago now presents in the ER with signs of fluid overload, low urinary output, hypertension, and tachycardia. Which of the following interventions/prescriptions would the nurse expect for this patient? Select all that apply.

❏ **(1)** Monitoring for signs of increased intracranial pressure

❏ **(2)** Implementing seizure precautions

❏ **(3)** Elevating the head of the bed to a maximum of 10 degrees

❏ **(4)** Instructing the client to avoid foods or liquids that produce diuresis

❏ **(5)** MD order for desmopressin acetate

Keywords in this question are *stroke two months ago; now presents in the ER; signs of fluid overload, low urinary output, hypertension, and tachycardia;* and *which of the following interventions/prescriptions would the nurse expect*. The correct answers are Choices (1), (2), and (3). The symptoms listed in the question indicate the syndrome of inappropriate antidiuretic hormone, which is caused by a stroke. Therefore, the appropriate measures are to watch for increased intracranial pressure, take seizure precautions, and raise the head of the bed no more than 10 degrees.

Doing damage control of the medical kind

Illness can be critical, acute, or chronic, and each of these types of illness can manifest itself in various ways. For example, individuals with a life-threatening critical illness have a realistic fear of death and permanent loss of function. The loss of control and sense of powerlessness can be overwhelming for clients. Chronic illness and disease, such as diabetes mellitus, may lead to loss of function or a body part, which necessitates adaptation to the changes that occur. Illness is a large focus area that can include many diseases and problems, so narrowing this subject area is a huge feat, but in this section I do my best.

NCLEX-RN questions in the vein of managing illness may resemble the following:

EXAMPLE

Which of the following tests is used to test for diabetes insipidus?

(1) Fluid deprivation test

(2) Urine glucose test

(3) Capillary blood glucose test

(4) Serum ketone test

The keyword for this question is *test for diabetes insipidus.* The correct answer is Choice (1). A fluid deprivation test involves withholding water for 4 to 18 hours and then checking urine and plasma osmolarity periodically. A client with diabetes insipidus will have an increased serum osmolarity of greater than 300 mOsm/kg; urine osmolarity will not increase. The urine glucose test measures glucose levels in the urine; diabetes insipidus doesn't affect urine glucose levels. A capillary blood glucose test allows rapid reading of blood glucose, and serum ketone tests will confirm diabetic ketoacidosis.

EXAMPLE

One hour after receiving pyridostigmine bromide, a client reports difficulty swallowing and excessive respiratory secretions. Which drug would the nurse prepare to give after notifying the physician?

(1) Additional pyridostigmine bromide

(2) Atropine

(3) Edrophonium

(4) Neostigmine

Keywords for this question are *pyridostigmine bromide, difficulty swallowing, excessive respiratory secretions,* and *which drug would the nurse prepare to give after notifying the physician.* The correct answer is Choice (2). These symptoms are indicative of a cholinergic crisis or an excess of acetyl-cholinesterase medication, typically happening 45 to 60 minutes after the last dose of acetylcholinesterase inhibitor. Atropine, an anticholinergic drug, is used to antagonize acetylcholinesterase inhibitors. The other drugs listed are acetylcholinesterase inhibitors. Edrophonium is a diagnostic drug, and pyridostigmine bromide and neostigmine are used for the treatment of myasthenia gravis.

Taking a Patient for Tests and Therapy

Patients undergoing tests and therapy require nursing care during and after their procedures. You need to know what's necessary to maintain safety during the exam and physiological integrity after the therapy.

Facing an MRI, the hot potato of medical tests

When you think of having an MRI, what's the first thing that comes to mind? If you thought "claustrophobia," you're on the same wavelength as many of your future patients. Many patients have a fear of being enclosed in an MRI, but claustrophobia isn't the only thing that can cause chaos in an MRI. Magnetic resonance imaging (MRI) uses magnetic and radio waves to create a detailed visualization of the brain, heart, and other body structures. Pacemakers and surgical or orthopedic clips can wreak havoc with the patient — and the equipment. (Shrapnel shouldn't be scanned, either, so be sure that you have a complete history!) Always remove jewelry and metal objects from the patient prior to the procedure, and always determine the patient's ability to lie still and the possibility that he or she may become claustrophobic.

Here's an example of questions related to patient tests:

EXAMPLE

A client is scheduled for magnetic resonance imaging (MRI) of the head. Which of the following areas is essential to assess before the procedure?

(1) Food and drink intake within the past eight hours

(2) The presence of metal fillings, prosthesis, or a pacemaker

(3) The presence of carotid artery disease

(4) Voiding before the procedure

Keywords for this question are *MRI of the head* and *essential to assess before the procedure*. The correct answer is Choice (2). Strong magnetic waves may dislodge metal in the client's body, possibly causing injury. Although the client may be told to restrict food intake for eight hours prior to the procedure, particularly if contrast will be used, metal is an absolute contraindication for this procedure because it's a safety issue. Voiding beforehand makes the client more comfortable and better able to remain still during the procedure, but it isn't essential for the test. And carotid artery disease isn't a contraindication.

Handling therapies, from dialysis to radiation

There's no end to therapy when you're a nurse. Types of therapy include chemotherapy, radiation, physical and occupational therapy, respiratory therapy, dialysis, and dozens of others. Every type of therapy has both an expected and unexpected outcome; you need to be aware of both the potential positive and negative outcomes so that you know what to look for when administering therapy to a patient. You also have to know the *what, why,* and *how* of therapy: What is this therapy expected to do for this patient? Why does the patient need it? What's gone wrong that needs to be corrected? And how does this therapy accomplish that?

Questions on therapies usually focus on radiation and chemotherapy. Tuck away the following facts, and you'll be well prepared for these types of questions:

>> When it comes to radiation:

- Side effects are cumulative. The effects appear after the total dose exceeds the body's ability to repair damage caused by radiation.

- Fatigue is one of the most common side effects of radiation and often isn't relieved by rest.

- Other side effects of radiation include skin problems, anorexia, nausea, vomiting, diarrhea, anemia, leucopenia, and thrombocytopenia.

- Physical therapy can be draining for the patient, and interventions are coordinated as necessary around patient needs.

>> When it comes to chemotherapy:

- Chemo is a balancing act based on the ability of a drug to kill cancer cells while damaging normal cells as little as possible.

- The destruction of normal cells leads to numerous side effects that affect body systems, including but not limited to GI, hematologic, integumentary, renal, reproductive, and neurologic systems.

- The effect of chemotherapy is greatest on rapidly dividing cells, such as bone marrow cells, GI tract, and hair.

Other therapies, such as wound therapy, may show up in questions related to pressure ulcers and nursing management. You can also expect questions on cardiovascular disorder interventions such as percutaneous transluminal coronary angioplasty (PTCA), coronary artery stents, atherectomy, coronary artery bypass graft (CABG), and cardiac transplant. I simply don't have the space to list all the main facts about all these therapies, so refer to your textbooks for a refresher.

The following are some examples of questions related to patient therapy:

EXAMPLE

The client is undergoing radiation therapy to treat lung cancer. Following the treatment, the nurse notes erythema on the client's chest and neck, and the client is complaining of pain at the radiation site. The nurse interprets this data to mean

(1) A superficial injury to the tissue from the radiation

(2) An allergic reaction to the radiation

(3) A cutaneous reaction to products formed by the lysis of the neoplastic cells

(4) An ischemic injury, much like decubitus formation, caused by pressure from the machine

Keywords for this question are *undergoing radiation therapy, treat lung cancer, erythema on the client's chest and neck, complaining of pain at the radiation site,* and *nurse interprets.* The correct answer is Choice (1). Superficial injury from radiation can manifest with erythema, hyperpigmentation, dry desquamation, or moist desquamation. Moist desquamation is comparable to a second-degree burn in histology, appearance, and sensation. Note the relationship between erythema in the question and the reference to *superficial* injury in the correct response.

EXAMPLE

A nurse is evaluating a client's response to cardioversion. Which of the following observations would be of the highest priority to the nurse?

(1) Oxygen flow rate

(2) Status of the airway

(3) Blood pressure

(4) Level of consciousness

Keywords in this question are *evaluating the client's response to cardioversion, observations,* and *the highest priority to the nurse.* The correct answer is Choice (2). Nursing responsibility after cardioversion is the maintaining of the airway first, followed by administering oxygen and assessing vital signs and level of consciousness. Noting the key phrase "highest priority" prompts you to refer to the ABCs and use the process of elimination to reach the correct answer.

EXAMPLE

A client is admitted to the emergency department with an active diagnosis of acute myocardial infarction. The patient is started on tissue plasminogen activator (tPA) by infusion. Which of the following parameters would a nurse determine requires the least frequent assessment to detect complications of therapy with tPA?

(1) Oxygen saturation

(2) Neurological signs

(3) Blood pressure and pulse

(4) Complaints of abdominal and back pain

Keywords in this question are *an active diagnosis of acute myocardial infarction, tissue plasminogen activator, which of the following parameters requires the least frequent assessment,* and *detect complications of therapy.* The correct answer is Choice (1). An acute myocardial infarction is due to a clot or plaque blockage, and the drug is given to break up clots. So your priority is bleeding. The key phrase here is *least frequent assessment.* Thrombolytic agents dissolve clots, and bleeding can occur anywhere in the body. The nurse monitors for any signs of bleeding and also for occult (hidden) signs of bleeding by taking hemoglobin and hematocrit values, blood pressure, and pulse; checking neurological signs; assessing abdominal and back pain; and checking for the presence of blood in the stool and/or urine. Bleeding is the primary complication of thrombolytic therapy.

REMEMBER

The preceding question requires you to set priorities. A change in neurological signs can indicate cerebral bleeding, abdominal and back pain can indicate abdominal bleeding, and change in blood pressure and pulse can be general indicators of hemorrhage. Oxygen saturation isn't an indicator of bleeding in the respiratory tract.

EXAMPLE

A client has moist saline dressings applied to an open ulcer of the foot. Ten days after ulcer development, the wound should have which appearance?

(1) Red, swollen tissue

(2) Dry, crusted scab

(3) Deep, wide keloid

(4) Warm, painful tissue

Keywords for this question are *moist saline dressings, open ulcer of the foot, ten days after ulcer development,* and *should have which appearance.* The correct answer is Choice (2). Ten days into healing, an ulcer should be at the end of the lag phase of healing, as indicated by a dry, crusted scab. The tissue is red, swollen, warm, or painful during the inflammatory period, which occurs two to seven days after the ulcer develops. A deep, wide keloid may appear three weeks to two years after ulcer development.

EXAMPLE

Which of the following treatments is a suitable surgical intervention for unstable angina?

(1) Cardiac catheterization

(2) Echocardiogram

(3) Nitroglycerin

(4) Percutaneous transluminal coronary angioplasty (PTCA)

The keywords for this question are *suitable surgical intervention* and *unstable angina.* The correct answer is Choice (4). Angina is caused by a blockage, so look for an answer choice that would open the blockage. PTCA can alleviate the blockage and restore blood flow and oxygenation. An echocardiogram is a noninvasive diagnostic test. Nitroglycerin is an oral or sublingual medication. Cardiac catheterization is a diagnostic tool, not a treatment.

EXAMPLE

A client has been to hemodialysis. Which of the following should the nurse be alert to for complications? Select all that apply.

❏ (1) Fluid volume excess

❏ (2) Disequilibrium

❏ (3) Hemorrhage

❏ (4) Shock

❏ (5) Air emboli

Keywords for this question are *has been to hemodialysis* and *alert to for complication*. The correct answers are Choices (2), (3), (4), and (5). Disequilibrium, hemorrhage, shock, and air emboli are all complications of hemodialysis. Hemodialysis takes fluid off, so Choice (1) is incorrect.

3

Just What You Were Looking For: A Full-Length Practice Test

Chapter **13**

A Story of Blood, Chills, and Pain: A Practice NCLEX-RN

You know your stuff — now's your chance to shine. The following is a 250-question sample exam. Read each question carefully, find your keywords, and choose the best answer or answers from the multiple-choice options and alternate item formats. Fill in your answers on the sheet that appears at the beginning of this chapter. (You may want to tear that two-sided answer sheet out of the book so that you don't have to keep flipping back and forth.) When you're finished with this exam, you can compare your answers with the answers and explanations provided in Chapter 14.

Although the questions for NCLEX-RN come up randomly, I've chosen to organize them into groups of similar subjects (except for the last few, which are random) so that you can see where your weak clinical areas are and can concentrate your study in those areas. After all, there's no sense in wasting time with stuff you already know!

TIP

Give yourself as much time as you need to complete this practice exam. After you get used to the types of questions that appear on the test, you can worry about timing.

Answer Sheet

1. ① ② ③ ④ ⑤	36. ① ② ③ ④	71. ① ② ③ ④	106. ① ② ③ ④
2. ① ② ③ ④	37. ① ② ③ ④	72. ① ② ③ ④	107. ① ② ③ ④
3. ① ② ③ ④	38. ① ② ③ ④	73. ① ② ③ ④	108. ① ② ③ ④
4. ① ② ③ ④	39. ① ② ③ ④	74. ① ② ③ ④	109. ① ② ③ ④
5. ① ② ③ ④	40. ① ② ③ ④	75. ① ② ③ ④	110. ① ② ③ ④
6. ① ② ③ ④	41. ① ② ③ ④	76. ① ② ③ ④	111. ① ② ③ ④
7. ① ② ③ ④ ⑤	42. ① ② ③ ④	77. ① ② ③ ④	112. ① ② ③ ④
8. ① ② ③ ④	43. ① ② ③ ④	78. ① ② ③ ④	113. ① ② ③ ④
9. ① ② ③ ④ ⑤	44. ① ② ③ ④	79. ① ② ③ ④	114. ① ② ③ ④
10. ① ② ③ ④	45. ① ② ③ ④ ⑤	80. ① ② ③ ④	115. ① ② ③ ④
11. ① ② ③ ④	46. ① ② ③ ④	81. ① ② ③ ④	116. ① ② ③ ④
12. ① ② ③ ④	47. ① ② ③ ④ ⑤	82. ① ② ③ ④	117. ① ② ③ ④
13. ① ② ③ ④ ⑤	48. ① ② ③ ④	83. ① ② ③ ④	118. ① ② ③ ④
14. ① ② ③ ④	49. ① ② ③ ④	84. ① ② ③ ④	119. ① ② ③ ④
15. ① ② ③ ④	50. ① ② ③ ④ ⑤	85. ① ② ③ ④	120. ① ② ③ ④
16. ① ② ③ ④	51. ① ② ③ ④	86. ① ② ③ ④	121. ① ② ③ ④
17. ① ② ③ ④ ⑤	52. ① ② ③ ④	87. ① ② ③ ④	122. ① ② ③ ④
18. ① ② ③ ④	53. ① ② ③ ④	88. ① ② ③ ④	123. ① ② ③ ④
19. ① ② ③ ④	54. ① ② ③ ④	89. ① ② ③ ④	124. ① ② ③ ④
20. ① ② ③ ④	55. ① ② ③ ④	90. ① ② ③ ④	125. ① ② ③ ④
21. ① ② ③ ④	56. ① ② ③ ④	91. ① ② ③ ④	126. ① ② ③ ④
22. ① ② ③ ④	57. ① ② ③ ④	92. ① ② ③ ④	127. — — — — —
23. ① ② ③ ④	58. ① ② ③ ④	93. ① ② ③ ④ ⑤	128. ① ② ③ ④
24. ① ② ③ ④	59. ① ② ③ ④	94. ① ② ③ ④	129. ① ② ③ ④
25. ① ② ③ ④	60. ① ② ③ ④	95. ① ② ③ ④	130. ① ② ③ ④
26. ① ② ③ ④	61. ① ② ③ ④	96. ① ② ③ ④	131. ① ② ③ ④
27. ① ② ③ ④	62. ① ② ③ ④	97. ① ② ③ ④	132. ① ② ③ ④
28. ① ② ③ ④	63. ① ② ③ ④	98. ① ② ③ ④	133. ① ② ③ ④
29. ① ② ③ ④	64. ① ② ③ ④	99. ① ② ③ ④	134. ① ② ③ ④
30. ① ② ③ ④	65. ① ② ③ ④	100. ① ② ③ ④	135. ① ② ③ ④
31. ① ② ③ ④	66. ① ② ③ ④	101. ① ② ③ ④	136. ① ② ③ ④
32. ① ② ③ ④	67. ① ② ③ ④ ⑤	102. ① ② ③ ④	137. ① ② ③ ④
33. ① ② ③ ④ ⑤	68. ① ② ③ ④	103. ① ② ③ ④	138. ① ② ③ ④
34. ① ② ③ ④	69. ① ② ③ ④	104. ① ② ③ ④	139. ① ② ③ ④
35. ① ② ③ ④	70. ① ② ③ ④	105. ① ② ③ ④	140. ① ② ③ ④

Answer Sheet

141. ① ② ③ ④	176. ① ② ③ ④	201. ① ② ③ ④	236. ① ② ③ ④
142. ① ② ③ ④	177. ① ② ③ ④	202. ① ② ③ ④	237. ① ② ③ ④
143. ① ② ③ ④	178. ① ② ③ ④	203. ① ② ③ ④	238. ① ② ③ ④
144. ① ② ③ ④	179. ① ② ③ ④	204. ① ② ③ ④	239. ① ② ③ ④
145. ① ② ③ ④	180. ① ② ③ ④	205. ① ② ③ ④	240. ① ② ③ ④
146. ① ② ③ ④	181. ① ② ③ ④	206. ① ② ③ ④	241. ① ② ③ ④
147. ① ② ③ ④	182. ① ② ③ ④	207. ① ② ③ ④	242. ① ② ③ ④
148. ① ② ③ ④ ⑤	183. ① ② ③ ④	208. ① ② ③ ④	243. ① ② ③ ④
149. ① ② ③ ④	184. ① ② ③ ④	209. ① ② ③ ④	244. ① ② ③ ④
150. ① ② ③ ④ ⑤	185.	210. ① ② ③ ④	245. ① ② ③ ④
151. ① ② ③ ④		211. ① ② ③ ④	246. ① ② ③ ④
152. ① ② ③ ④		212. ① ② ③ ④	247. ① ② ③ ④
153. ① ② ③ ④		213. ① ② ③ ④	248. ① ② ③ ④
154. ① ② ③ ④		214. ① ② ③ ④	249. ① ② ③ ④
155. ① ② ③ ④		215. ① ② ③ ④	250. ① ② ③ ④
156. ① ② ③ ④		216. ① ② ③ ④	
157. ① ② ③ ④		217. ① ② ③ ④	
158. ① ② ③ ④		218. ① ② ③ ④	
159. ① ② ③ ④		219. ① ② ③ ④	
160. ① ② ③ ④		220. ① ② ③ ④ ⑤	
161. ① ② ③ ④	186. ① ② ③ ④	221. ① ② ③ ④	
162. ① ② ③ ④	187. ① ② ③ ④	222. ① ② ③ ④	
163. ① ② ③ ④	188. ① ② ③ ④	223. ① ② ③ ④	
164. ① ② ③ ④	189. ① ② ③ ④	224. ① ② ③ ④	
165. ① ② ③ ④	190. ① ② ③ ④ ⑤	225. ① ② ③ ④	
166. ① ② ③ ④	191. ① ② ③ ④	226. ① ② ③ ④	
167. ① ② ③ ④	192. ① ② ③ ④	227. ① ② ③ ④	
168. ① ② ③ ④	193. ① ② ③ ④	228. ① ② ③ ④	
169. ① ② ③ ④	194. ① ② ③ ④	229. ① ② ③ ④	
170. ① ② ③ ④	195. ① ② ③ ④	230. ① ② ③ ④	
171. ① ② ③ ④ ⑤	196. ① ② ③ ④	231. ① ② ③ ④	
172. ① ② ③ ④	197. ① ② ③ ④	232. ① ② ③ ④	
173. ① ② ③ ④	198. ① ② ③ ④	233. ① ② ③ ④	
174. ① ② ③ ④	199. ① ② ③ ④	234. ① ② ③ ④	
175. ① ② ③ ④	200. ① ② ③ ④	235. ① ② ③ ④	

1. A 75-year-old male has been admitted to the emergency department. Upon arrival, he is complaining of dyspnea, peripheral edema, fatigue, and having only gone to the bathroom three times in the past 24 hours, producing a very small amount of urine each time. The history of the patient reveals that he has type 1 diabetes and has a history of hypertension. He has just finished his antibiotic for sepsis yesterday. Which of the following diagnostic tests would the nurse expect to see on the physician's orders to confirm the diagnosis of acute kidney injury? Select all that apply.

   ❏ (1) Chest X-ray
   ❏ (2) UA
   ❏ (3) UA culture and sensitivity
   ❏ (4) Ultrasound of the heart
   ❏ (5) CT scan of the kidneys

2. A patient is undergoing diagnostic testing for chronic renal failure. Which of these laboratory values would support a diagnosis of chronic renal failure?

   (1) Blood glucose of 115 mg/dl
   (2) Serum creatinine of 1.1 mg/dl
   (3) Serum potassium of 6.1 mEq/L
   (4) Blood urea nitrogen of 20 mg%

3. The client is being given oxybutynin chloride. The nurse needs to monitor for which therapeutic effect?

   (1) The client is able to go to the bathroom without having any urinary incontinence.
   (2) The client is able to breathe more easily when doing activities of daily living.
   (3) The client is able to have a bowel movement with no straining.
   (4) The client is able to maintain blood glucose within the acceptable range.

4. While undergoing hemodialysis, a patient develops painful muscle cramps. The nurse should know that this symptom is due to

   (1) Fluid rapidly leaving the extracellular space
   (2) Disturbed insulin-glucose metabolism
   (3) Impaired perfusion due to poor arterial blood gases
   (4) An increase in serum sodium and potassium levels

5. A male patient is scheduled for a transurethral prostatectomy (TURP) with spinal anesthesia. Prior to the procedure, the nurse plans to reinforce the teaching the patient has already received about the anesthesia. What should the nurse include in the teaching?

   (1) The patient will have an endotracheal tube with breathing assistance from a ventilator.
   (2) The patient will be unable to move his arms and legs for several hours after the procedure.
   (3) The patient may experience a headache after the procedure and should remain supine post-procedure.
   (4) The patient will be unconscious until the procedure is completed and will be able to move when fully alert.

6. A patient is in intensive care for multiple internal injuries and fractures due to a motor vehicle accident. Which parameter would alert the nurse that the patient may be undergoing acute renal failure due to the injury?

   (1) A urine creatinine clearance of 125 ml/ minute
   (2) Urinalysis showing tubular epithelial cells and casts
   (3) BUN/creatinine ratio of 10:1
   (4) A urine specific gravity of 1.020

7. A nurse is teaching a patient about how to avoid recurrences of urinary tract infections. Which of these measures should the nurse include in the teaching plan? Select all that apply.

☐ **(1)** Wipe the perineal area from back to front after voiding.

☐ **(2)** Limit fluid intake to decrease voiding.

☐ **(3)** Avoid tight-fitting slacks and underwear.

☐ **(4)** Douche twice a week with a commercial preparation.

☐ **(5)** Wear cotton underwear.

8. A patient is hospitalized with severe right flank pain related to suspected renal calculi. During the diagnostic period, the nurse should first

(1) Prepare the patient for urinary catheterization

(2) Teach the patient about which foods to eat to avoid calculi recurrence

(3) Institute high fluid volume intake measures

(4) Administer analgesics as ordered to control pain

9. A nurse is caring for a patient who is in skeletal traction for a left femur fracture. Which of the following would the nurse do if the client were experiencing a fat embolus? Select all that apply.

☐ **(1)** Notify the healthcare provider

☐ **(2)** Document the event and actions that are taken

☐ **(3)** Give intravenous fluids as prescribed

☐ **(4)** Provide oxygen

☐ **(5)** Place the client in Trendelenburg

10. A patient who has a left leg fracture and is in skeletal traction is being closely monitored for the development of fat emboli. What manifestation should alert the nurse to the development of fat emboli?

(1) Chest pain

(2) Paralytic ileus

(3) Sweating below the level of the injury

(4) Paresthesias in both feet

11. A nurse is repositioning a patient in the immediate postoperative period following hip surgery for a right hip fracture. The nurse should position the patient

(1) On the right side with legs abducted with an abduction pillow

(2) Prone, with legs adducted and head turned to the side

(3) On the left side with legs slightly flexed with an abduction pillow

(4) Supine, with legs adducted and one foot resting over the other foot

12. A patient has been diagnosed with a hip fracture and has been placed in Buck's traction prior to surgery. The nurse should know that while waiting for surgery, the patient should be frequently assessed for

(1) Pin site infection

(2) Skin pressure

(3) Arthritis

(4) Intracranial pressure

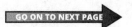

13. A patient is being treated for osteoarthritis. Which of the following signs and symptoms would the nurse most likely anticipate observing in this patient? Select all that apply.

   ❑ **(1)** Pain that gets better after rest and worsens after exercise

   ❑ **(2)** Pain that gets worse in cold temperature and changes in humidity

   ❑ **(3)** Swollen, hot joints with pain on movement

   ❑ **(4)** Presence of Heberden's nodes

   ❑ **(5)** Difficulty getting up after sitting for a prolonged time

14. A nurse is caring for a patient who has had a below-the-knee amputation of her right leg. During the immediate postoperative period, what is the most important assessment parameter the nurse should monitor?

   (1) Blood saturation of the stump dressings

   (2) Presence of phantom limb symptoms

   (3) Mobility of the patient from bed to chair

   (4) The psychological impact of the surgery

15. A patient is experiencing an exacerbation of her rheumatoid arthritis (RA). Which finding is characteristic of RA?

   (1) A unilaterally boggy and painful weight-bearing joint

   (2) A decreased serum erythrocyte sedimentation rate (ESR)

   (3) Fatigue and limited joint function

   (4) Heberden's nodes on distal finger joints

16. A nurse is teaching a three-point gait to a patient on crutches. Which of these actions, if taken by the patient, shows understanding and use of a three-point gait?

   (1) The patient alternates the right crutch, then the left foot, then the left crutch, and then the right foot.

   (2) The patient moves the affected leg and crutches at the same time followed by the unaffected leg.

   (3) The patient puts the crutches forward and swings both legs through.

   (4) The patient puts both crutches ahead and then brings both feet to the crutches.

17. A nurse is caring for a client who has a lumbar disc herniation, which normally occurs in the L4-L5 interspace. Which of the following interventions would the nurse expect to put in place? Select all that apply.

   ❑ **(1)** Apply heat to decrease the muscle spasms.

   ❑ **(2)** Apply ice to decrease inflammation and swelling.

   ❑ **(3)** Apply skeletal traction as prescribed.

   ❑ **(4)** Apply pelvic traction as prescribed.

   ❑ **(5)** Begin progressive ambulation as inflammation edema in pain decrease.

18. A nurse is monitoring a patient who has had a cervical discectomy at C-6. Which of these findings would alert the nurse to the development of a serious potential complication?

   (1) Pain at the suture site

   (2) Blood pressure of 140/82

   (3) Temperature of 100.2 degrees Fahrenheit

   (4) Drooling and inability to swallow

19. A nurse is caring for a patient with a spinal cord injury at level C-5. Which of these symptoms, if exhibited by the patient, would be typical of autonomic hyperreflexia?

    (1) Profound hypotension

    (2) Dry nose and mouth

    (3) Severe headache

    (4) Tachycardia

20. A patient who has a spinal cord injury at level C-7 has been diagnosed with Brown-Sequard syndrome. The nurse would expect which of these assessment findings?

    (1) Loss of function on the same side as the lesion, and loss of pain and temperature below the injury level on the opposite side of the lesion

    (2) Loss of pain, temperature, and position sense on both sides below the level of the injury

    (3) Loss of sensation, pain, and motor function on the opposite side of the injury, with the same side of the injury intact

    (4) Seizure with loss of consciousness and increased sweating above the injury level

21. A nurse is caring for a patient who had a complete transection of the spinal cord at the T-5 level. The patient is to receive leg braces for use in physical therapy. When applying and monitoring the leg braces, the nurse must

    (1) Check for pressure points on the extremities.

    (2) Have the patient perform active range of motion before the braces are on.

    (3) Be sure the patient can ambulate without help.

    (4) Massage the legs before the application of the braces.

22. A nurse is caring for a patient who was admitted to the hospital with a spinal cord injury. The patient is stabilized, and steroid therapy is initiated. What is the priority of care the nurse must address next?

    (1) The potential for skin breakdown

    (2) The patient's risk for seizures

    (3) Encouraging active ROM of the lower extremities

    (4) Signs of secondary extending injury

23. A patient has been diagnosed with a complete spinal cord injury at C-4. What is this patient's rehabilitative potential, based on the injury level?

    (1) Ability to transfer self from bed to wheelchair without assistance

    (2) Eventual ambulation with long leg braces

    (3) Ability to drive electric wheelchair with mouth stick and head support

    (4) Adequate sitting balance while self-feeding

24. A nurse is assessing a patient for signs of neurogenic shock following a severe spinal cord injury at T-6. Which of these manifestations should the nurse anticipate seeing in this patient?

    (1) Drop in blood pressure and heart rate

    (2) Flaccid paralysis of skeletal muscles below the level of injury

    (3) Hyperactive bowel sounds

    (4) Urinary urgency and frequency

GO ON TO NEXT PAGE

25. A nurse is conducting an initial assessment for a newly admitted 83-year-old female patient. The nurse documents that the patient demonstrates "significant kyphosis." The nursing student should know that this means that the

(1) Patient demonstrates mild hemiplegia when walking

(2) Patient's spine has slowly collapsed due to microfractures

(3) Patient will need a wheelchair for mobility

(4) Patient will be incontinent of urine

26. A patient has an intracranial pressure (ICP) reading of 22 mm Hg. Which of the following interventions should the nurse provide this patient?

(1) Have the lights on and the TV showing the patient's favorite show.

(2) Give the patient a sedative to promote rest.

(3) Place the head of the bed at 30 degrees and the patient's head in the midline position.

(4) Provide a regular diet to help with healing.

27. A patient is having atonic seizures. The nurse should know that these seizures are identified by

(1) A brief cessation of motor activity with a blank stare and unresponsiveness

(2) Alternating contraction and relaxation of extremity muscles and hyperventilation

(3) Motor activity that spreads sequentially to adjacent parts, finger to arm

(4) A sudden drop attack with an extended loss of consciousness

28. A nurse observes a patient having a grand mal seizure. Which action should the nurse not attempt to do?

(1) Protect the patient from harming herself.

(2) Force an airway open with a bite stick.

(3) Notify a physician for a medication order.

(4) Get help to protect the patient from falling or injuring herself.

29. A nurse observes a patient having a tonic-clonic seizure from the beginning. The patient's arm and leg muscles stiffen and relax alternately for about a minute as the patient begins to hyperventilate. The patient loses consciousness and then arouses and opens his eyes. Two minutes later he falls asleep. Which of the following statements should the nurse document about this seizure?

(1) The patient had contracting and relaxing of the arm and leg muscles.

(2) The seizure lasted two minutes.

(3) The patient opened his eyes and then fell asleep immediately.

(4) The patient lost consciousness during the seizure, which lasted for five minutes.

30. A nurse is planning to conduct a mental status exam on a patient. What is the best way to assess the state of consciousness during this assessment?

(1) Conduct a depression inventory to check for mood problems.

(2) Assess the patient's long-term memory functioning by asking for details about the patient's childhood.

(3) Observe the patient's manner of dress, posture, motor activity, and general grooming.

(4) Ask the patient to state name, current location, and the last three presidents.

31. A nurse is caring for a patient with a head injury who is being monitored for potential increasing intracranial pressure (ICP) due to a head injury. The patient's readings are temperature 101.4 degrees Fahrenheit, blood pressure 130/80, pulse 80, respirations 18, ICP 15 mm Hg. Which of these readings requires the nurse's immediate intervention?

    (1) Temperature

    (2) Pulse

    (3) Blood pressure

    (4) Intracranial pressure

32. A patient who has had a cerebrovascular accident (CVA) is being assessed for her ability to undertake her first oral feeding. Which action is most important for the nurse to take first before the patient attempts to eat?

    (1) Provide mouth care before the meal.

    (2) Teach the patient to feed herself.

    (3) Place the food on the unaffected side of the mouth.

    (4) Stroke the back of the tongue with a tongue blade.

33. A patient is scheduled to receive an electroencephalogram (EEG). For which of the following conditions would the nurse expect to see an order for an EEG? Select all that apply.

    ❑ (1) Head injury

    ❑ (2) Sleep disorder

    ❑ (3) Myocardial infarction

    ❑ (4) Seizures

    ❑ (5) Deep vein thrombosis

34. A nurse is caring for a patient who has a diagnosis of bacterial meningitis. The nurse's priority of care is to

    (1) Monitor intake and output every four hours

    (2) Apply a vest restraint to prevent falling out of bed

    (3) Institute seizure precautions

    (4) Observe for leaking cerebrospinal fluid

35. Which of the following goals would be achieved by performing a craniotomy on a client with Reye's syndrome?

    (1) Decrease carbon dioxide levels

    (2) Determine the extent of brain injury

    (3) Reduce pressure from an edematous brain

    (4) Allow continuous monitoring of intracranial pressure (ICP)

36. Which of the following patients is least likely to have skin breakdown?

    (1) A patient who can't move and is confined to bed

    (2) An incontinent patient

    (3) A patient with chronic nutritional deficiencies

    (4) A patient with decreased mental status

37. The nurse is preparing to give cyclobenzaprine to a client. The nurse knows that which of the following is true about the administration of cyclobenzaprine?

    (1) Cyclobenzaprine can be given with MAOIs or monoamine oxidase inhibitors.

    (2) Cyclobenzaprine has a cholinergic effect.

    (3) Cyclobenzaprine is an antigout medication.

    (4) Cyclobenzaprine is used only for short-term therapy.

38. A patient is receiving methylprednisolone to treat a spinal cord injury at L-1. What action should the nurse anticipate to monitor one of the adverse side effects of this medication?

    (1) Monitor level of consciousness every hour.

    (2) Conduct a 24-hour creatinine clearance.

    (3) Take a blood glucose reading every four hours.

    (4) Check skin turgor every two hours.

GO ON TO NEXT PAGE ➤

39. Mannitol has been ordered to help reduce a patient's intracranial pressure. The nurse would anticipate that a therapeutic response to the medication would be

    (1) An increase in the patient's urinary output

    (2) An increase in the patient's diastolic blood pressure

    (3) Lessening of the patient's nausea

    (4) Patient's report of reduced muscular pain

40. Sodium polystyrene sulfonate is ordered for immediate administration to a 65-year-old patient with renal disease. The nurse should anticipate which of these therapeutic responses to this medication?

    (1) Reduction in blood serum ammonia

    (2) Elevation of red blood cell count

    (3) Reduction in blood serum potassium

    (4) Elevation in arterial blood pH

41. A patient who has glaucoma of the left eye is receiving carbachol eyedrops. The nurse should explain to the patient that the purpose of this medication is to

    (1) Facilitate the outflow of aqueous humor

    (2) Dilate the pupil of the eye

    (3) Increase lens accommodation

    (4) Anesthetize the eye muscles

42. A nurse is teaching a group of older adults about open-angle glaucoma. Which of these statements, if made by the nurse, describes this type of glaucoma?

    (1) "Your affected eye will be red and constantly tearing."

    (2) "You will have a sudden onset of eye pain."

    (3) "Straight lines will appear wavy to you."

    (4) "There are very few early symptoms."

43. A nurse has an order to give eyedrops. Which of the following would the nurse do first in giving the eyedrops?

    (1) Pulling down on the cheek to expose the lower conjunctival sac

    (2) Giving the client a tissue so she can wipe away excess medication

    (3) Holding the dropper above the eyeball

    (4) Tilting the head back slightly and asking the client to look up

44. A nursing student is teaching a patient newly diagnosed with macular degeneration about the disease. Which of the following statements, if made by the student, would be correct?

    (1) "It occurs when the layers of the retina separate because of accumulation of fluid between them."

    (2) "It occurs when the lens gets thick and loses its clarity."

    (3) "It's an eye disease that results in increased ocular pressure."

    (4) "It occurs when the macula deteriorates, which leads to central vision loss."

45. A 40-year-old female patient who has just been diagnosed with Ménière's disease asks the nurse how to manage the symptomatic episodes. Which of the following interventions would the nurse expect to use with this patient? Select all that apply.

    ❏ (1) Have her try to overcome the symptoms by following her normal routine

    ❏ (2) Instruct her to stop smoking

    ❏ (3) Have her initiate weight-bearing exercise for at least one hour daily

    ❏ (4) Instruct her to lie down in a quiet, dark room during the peak exacerbation

    ❏ (5) Give her a prescription for nicotinic acid for its vasodilatory effect

46. A 60-year-old patient has been diagnosed with presbyopia. This means that due to the loss of lens elasticity, the patient is

    (1) Unable to see objects at a distance
    (2) Seeing double objects
    (3) Having difficulty reading
    (4) Seeing wavy lines instead of straight ones

47. Which of the following test(s) would be used for glaucoma? Select all that apply.

    ❑ (1) Tonometry
    ❑ (2) CT scan
    ❑ (3) Peripheral vision test
    ❑ (4) A complete eye exam
    ❑ (5) Corneal staining

48. A patient has been diagnosed with macular degeneration (dry type). Which of these techniques would be used to identify extending areas of visual distortion?

    (1) Laser photocoagulation
    (2) Magnifying glass
    (3) Amsler grid
    (4) Tonometry

49. Following a cerebral vascular accident, a patient tells the nurse that he is lacking the right half of his visual field in both his right and left eyes. The nurse informs the health-care team that the patient is complaining of

    (1) Akinesthesia
    (2) Homonymous hemianopia
    (3) Apraxia
    (4) Presbyopia

50. A patient asks the nurse whether his medications could cause damage to his hearing. Which of this patient's medications are potentially ototoxic and should be discussed with him? Select all that apply.

    ❑ (1) Furosemide
    ❑ (2) Aspirin
    ❑ (3) Nitroglycerine
    ❑ (4) Pilocarpine
    ❑ (5) Amikacin

51. A patient states to the nurse that life is useless and she wants to "put an end to her misery." What is the nurse's first priority in response to this statement?

    (1) Determining the patient's suicide potential
    (2) Checking the patient regularly during the night
    (3) Placing the patient in a room near the nurse's station
    (4) Observing the patient for sudden changes in affect

52. A nurse is working with a couple who have sought treatment related to the woman's excessive alcohol consumption and episodes of intoxication. In assessing the role of alcohol in this relationship and the dynamics between the couple, what interaction would indicate codependence?

    (1) The woman openly discusses her inability to meet her husband's needs.
    (2) The man focuses on his wife's needs and does not discuss his own needs.
    (3) The couple discusses how they are able to meet each other's needs.
    (4) The man openly discusses his inability to meet his wife's needs.

GO ON TO NEXT PAGE ▶

53. A nurse is planning care for a patient who is in the acute stage of a manic episode. Which of these approaches would be most therapeutic for the patient?

(1) Expend the patient's excessive energies in competitive group activities.

(2) Put the patient in charge of a discussion group so she can express her feelings.

(3) Shadow the patient and remind her to control her hyperactive behavior.

(4) Interact with the patient one-on-one until she can control environmental input.

54. A nurse is planning care for a patient who has a diagnosis of depression. The nurse should recognize that the patient is at risk for suicide if he

(1) Is not permitted to engage in his compulsive rituals

(2) Has a number of recurring somatic complaints

(3) Gives other patients gifts of his personal possessions

(4) Tells the staff he is very angry about new day room restrictions

55. A patient who was admitted to a psychiatric unit with a diagnosis of schizophrenia tells the nurse, "I'm getting transmissions from my teeth that a plane will drop a bomb on us very soon." Which of these responses is the most therapeutic for the nurse to make?

(1) "When was the last time you saw your dentist?"

(2) "Nothing will happen to you here because the roof is very strong."

(3) "It sounds as if you are feeling afraid today."

(4) "Where is the plane coming from, and who is dropping the bomb?"

56. A patient on a psychiatric unit who has a diagnosis of borderline personality disorder compliments staff members and then requests special favors. What is the most important measure the nurse should take when managing this patient?

(1) Offer the patient a variety of recreational activities.

(2) Give the patient leadership responsibilities on the unit.

(3) Place the patient in a quiet room and limit visitors.

(4) Provide the patient with consistent boundaries.

57. A nurse is taking a health history from a patient in a psychiatric unit. During the interview, the patient asks the nurse whether she has any children. What is the nurse's best reply?

(1) "Why do you want to know that information?"

(2) "You are trying to avoid my questions by asking me questions."

(3) "We need to get to know more about you and what brought you here."

(4) "I'm the nurse; I get to ask the questions, and you will answer them."

58. A nurse is evaluating the affect of a patient who has been admitted to the psychiatry unit. Which of these questions should the nurse ask the patient?

(1) "Are your medications working yet?"

(2) "How do you feel today?"

(3) "What did you eat for breakfast today?"

(4) "Would you repeat a sequence of numbers?"

59. A nurse is planning care for a depressed patient who is withdrawing from most social contacts on the psychiatric unit. Which intervention is the most appropriate for this patient?

(1) Establishing a schedule of daily activities for the patient

(2) Allowing the patient to stay in her room until she feels better

(3) Encouraging the patient to make her own activity decisions

(4) Requiring the patient to sit in the day room for social stimulation

60. A nurse is caring for a patient on the psychiatric unit who has been diagnosed with an antisocial personality disorder. Which behaviors would the nurse expect the patient to exhibit?

(1) Isolation from most social interactions on the unit

(2) Colorful descriptions of his auditory hallucinations

(3) Disorganized conversation with loose associations

(4) Charming manipulation of staff to foster alliances

61. A patient who admits to drinking a gallon of beer per day for several years has been admitted to the hospital for treatment of esophageal varices. The nurse should be alert to which of the following early signs of alcohol withdrawal (3 to 36 hours post last drink)?

(1) Anxiety, tremors, and tachycardia

(2) Depression, fever, and vomiting

(3) Delusions, bradycardia, and dyspnea

(4) Flat affect, drowsiness, and coma

62. A nurse is explaining the addictive qualities of narcotics to a group of high school students as part of an anti-drug project. Which explanation accurately describes the effect narcotics have on the brain?

(1) The brain's pain threshold is decreased.

(2) Bodily functions become accelerated.

(3) Dependence is gradual and mild.

(4) Endorphin receptors are stimulated.

63. A nurse is teaching a women's group about violence in the family. Which of these statements, if made by one of the women, would indicate to the nurse that she needs further instruction?

(1) "Spouses who abuse have low self-esteem."

(2) "Abusive behavior typically follows a cyclical pattern."

(3) "Violence occurs primarily in low-income families."

(4) "Abused spouses suffer from guilt and helplessness."

64. A patient has been admitted to the psychiatric unit with the paranoid delusion that people are trying to poison her. The patient states, "I'm not going to eat this hospital food — do you think I want to die?" What should the nurse say to this patient?

(1) "No one is poisoning your food; it's important to eat."

(2) "Perhaps you don't like the way the food is prepared."

(3) "I used to think that way sometimes."

(4) "You sound very worried."

GO ON TO NEXT PAGE

65. A home health nurse is caring for an 80-year-old woman who is taking several medications for a variety of disorders. During this visit, the patient's behavior is markedly different. The nurse notes that the patient seems agitated at first, then sleepy. The patient can't remember what day it is or her address, and she seems uncooperative in following the nurse's instructions. What action is most important for the nurse to take?

   (1) Investigate the home for bottles of alcohol.

   (2) Do a 24-hour recall of the patient's diet.

   (3) Ask the patient to cough and deep breathe.

   (4) Call the patient's physician and report her condition.

66. A patient on the psychiatric unit who has recently had an increase in his prescribed haloperidol dose tells the nurse that he is having chills and feeling "stiff." The nurse should immediately assess the patient for which complication of drug therapy?

   (1) Dystonia

   (2) Aphasia

   (3) Neuroleptic malignant syndrome

   (4) Tardive dyskinesia

67. A nurse is administering haloperidol to a patient who has been admitted to the psychiatric unit. The nurse should watch for which of the following side effects of this medication? Select all that apply.

   ❑ (1) Rigidity

   ❑ (2) Drooling

   ❑ (3) Hypotension

   ❑ (4) Dysphagia

   ❑ (5) Parkinsonism

68. A nurse is teaching a patient who has bipolar disorder about toxic side effects of lithium carbonate, which she will be taking to stabilize her mood. The nurse should tell the patient that she may experience which of these signs/symptoms/labs of moderate toxicity?

   (1) Serum lithium level of 1.5

   (2) Mild to moderate ataxia and incoordination

   (3) Nystagmus

   (4) Tonic-clonic seizures or coma

69. A patient who is taking chlorpromazine reports to the nurse that he is having difficulty with his neck muscles after arising in the morning. What action should the nurse take next?

   (1) Prepare a warm compress for the patient's neck.

   (2) Instruct the patient to do range of motion movements for the neck.

   (3) Ask the patient to show and describe the neck and head problems.

   (4) Check the patient's room for cold air conditioning drafts.

70. A nurse instructs a patient who has just been prescribed phenelzine for depression about how to manage the medication. Which of these statements is most important for the nurse to emphasize to the patient?

   (1) "Avoid foods such as bananas, eggplant, papaya, and sauerkraut."

   (2) "Drink eight glasses of fluid each day, and eat green vegetables."

   (3) "Limit your intake of citrus and berry fruits."

   (4) "Anticipate that you may have episodes of diarrhea."

71. A patient who has chronic liver failure and increasing ascites is now dyspneic. The nurse has been asked to prepare the patient for a procedure that will temporarily relieve the patient's respiratory symptoms. For which procedure should the nurse prepare the patient?

(1) Thoracentesis

(2) Kayexalate enema

(3) Sengstaken–Blakemore tube placement

(4) Paracentesis

72. A patient whose liver is failing has developed spider angiomas and platelet abnormalities. What assessment parameter is most important for the nurse to monitor to check for impending hepatic coma?

(1) Mental status

(2) Abdominal girth

(3) Urine specific gravity

(4) Hemoglobin and hematocrit

73. A patient who has cirrhosis and is having an episode of bleeding esophageal varices would have which of the following tubes placed to treat the episode?

(1) Sengstaken–Blakemore tube

(2) Salem Sump/double lumen tube

(3) Miller–Abbott tube

(4) Cantor tube

74. A nurse is teaching a patient with esophageal varices about how to avoid rupture of the varices after discharge to home. Which of these measures is correct?

(1) "Observe your neck and shoulders for swelling."

(2) "Do coughing and deep breathing several times a day."

(3) "Do not lift heavy objects or strain at stool."

(4) "Take an aspirin every day."

75. The nurse is preparing to give a patient an enteric tube. The tube has a weight at the end to assist in placement in the small intestine. In which position should the nurse place the patient after tube insertion?

(1) Supine

(2) Head of the bed elevated 30 degrees

(3) On the right side

(4) On the left side

76. A nurse is caring for a patient who has been diagnosed with hepatitis C. Which of these measures should the nurse institute for this patient?

(1) Instruct the patient to use disposable dinnerware for meals.

(2) Advise the patient to limit fluid intake.

(3) Assist the patient in developing a nutritional plan.

(4) Immunize with the HAV vaccine.

77. A patient who has a hepatitis B infection is progressing from the preicteric to the icteric phase. What manifestation is a cardinal sign of entering this phase?

(1) Weight loss

(2) Dark urine

(3) Decreased sense of smell and taste

(4) Anorexia

78. A nurse is caring for a patient with cirrhosis of the liver who requires a diuretic to reduce fluid retention. The patient is receiving spironolactone 50 mg PO (by mouth) once a day. Which of these responses would the nurse recognize as a side effect of this medication?

(1) Hypertension

(2) Depression

(3) Constipation

(4) Tachycardia

GO ON TO NEXT PAGE

79. Lactulose is ordered for a patient who has a diagnosis of cirrhosis of the liver. Which of these expected outcomes should the nurse expect to see?

    (1) Relief from diarrhea

    (2) Decrease in the ammonia level

    (3) Relief of epigastric pain in the right upper quadrant

    (4) Relief of vomiting

80. A patient who is having an esophageal bleed from ruptured varices is prescribed medication to control the bleeding episodes. What medication should the nurse prepare for this patient?

    (1) Cyclosporine

    (2) Omeprazole

    (3) Pancreatin

    (4) Vasopressin

81. A nurse is caring for a patient who is at high risk for developing sepsis following major burns to his trunk and legs. Which of these signs would alert the nurse to the development of sepsis?

    (1) Pulse rate of 108

    (2) WBC count of 9,000/µl

    (3) Urine output of 50 ml/hour

    (4) Blood pressure of 116/64

82. A patient has sustained a major electrical burn following an injury while working on a telephone pole. What would be the nurse's immediate concern on the patient's arrival to the emergency department?

    (1) The patient's pain level

    (2) The entry and exit wounds on the patient's body

    (3) Preventing the patient from moving his extremities

    (4) Establishing the patient's respiratory status

83. During a fire, a family was exposed to excessive levels of carbon monoxide. The nurse should know the signs of moderate carbon monoxide poisoning. Which of these indicates moderate CO poisoning?

    (1) Fruity breath odor

    (2) Hallucinations

    (3) Confusion

    (4) High anxiety level

84. While assessing a 300-pound patient who has full-thickness burns to his right leg, a nurse notes that the pedal pulse cannot now be palpated or located by Doppler. What determination should the nurse make about this finding?

    (1) The patient has a preexisting peripheral vascular disease.

    (2) Obesity is preventing the nurse from palpating the pulse.

    (3) Eschar is creating a compartment syndrome in the leg.

    (4) Pulses are never palpable after a severe burn to an extremity.

85. A nurse is caring for a severely burned patient who is 12 hours post-injury and now has fluid and electrolyte imbalance. What would the nurse most likely encounter in this patient?

    (1) Decreased hematocrit

    (2) Increased renal blood flow

    (3) Hypertension

    (4) Low serum protein

86. A nurse is teaching a patient who has hypo-thyroidism about her newly prescribed medication, levothyroxine sodium, to treat the disorder. Which of these statements, if made by the patient, would indicate that the patient's knowledge of the instructions is correct?

    (1) "I will probably gain weight while I take this medication."

    (2) "I will take this medication until my condition improves."

    (3) "I should stop the medication if my appetite decreases."

    (4) "I may not see the overall improvement for several weeks."

87. A nurse is conducting an assessment of a patient with an unconfirmed diagnosis of hyperthyroidism. Which of these manifesta-tions would support this diagnosis?

    (1) Bradycardia

    (2) Cool, dry skin

    (3) Weight gain

    (4) Insomnia

88. A patient asks the nurse how she acquired Graves' disease. The nurse should explain to the patient that the disease

    (1) Is a result of a bacterial infection that is treated with antibiotics

    (2) May be caused by genetic, stress, dietary, and infective factors

    (3) Occurs as a result of exposure to heavy metals

    (4) Results from a history of diabetes mellitus

89. A nurse is teaching a patient who has hypo-parathyroidism about maintenance therapy for this disorder. What should the nurse advise the patient to do?

    (1) Take calcium supplements.

    (2) Consume a diet high in oxalic acid.

    (3) Drink large quantities of water.

    (4) Add extra phosphorus to her diet.

90. A patient with Cushing syndrome is recovering following adrenalectomy. During the immedi-ate postoperative period, the nurse's priority of care would be to

    (1) Frequently assess the patient for signs of infection

    (2) Take additional measures to protect the patient from skin breakdown

    (3) Monitor the patient's fluid and electro-lyte balance

    (4) Prevent disruptive emotional responses

91. A nurse checks the patient's cardiac monitor when it alarms and finds that the patient has developed ventricular fibrillation. What is the nurse's next action after bringing the defibril-lator to the bedside?

    (1) Shave the patient's chest where the paddles will be placed.

    (2) Place the gel or defibrillator pads on the patient's chest.

    (3) Turn on the defibrillator synchronizer switch.

    (4) Tell the staff, "All clear."

92. A patient who is in cardiogenic shock has developed pulmonary edema. The nurse should anticipate which of these findings typical of pulmonary edema?

    (1) Knife-like chest pain

    (2) Hyperthermia

    (3) Sleepiness

    (4) Pink, frothy sputum

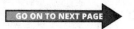

GO ON TO NEXT PAGE

93. A patient has been admitted to the unit with the diagnosis of right-sided heart failure. The nurse knows the client should be experiencing which signs and symptoms? Select all that apply.

    ❑ (1) Dependent edema

    ❑ (2) Abdominal distention

    ❑ (3) Jugular vein distention

    ❑ (4) Dry hacky cough

    ❑ (5) Weight gain

94. A nurse is caring for a patient with acute pericarditis. What sign would alert the nurse to the development of cardiac tamponade in this patient?

    (1) Jugular vein distention

    (2) Widening pulse pressure

    (3) Bradycardia

    (4) Respiratory rate less than 12 breaths/minute

95. A nurse walks into a patient's room and sees the patient sitting upright in his chair. When he does not respond to the nurse's question, the nurse shakes his shoulder and asks, "Are you okay?" When the patient does not respond to a repeated attempt to arouse him, the nurse's next action should be to

    (1) Administer four sharp, upward abdominal thrusts to the patient

    (2) Pull back the patient's head, open his mouth, and do a finger sweep

    (3) Lower the patient to the floor while calling out for help

    (4) Run down the hall and look for help to lift the patient to the bed

96. Following a percutaneous transluminal coronary angioplasty (PTCA), with femoral access, the nurse should notify the doctor of which of the following complaints?

    (1) Warm feeling of the leg

    (2) Numbness and tingling in the leg

    (3) Peripheral pulses

    (4) Diarrhea

97. A nurse is caring for a patient in cardiogenic shock. The physician adds nitroglycerine to augment the dopamine drip the patient is receiving. The nurse knows that the purpose of this action is to

    (1) Dilate coronary arteries

    (2) Restore electrolyte imbalance

    (3) Reduce peripheral edema

    (4) Prevent dysrhythmias

98. A patient has sustained an anterior wall myocardial infarction, and an intraaortic balloon pump has been inserted to support heart function. Nursing care of this patient would include

    (1) Elevating the head of the bed to 60 degrees

    (2) Providing an equal balance of activity and rest

    (3) Frequently checking the warmth and color of extremities

    (4) Administering antihypertensives

99. A nurse is admitting a patient who has a diagnosis of acute myocardial infarction. How should the nurse initially position the patient in bed?

    (1) Flat in bed with legs elevated

    (2) On back with the head elevated 30 degrees and legs elevated

    (3) On back with the head of the bed at 60 degrees

    (4) Completely flat with no head or leg elevation

100. A nurse is caring for a patient who is experiencing cardiogenic shock. The cardiac monitor shows ventricular fibrillation that has not responded to one attempt at defibrillation. The nurse should know that which of these drugs will make the heart muscle more responsive to defibrillation?

(1) Atropine

(2) Epinephrine

(3) Dopamine

(4) Nitroglycerine

101. A patient has been placed on warfarin sodium following a postsurgical pulmonary embolus. Which food would interact with the warfarin sodium by reducing its effect?

(1) Chocolate cake

(2) Sweet potato

(3) Brussels sprouts

(4) Scrambled eggs

102. A nurse is making a health assessment visit and observes a group of 2-year-old children playing in a day-care center. The nurse should know that, developmentally, it would be typical of toddler play patterns to see

(1) Five children playing a softball game

(2) Three children playing an interactive board game

(3) Two children making towers in the sandbox side-by-side

(4) One child watching a videotape and another child sleeping

103. A nurse is caring for a 10-year-old who has rheumatic heart disease. The nurse would expect the boy to make which of these statements?

(1) "I don't know where I belong in this world."

(2) "I live for my girlfriend."

(3) "My friends and my mom are most important to me."

(4) "I come first, and I let everyone know that."

104. A nurse is evaluating an 8-month-old infant during a routine pediatric clinic visit. Which of these findings would be developmentally normal at this infant's age?

(1) The infant cries when the nurse tries to pick him up.

(2) The infant has gained 6 pounds since birth.

(3) The infant abducts his extremities and fans his fingers when startled.

(4) The infant stands without support.

105. A 10-year-old child is prescribed Amoxicillin in the hospital. The child has refused the last dose, which the mother tried to help administer. What comment would be the best approach for the nurse to take?

(1) "This medicine tastes just like candy."

(2) "If you take this medicine, I will let you go to the gift shop."

(3) "This medicine will help you get well so that you can go home."

(4) "If you don't take this medicine, you'll get much sicker."

106. A nurse is counseling the parents of a 2-month-old infant who is being assessed for pyloric stenosis. Which of these instructions should the nurse give the parents?

(1) "Offer the infant thickened rice cereal mixed with formula each morning."

(2) "Document and report any episodes of forceful vomiting."

(3) "Place the infant in a lying position during feedings."

(4) "Cut back on the number of feedings until a diagnosis is determined."

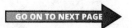
GO ON TO NEXT PAGE

107. A nurse is planning care for a 7-year-old child who has sickle cell anemia. The child is complaining of pain at the joint sites. Which of these measures should the nurse take for this client?

   (1) Start a continuous schedule of pain medications for pain prevention when a crisis begins.

   (2) Reduce daily fluid intake to half the usual amount.

   (3) Reduce physical activity during the crisis phase and place extremities in a dependent position.

   (4) Maintain the child on daily oxygen therapy as a preventive measure.

108. A 2-year-old child is in the emergency department for a crush injury of her right leg. Laboratory studies indicate that her potassium level is 6.2 mEq/L. What clinical manifestation should the nurse be especially alert to in this child?

   (1) Laryngospasm

   (2) Tetany

   (3) Ventricular fibrillation

   (4) Hyperthermia

109. The nurse is assessing a 10-month-old infant who has a suspected diagnosis of acute epiglottitis. Which of the following findings would need immediate intervention?

   (1) Inspiratory crackles over both lung fields

   (2) Purulent nasal secretions

   (3) Excessive oral drooling

   (4) A barking cough

110. A nurse is reviewing signs and symptoms of hypoglycemia with a 12-year-old boy who recently has been diagnosed with diabetes mellitus. Which of these signs and symptoms, if stated by the boy, would the nurse have to correct?

   (1) Shaky feeling

   (2) Fruity breath

   (3) Headache

   (4) Irritability

111. A 19-year-old young man who has a previous diagnosis of glomerulonephritis is having a renal workup for suspected chronic renal failure. Which of these signs would support a diagnosis of chronic renal failure?

   (1) Reddish-brown urine

   (2) Yellowish cast to palate and conjunctiva

   (3) Trouble initiating a urine stream

   (4) Weight loss of seven pounds

112. The nurse is caring for a 5-year-old who has a fractured right tibia. The temporary application of Buck's traction is ordered. Which of the following is a priority of the nurse caring for a child in Buck's traction?

   (1) Site and pin care

   (2) Assessment of the skin for pressure

   (3) Prevention of infection

   (4) Preventing contractures

113. A 17-year-old patient has been diagnosed with Guillain-Barré syndrome. The nurse's most immediate concern would be to

   (1) Check for distal muscular paresthesias

   (2) Watch for facial weakness and ataxia

   (3) Provide pain relief for trigeminal neuralgia

   (4) Monitor respiratory rate, depth, and vital capacity

114. A 3-year-old child who was adopted from another country is admitted to the hospital for heart surgery to repair an untreated tetralogy of Fallot. The nurse observes that the child has clubbed fingers and should know that this clubbing is due to

(1) Delayed physical growth

(2) Iron-deficiency anemiah

(3) Peripheral hypoxia

(4) Altered immune response

115. An 18-month-old child has been diagnosed with intussusception. Which of these findings would alert the nurse that the condition may have resolved?

(1) The child has had 24 hours without colicky abdominal pain.

(2) The child has passed several raisin-sized, jelly-like stools.

(3) The child has expelled long, ribbon-like brown stools.

(4) The child has passed a typical brown stool.

116. A 4-year-old child has been admitted to the pediatric unit with a diagnosis of hepatitis A. In order to prevent the spread of this disease, the nurse should

(1) Have visitors wear masks, gowns, and gloves when visiting this child

(2) Be certain that staff thoroughly wash their hands when working with this child

(3) Test all children on the unit for hepatitis A within 48 hours

(4) Obtain permission to immunize all children on the unit with HAV

117. An 18-year-old young man has been placed in balanced suspension traction with a Thomas splint and Pearson attachment for a fractured left leg following a motor vehicle accident. Within the first 24 hours, the nurse should carefully observe the patient for which of these complications?

(1) Avascular necrosis

(2) Fat embolism

(3) Malunion of bone

(4) Osteomyelitis

118. An 8-year-old child has been diagnosed with a cerebellar brain tumor. Which sign would the nurse anticipate seeing in this child?

(1) Periorbital edema

(2) Homonymous hemianopia

(3) Ataxia

(4) High-pitched cry

119. A 12-year-old child who has a head injury is being observed for signs of increasing intracranial pressure. Which of these situations involving the child needs the nurse's immediate intervention?

(1) Glasgow coma scale is assessed at 13 for 8 hours.

(2) Head of the child's bed is placed at 30 degrees.

(3) Vest restraints are placed on the child when he becomes restless.

(4) Intracranial pressure is at 12 mm Hg for 12 hours.

120. A 10-year-old child is in acute respiratory failure. His arterial blood gases are pH 7.20, pCO_2 60, PO_2 45, HCO_3 25, and O_2 saturation of 87%. The nurse should know that this arterial blood gas indicates

(1) Metabolic acidosis

(2) Respiratory acidosis

(3) Metabolic alkalosis

(4) Respiratory alkalosis

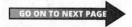

121. A nurse is preparing a 7-year-old child for an electroencephalogram (EEG). The nurse knows that an EEG is conducted to determine brain death and to diagnose

   (1) Myasthenia gravis disease

   (2) Pituitary tumors

   (3) Meningitis

   (4) Seizure disorders

122. A 13-year-old child is on a ventilator due to complications related to septic shock. When the high pressure alarm sounds, the nurse's first action would be to

   (1) Reset the ventilator alarm

   (2) Suction the endotracheal tube

   (3) Look for loose connections in the tubing

   (4) Draw arterial blood gases

123. Which of these signs should a nurse identify as early dehydration in an infant who has had diarrhea for 48 hours?

   (1) Increased blood pressure

   (2) Bradycardia

   (3) Bulging anterior fontanel

   (4) Decreased urination

124. A 2-year-old child has arrived in the emergency department after being removed from her burning apartment. Her face is smoke-tinged, and her hair is singed. Which of these measures would be the nurse's first priority?

   (1) Start an intravenous line and replace fluids.

   (2) Establish and maintain an airway.

   (3) Administer tetanus prophylaxis.

   (4) Obtain baseline laboratory studies.

125. A 12-year-old boy is undergoing diagnostic studies to determine a diagnosis of acute poststreptococcal glomerulonephritis (APSGN). Which of these tests would help confirm a diagnosis of APSGN?

   (1) Blood urea nitrogen (BUN)

   (2) Anti-streptolysin O titer

   (3) Complete blood count (CBC)

   (4) Intravenous pyelogram (IVP)

126. A school nurse is conducting a class on disease prevention to a group of seventh grade students. The nurse should know that the students require additional teaching if the students tell the nurse that Lyme disease is

   (1) Preventable by avoiding wooded areas and using insect repellents

   (2) A disease that can become chronic and cause heart and joint problems

   (3) Characterized by a fine, raised rash over the palms, soles, and extremities

   (4) Caused by the bite of a tick that lives on deer and mice

127. A nurse is preparing a patient for endotracheal extubation. Using numbers 1 through 5, indicate the order in which the nurse should implement the extubation.

   _____ Deflate the endotracheal tube cuff.

   _____ Ask the patient to deep inhale then extubate during exhale

   _____ Suction the tracheobronchial tree and oropharynx.

   _____ Explain the procedure to the patient.

   _____ Administer oxygen to the patient by a mask.

128. A nurse is caring for a patient who has the following arterial blood gas values: pH 7.28, $PaCO_2$ 56, PaO_2 60, HCO_3 22, O_2 Sat. 88%. The nurse should know that these findings are related to

   (1) Hyperventilation
   (2) COPD
   (3) Diabetic acidosis
   (4) Excessive ingestion of antacids

129. A patient on a ventilator is on SIMV. When the high pressure alarm sounds, the nurse's next action should be to

   (1) Turn the alarms off and give a manual sigh
   (2) Review the chart for the last arterial blood gas values
   (3) Oxygenate the patient and prepare to suction
   (4) Ask the respiratory therapist to see the patient

130. A nurse is caring for an intubated patient who is in acute respiratory failure and maintained on a ventilator. Of these nursing measures, which one is most important when managing a patient on a ventilator?

   (1) Drain condensed moisture in the ventilator tubing toward the patient.
   (2) Increase IV fluids to prevent orthostatic hypotension.
   (3) Administer morphine when transitioning from CMV to SIMV mode.
   (4) Establish a communication system with the patient.

131. A patient has been intubated and placed on ventilatory support. Which complication should the nurse anticipate for this patient?

   (1) Rising levels of BUN and creatinine
   (2) Gastrointestinal ulcers
   (3) Premature ventricular contractions (PVCs)
   (4) Focal seizures

132. A patient who has a chronic obstructive pulmonary disease and who was admitted to the hospital for treatment of respiratory failure tells the nurse that he doesn't "feel well." His vital signs are BP 90/50, heart rate 140 beats/minute, respiratory rate 36/minute. The nurse's next action should be to

   (1) Increase the patient's IV rate from 60 gtts/minute to 200 gtts/minute
   (2) Increase the patient's oxygen level from 2 L/minute to 10 L/minute
   (3) Obtain an immediate pulse oximetry reading
   (4) Check the patient's peripheral pulses and capillary refill

133. A nurse is caring for an intubated patient who is in acute respiratory failure and is on a ventilator. If the low pressure alarm sounds, what should the nurse check first?

   (1) The patient's blood pressure
   (2) Whether the patient needs to be suctioned
   (3) The endotracheal cuff pressure and tubing connections
   (4) Whether there is ample humidification in the system

134. A nurse is teaching a patient how to use the prescribed metered-dose albuterol inhaler. Which of these instructions, if taught by the nurse, is correct?

   (1) "Exhale completely before putting the inhaler in your mouth, pressing the cartridge, and then inhaling."
   (2) "Cough and blow your nose immediately after inhaling the medication."
   (3) "Inhale a little just before putting the inhaler in your mouth and pressing the cartridge; then exhale immediately."
   (4) "Breathe deeply and exhale five times before inhaling the medication."

GO ON TO NEXT PAGE ▶

135. A patient who has just had surgery under general anesthesia arrives in the postsurgical unit with an oral airway in place. The oral airway is removed. What would indicate to the nurse that the patient is not tolerating having the airway removed?

   (1) The patient has a respiratory rate of 20.
   (2) Crackles heard bilaterally turn alarms.
   (3) The nurse hears the sound of stridor.
   (4) The patient's blood pressure is 130/88.

136. A nurse is caring for a patient who was admitted to the hospital for observation following a severe asthmatic episode. The patient tells the nurse that he feels that he is again becoming "unable to catch his breath." Of these assessment parameters, which one is most important for the nurse to perform immediately?

   (1) Check the patient's chest for signs of retraction with each breath.
   (2) Observe the patient's mucous membranes and palate.
   (3) Take the patient's blood pressure.
   (4) Listen to the patient's breath sounds.

137. A patient who has acquired immune deficiency syndrome (AIDS) has been admitted to the hospital with a preliminary diagnosis of Kaposi's sarcoma. Which of these tests would best indicate the patient's immune status related to the development of opportunistic infections?

   (1) CD4+ T cell count
   (2) Western blot
   (3) ELISA
   (4) P24 assay

138. A patient is experiencing an exacerbation of her rheumatoid arthritis (RA). Which finding is characteristic of RA?

   (1) A unilateral swollen weight-bearing joint
   (2) A decreased serum erythrocyte sedimentation rate (ESR)
   (3) Fatigue and limited joint function
   (4) Heberden's nodes on distal finger joints

139. A patient with acquired immune deficiency syndrome (AIDS) has been diagnosed with *Cryptosporidium*. What symptoms would the nurse expect to assess during home visits to the patient?

   (1) Partial blindness
   (2) Mental status changes
   (3) Productive cough
   (4) Diarrhea

140. A nurse is caring for a patient who has been admitted to the unit with an exacerbation of systemic lupus erythematosus (SLE). The nurse should tell the patient that possible triggers for exacerbations of the disease may include

   (1) Surgery to repair a fractured leg
   (2) Fat-soluble vitamins
   (3) High-protein diet
   (4) Mild exercise

141. A patient who has *Mycobacterium avium* complex due to AIDS is having severe symptoms characteristic of wasting syndrome. The nurse should know that this patient likely contracted the illness from organisms in

   (1) Pigeons or other birds
   (2) Food or water in the environment
   (3) Cat litter
   (4) The respiratory tracts of young children

142. A nurse working in an *AIDS out*reach clinic should know that the child least likely to test positive for HIV infection is

   (1) A 4-month-old infant born to a chronic IV drug-using mother
   (2) A 17-year-old adolescent treated for hemophilia for 15 years
   (3) A sexually active 16-year-old female who wants to be a mother
   (4) A 9-year-old boy whose best friend is HIV positive

143. A patient is experiencing an exacerbation of her rheumatoid arthritis (RA). Which finding is characteristic of RA?

(1) Accelerated pedal pulses and normal heart rate

(2) A decreased serum erythrocyte sedimentation rate (ESR)

(3) Fatigue and bilateral swollen joints with pain on movement

(4) Unilateral hip and groin pain that lasts more than two hours

144. A young man is brought to the clinic with a fever of 104 degrees Fahrenheit (40 degrees Celsius). The nurse's first action should be to

(1) Administer an antipyretic as ordered

(2) Expose the patient's skin to the air

(3) Give the patient a bath with iced water

(4) Order a cooling (hypothermia) blanket

145. A nurse is caring for a patient who has been diagnosed with acute lymphocytic leukemia (ALL). Which of these nursing diagnoses would be the nurse's first priority?

(1) Alteration in activity level due to fatigue

(2) Risk for bleeding related to thrombocytopenia

(3) Altered nutrition related to anorexia and stomatitis

(4) Anxiety related to disturbance in body image

146. A patient who has received a kidney transplant is placed on immunosuppressive therapy. Which of these medications will the patient receive for this therapy?

(1) Zidovudine

(2) Ceftriaxone

(3) Hydroxyzine

(4) Cyclosporine

147. Which of these side effects of cancer chemotherapy treatment, if assessed in a 50-year-old patient, should the nurse consider potentially serious and an indication of toxicity?

(1) Anorexia and nausea

(2) White patches in the mouth

(3) Fatigue and malaise

(4) Shortness of breath

148. A nurse has called the doctor and stated the patient has an oncological emergency. Which of the following are manifestations of an oncological emergency? Select all that apply.

❏ (1) Calcium of 12.5

❏ (2) Periorbital edema in the morning

❏ (3) Spinal cord compression

❏ (4) Diabetes insipidus

❏ (5) Syndrome of inappropriate antidiuretic hormone (SIADH)

149. A nurse is teaching a patient who has recently had a mastectomy about tamoxifen. The nurse should emphasize that a potentially dangerous side effect of this drug is

(1) Deep vein thrombosis

(2) Lymphedema

(3) Infection at incision site

(4) Weight loss

GO ON TO NEXT PAGE

150. A patient has been diagnosed with a primary cerebral brain tumor. The nurse would expect to see which of these signs/symptoms? Select all that apply.

❑ **(1)** Aphasia

❑ **(2)** Ataxia

❑ **(3)** Personality changes

❑ **(4)** Blindness

❑ **(5)** Headache

151. A nurse is explaining sentinel node mapping to a woman who is planning to have breast cancer surgery. Which statement reflects correct information that the nurse should include in the explanation?

(1) "This is a hormonal therapy that destroys estrogen receptors in breast tissue."

(2) "High-dose radioactive seeds are placed in the breast to destroy cancer cells."

(3) "Genetic testing checks the potential for breast cancer recurrence."

(4) "This procedure analyzes the presence of cancer by injecting blue dye into the tumor."

152. A man has received a course of chemotherapy with intravenous 5-Fluorouracil (5-FU) for colon cancer. After three months of therapy, the nurse would expect which of the following?

(1) Hematocrit 55%

(2) Agnosia

(3) Hypertension

(4) Platelet count 50,000/mm^3

153. A woman must undergo radiation therapy after a lumpectomy of the left breast. Which of the following statements, if made by the woman, indicates that she understands self-care during the therapy?

(1) "It's best to wear a well-fitting bra that's 100% cotton."

(2) "Cream should be applied to my left chest."

(3) "My left breast area should be exposed to air and sun."

(4) "Cold compresses should be applied to the left chest area."

154. A 63-year-old client returns to the outpatient clinic four days after starting chemotherapy for the treatment of colon cancer. To plan care for this client, the nurse should recognize that an early side effect of chemotherapy is

(1) Weight loss

(2) Skin ulcers

(3) Malnutrition

(4) Mouth ulcerations

155. A young man who has just learned how to do a testicular self-exam asks the nurse how often he should perform the exam. The nurse should respond

(1) "It's most important after you reach age 35."

(2) "You should do the exam every month."

(3) "It is necessary about once a year."

(4) "Only when you feel pain or swelling in the area."

156. A client with lung cancer is taking vincristine and allopurinol. The nurse should explain to the client that allopurinol is used to

(1) Strengthen the action of vincristine

(2) Help destroy rapidly multiplying cells

(3) Prevent uric acid neuropathy

(4) Suppress the bone marrow

157. The nurse evaluates a diabetic patient's compliance with the diabetic diet, insulin, and activity regimens over a two-month period. Which of the following is the best way for the nurse to collect this data?

   (1) Ask the patient to keep a written record of activities at home.

   (2) Obtain a glycosylated hemoglobin level.

   (3) Take a post-prandial blood glucose test.

   (4) Check the patient's shopping receipt to see what's purchased.

158. The nurse is teaching a woman how to perform self-monitoring blood glucose (SMBG) using a blood glucose monitor. Which of the following actions, if performed by the patient, would indicate that the teaching was successful?

   (1) The patient elevates her hand above her heart before the procedure.

   (2) The patient lets a large drop of blood fall to the test strip.

   (3) The patient soaks her fingers in cold water before the procedure.

   (4) The patient sticks the center of the right middle phalanx.

159. A 26-year-old man with type 1 insulin-dependent diabetes mellitus (IDDM) contacts his home-care nurse with complaints of nausea and abdominal pain. The nurse should advise the client to

   (1) Hold his regular dose of insulin

   (2) Check his glucose level frequently

   (3) Eat foods high in simple sugars

   (4) Increase his activity level

160. A 19-year-old man is diagnosed with type 1 insulin-dependent diabetes mellitus (IDDM). The physician orders NPH daily and regular insulin on a sliding scale. The nurse should tell the family members that if the client should suddenly become unconscious, they should

   (1) Inject regular insulin according to the sliding scale

   (2) Give him 8 ounces of orange juice to drink

   (3) Inject glucagon according to the package directions

   (4) Take him to the hospital immediately

161. The husband of a 76-year-old client with type 1 insulin-dependent diabetes mellitus (IDDM) calls the clinic nurse to report that his wife experiences trembling and headaches every afternoon around 4 p.m. Which of the following statements, if made by the husband, should the nurse consider most significant?

   (1) "She awakens at 7 a.m., walks the dog at 8:30 a.m., and naps for half an hour at 1 p.m."

   (2) "I give her the NPH insulin at 8 a.m., she eats lunch at noon, and she eats dinner at 7 p.m."

   (3) "She eats eggs, toast, and coffee for breakfast and a sandwich for lunch."

   (4) "She takes her blood pressure medication at lunchtime."

GO ON TO NEXT PAGE ➤

162. A man with insulin-independent diabetes mellitus (IDDM) comes to the clinic with complaints of pain in his left leg and foot. A diagnosis of peripheral arterial disease (PAD) is made. Which of the following symptoms would the nurse anticipate?

(1) The left lower leg appears flushed and feels warm.

(2) The patient does not feel sharp and dull pressure on his left leg.

(3) The patient obtains pain relief when the legs are elevated.

(4) The patient has moderate swelling distal to the malleolus on his left foot.

163. A woman who has a vascular access device has developed a subclavian vein thrombosis. Which of the following symptoms would the nurse expect to see?

(1) Pale, cold skin around the area

(2) Bounding erratic radial pulse

(3) Hard, cord-like vein at the site

(4) Tingling and numbness in the area

164. A woman is admitted to the hospital for treatment of recurrent deep vein thrombosis (DVT) in her right leg. A student nurse is going to be taken care of this patient. Which of the following actions by the student nurse would require the RN to intervene?

(1) Placing a pillow under the knee

(2) Providing thigh-high or knee-high TED hose

(3) Administering continuous warm, moist compresses

(4) Measuring the circumference of the thigh and calves and recording it in the chart

165. A man with arterial insufficiency informs the clinic that he is often unable to sleep due to pain in his lower legs. When pain occurs as the patient lays in bed, the nurse should advise the patient to

(1) Elevate both legs on two or more pillows

(2) Dangle the painful leg in a dependent position

(3) Avoid using blankets over his legs

(4) Wear thermal pants to keep his legs warm

166. For a patient in Bed A, a nurse hangs an intravenous fluid and sets the rate that was ordered for the patient in Bed B in the same room. This mistake results in hyperglycemia and fluid overload for the patient in Bed A, who received the incorrect IV fluid. The nurse could be served with a lawsuit for

(1) Assault

(2) Battery

(3) Malpractice

(4) Libel

167. A nurse receives an order to administer a sedative preoperatively to a patient who is to undergo eye surgery within the next hour. What should the nurse do before giving this medication?

(1) Start the intravenous line for the patient.

(2) Be certain that the surgical consent is signed.

(3) Take and record the patient's vital signs.

(4) Bring the family members into the holding area.

168. A nurse manager overhears a staff nurse telling a patient that a certain nursing assistant is unprofessional and incompetent. The nurse manager should know that this action is an example of

 (1) Breach of duty

 (2) Libel

 (3) Violation of patient's confidentiality

 (4) Slander

169. A nurse manager is analyzing the tasks performed by the hospital unit staff. Which of these actions would be most appropriate for a registered nurse to perform?

 (1) Transferring a patient who has had a cerebrovascular accident (CVA) from the bed to a chair using a Hoyer lift

 (2) Changing the bed sheets for a stuporous patient who has a tracheostomy and is on mechanical ventilation

 (3) Taking the temperature of a patient who is in a negative pressure isolation room and is being treated for tuberculosis

 (4) Checking the apical pulse of a patient following a detected irregularity in the radial pulse

170. A nursing team leader delegates a simple wound irrigation and dressing to a licensed practical nurse (LPN). The LPN tells the RN that she has not done that procedure for over a year and feels unsure about performing this task. The RN team leader's best response is to

 (1) Assign the procedure to another staff member

 (2) Direct the LPN to read the procedure manual before performing the skill

 (3) Have the LPN explain and demonstrate the procedure to the RN

 (4) Ask a nursing assistant to assist the LPN with the procedure

171. When delegating a series of tasks to a unlicensed assistive personnel, the RN should make it a priority that the unlicensed assistive personnel can do which of the following? Select all that apply.

 ❏ **(1)** Empty catheter bags of urine

 ❏ **(2)** Explain what a myocardial infarction is to a new patient

 ❏ **(3)** Start IV fluids when the IV has been inserted

 ❏ **(4)** Ambulate a postoperative patient for the second day postoperative

 ❏ **(5)** Take vital signs on a client returning from surgery

172. A post-surgical patient is being transferred from an intensive care unit to a general nursing unit. The team leader should avoid transferring the patient into a room in which the roommate

 (1) Speaks a language different from the transferring patient

 (2) Has a fever of unknown origin (FUO)

 (3) Has had a cerebrovascular accident (CVA) and is being weaned from a ventilator

 (4) Is being treated for depression as well as bone cancer

173. An RN is planning the day shift care for a group of patients on the nursing unit. Which of the following patients should the nurse prioritize to see first?

 (1) A heart failure patient who has furosemide ordered for 9 a.m.

 (2) A patient receiving captopril who complains of a cough

 (3) A patient who is to receive alteplase for a myocardial infarction

 (4) An atrial fibrillation patient who has phytonadione ordered for INR of 2.9

GO ON TO NEXT PAGE ➤

174. A nurse arrives to work 15 minutes late for the second time in a week during a unit meeting at the change of shift. The nurse manager should

    (1) Privately ask the nurse for a one-on-one meeting when the unit meeting is over

    (2) Ignore the lateness and assume the situation will resolve itself

    (3) Say, "Thank you for joining us," and resume the meeting

    (4) Make a note of the lateness and put it in the nurse's annual evaluation

175. The nurse has to assign beds to four patients who are being admitted to an acute care nursing unit at the hospital. Three semiprivate rooms and one private room are available. Each of the semiprivate rooms has a female patient over the age of 60, postoperative with no complications. Which of the four patients being admitted should the nurse assign to the private room?

    (1) A 75-year-old woman with terminal breast cancer and congestive heart failure

    (2) A 19-year-old woman with a suspected ectopic pregnancy and abdominal pain

    (3) A 69-year-old woman with Alzheimer's disease, hepatitis A, and jaundice

    (4) A bedfast 95-year-old woman with a urinary tract infection who came from a nursing home

176. A patient's blood pressure has been rising for 48 hours, and he is showing a 2-pound weight gain in two days. The nurse should assess this patient further for

    (1) Bradycardia

    (2) A decrease in pulse pressure

    (3) Full, bounding pulses

    (4) Paralytic ileus

177. A patient is receiving continuous enteral feedings and develops diarrhea. The nurse should know that the diarrhea is related to the

    (1) High Fowler's position during the feeding

    (2) High osmolarity of the feeding

    (3) Vitamins and minerals in the feeding

    (4) Intermittent administration of the feeding

178. A patient who is A– is to receive a unit of packed cells. Four units of packed red blood cells are available from the blood bank. The nurse knows the patient can receive which unit of blood?

    (1) AB+

    (2) AB–

    (3) O–

    (4) O+

179. A patient with Alzheimer's disease is hospitalized for surgery. The nurse notes that the settings on the IV infusion pump are incorrect. The patient's order is for 125 ml/hour of 0.9% NaCl, but the patient receives 250 ml of IV fluid in one hour. The nurse should assess the patient for

    (1) Distended neck veins and moist crackles

    (2) Postural hypotension and hyperthermia

    (3) Warm, dry skin and an irregular pulse

    (4) Decreased urinary output and thirst

180. A client has been diagnosed with hypocalcemia. Her healthcare provider has asked her to increase her consumption of calcium. Which of the following meals best supports that goal?

    (1) Pork, spinach greens, and yogurt

    (2) Pot roast, potatoes, and rhubarb pie

    (3) Ham and cheese sandwich and coffee

    (4) Canned salmon, a lettuce salad with tofu, and milk

181. An 86-year-old man is admitted to the hospital from a nursing home. The nurse establishes a nursing diagnosis of fluid volume deficit related to decreased intake and fever. Which of the following symptoms would substantiate this nursing diagnosis?

(1) The patient's pulse is 120, BP 90/60, temperature 101.2 degrees F (38.4 degrees C), respirations 22 and deep.

(2) The patient has difficulty breathing in a low Fowler's position or with minimal activity.

(3) The patient's skin is pale and cool to touch with pitting edema in dependent areas.

(4) The patient complains of headache and appears lethargic.

182. A patient is started on total parenteral nutrition (TPN). Upon entering the room, the nurse notes the patient is apprehensive and has a rapid, weak pulse. The patient is sitting on the side of the bed struggling to breathe. Which of the following actions is the priority of the nurse?

(1) Obtain a blood glucose level immediately.

(2) Check the tubing connections.

(3) Place the client in a left side-lying position with the head lower than the feet.

(4) Reassure the client that nothing is wrong.

183. A nurse is assessing the skin turgor of an older patient. Where is the preferred site for assessing turgor in the older patient?

(1) Forearm

(2) Sternum

(3) Ankle

(4) Cheek

184. A patient who is being treated for renal failure has been diagnosed with hyperphosphatemia. Which of these measures would the nurse know should not be included in the patient's plan of care?

(1) Calcium supplements

(2) Sevelamer

(3) Dairy products such as ice cream, milk, and yogurt

(4) Calcium carbonate

185. When taking a patient's carotid pulse, where do you place your fingers?

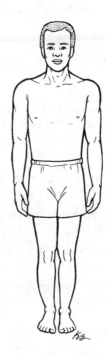

186. A woman who is 38 weeks pregnant tells the nurse that for the past few days she feels like she is urinating every ten minutes. The nurse should first assess the woman for

(1) Rupture of membranes

(2) Quickening

(3) Lightening

(4) Effacement

GO ON TO NEXT PAGE

187. A mother with gestational diabetes has just given birth at 37 weeks. The nurse is performing the one-minute Apgar scoring. Which of the following scores would require immediate resuscitation?

  (1) Heart rate of 110, weak cry with irregular respirations, very little flexion of lower extremities, prompt crying with stimulation, and normal body color

  (2) Heart rate of 80, weak cry, minimal response to slap on the sole of the foot, and blue extremities

  (3) Heart rate of 112, vigorous cry and respiratory rate of 50, flexion of all extremities with stimuli, and normal color

  (4) Heart rate of 60, irregular respirations, cyanosis, no reaction to stimuli, flaccidity

188. A woman has been in early labor for 14 hours. The nurse notes an initial episode of variable decelerations on the fetal monitor strip. The nurse should first

  (1) Prepare the woman for an immediate Cesarean delivery

  (2) Assist the woman to change her position to her left side

  (3) Increase the intravenous flow rate into the woman's left arm

  (4) Intervene only if the decelerations continue for several hours

189. A client comes in to be induced, and the oxytocin infusion is started. The next shift, the nurse finds that the patient is having contractions every 1½ minutes and the fetal heart rate is 110. Which of the following should the nurse place as the priority?

  (1) Administering oxygen at 8 to 10 liters per minute

  (2) Obtaining vital signs on the mother and the fetal heart rate

  (3) Documenting the signs and symptoms observed

  (4) Stopping the oxytocin infusion

190. A woman who is 33 weeks pregnant has been admitted to the labor and delivery unit with a diagnosis of gestational hypertension. Which of the following are predisposing conditions for pre-eclampsia? Select all that apply.

  ❏ (1) Being an 18-year-old female

  ❏ (2) Diabetes mellitus

  ❏ (3) Family history of gestational hypertension

  ❏ (4) Chronic renal disease

  ❏ (5) Epilepsy

191. A woman tells the nurse that she and her husband are planning their first pregnancy. Which instruction is the most appropriate for the nurse to give at this time?

  (1) "Eat more foods with folic acid, and take a prenatal vitamin."

  (2) "It's best to avoid having cats in the home during pregnancy."

  (3) "Don't have any dental work done until after delivery."

  (4) "Try to stop drinking alcohol by the 20th week."

192. A patient who is Rh– is pregnant with her second baby. The patient is scheduled to receive Rho (D) immune globulin (RhoGAM). The nurse knows that the purpose of RhoGAM is to

  (1) Increase the woman's serum iron-binding capacity (TIBC)

  (2) Generate the production of fetal antibodies to counteract the mother's blood cells

  (3) Reduce the woman's production of maternal serum hemoglobin

  (4) Suppress the production of the mother's antibodies against Rh+ blood cells

193. The nurse is counseling a pregnant patient about nutrition. The nurse should advise the patient that the best fluid to take with ferrous sulfate is

(1) Skim milk

(2) Decaffeinated coffee

(3) Orange juice

(4) Water

194. A pregnant woman tells the nurse she had a reactive nonstress test. The nurse should know that this means that

(1) The fetus must be monitored more closely for possible complications

(2) It does not offer any information, and the test should be repeated shortly

(3) The fetal neurological system is functioning adequately

(4) The test indicates a measure of fetal well-being with no obvious signs of distress

195. The nurse offers a new mother contraception information the day she is going home from the hospital. The nurse should tell the mother that ovulation

(1) Will not recur until the uterus is completely involuted

(2) Will not occur until the client stops breastfeeding

(3) Can occur before menstrual periods return

(4) Only begins after the fourth month following delivery

196. A nurse is called to a woman's birthing room by a cry of "Hurry, I feel like the baby's coming out!" The nurse sees that the infant's head is beginning to crown. After the nurse puts on gloves, the next action should be to

(1) Tell the patient to take a deep breath, hold it, and push down hard

(2) Apply gentle pressure on the exposed fetal head toward the vagina

(3) Put her hands on the bulging perineum and firmly push the head back

(4) Assist the patient to a squatting position and have her hold her breath

197. A woman is pregnant with her first child and is trying to determine the due date. The woman is certain that the first day of her last menstrual period was June 11. The nurse should calculate that the client's estimated date of delivery (EDC) is

(1) February 11

(2) March 18

(3) April 11

(4) April 18

198. When assessing a postpartum patient, a nurse finds her lying in a pool of blood and complaining of feeling nauseated and dizzy. The patient's skin is pale and clammy, blood pressure is 88/55, pulse 120 beats per minute, and respirations 40 breaths/minute. What is the first action the nurse should take?

(1) Run to the nurse's station to get help and call the physician.

(2) Place the patient in a high Fowler's position and start oxygen.

(3) Gently massage the patient's uterus with two hands and call for help.

(4) Insert a Foley catheter and increase the patient's IV fluid rate.

GO ON TO NEXT PAGE ▶

199. A nurse asks a woman who is 36 weeks pregnant what to expect when labor begins. Which one of these statements, if made by the patient, should the nurse correct?

(1) "I will have a bloody show for at least a week before my labor starts."

(2) "My backache may become stronger and more painful when I am in labor."

(3) "I'll probably lose a few pounds in the days before I start labor."

(4) "I might expel the mucous plug before my labor starts."

200. A woman has been diagnosed with *chlamydia trachomatis* infection. What information should the nurse give to the patient about this infection?

(1) The patient's partner will have to be treated before further exposures.

(2) Older clients are at greater risk of infection than younger clients.

(3) This infection is usually symptomatic in women and easily detected.

(4) This infection is relatively benign and exposure renders immunity.

201. An expectant father is timing the frequency of his wife's contractions in the birthing room. The nurse knows that the contractions are being monitored correctly if the father is marking the time from the

(1) End of one contraction to the end of the next contraction

(2) Beginning of one contraction to the beginning of the next contraction

(3) End of one contraction to the beginning of the next contraction

(4) Beginning of a single contraction to its end, before the interval

202. The nurse is caring for a healthy newborn whose mother had a low-risk pregnancy. After establishing the neonate's airway and respiration, what is the nurse's next priority?

(1) Place the newborn in a warmer or wrap in a blanket.

(2) Check the infant's blood glucose level.

(3) Wash the infant and remove all blood and vernix.

(4) Monitor the infant's sensory functions, noting any deficits.

203. A new mother is breast-feeding her newborn baby but does not know how to tell if the baby is getting an adequate amount of milk. The nurse should advise the mother that she will know that the baby is getting enough milk if the baby

(1) Has six to eight wet diapers per day

(2) Feeds four to six times daily

(3) Rarely cries

(4) Sleeps through the night

204. During the transition phase of labor, a patient tells her husband, who is her coach, "Leave me alone, go away!" The husband begins to leave the room. The nurse's best response is to

(1) Warn the partner that it would be a big mistake to leave the room

(2) Agree that the husband should leave and send in another visitor

(3) Advise the patient that her behavior is out of control and she needs to relax

(4) Let the partner know that this is a normal response and is to be expected

205. A woman in active labor has just had an amniotomy. Which parameter should the nurse monitor immediately?

(1) The woman's pain level

(2) The woman's blood pressure and pulse

(3) The fetus's heart rate

(4) The frequency of uterine contractions

206. The parents of a 4-year-old child have been advised to have their child tested for cystic fibrosis. The clinic nurse knows that the child will undergo which of the following tests?

(1) Bone marrow aspiration

(2) Lung scan

(3) Renal biopsy

(4) Sweat chloride test

207. The nurse is preparing a patient for surgery to establish an ileal conduit. Which of the following statements, if made by the patient, indicates to the nurse that the patient understands the possible complications of this procedure?

(1) "I'm going to be embarrassed about the stoma on my abdomen."

(2) "I should have a bowel movement within two to three days."

(3) "I could develop pyelonephritis from this procedure."

(4) "I will always have to self-catheterize myself to drain the reservoir."

208. A woman is admitted to the emergency room with a pneumothorax. The nurse would expect the patient to exhibit

(1) Breath sounds bilaterally

(2) Bradycardia

(3) Tracheal deviation

(4) Hypertension

209. A man is diagnosed with a malignant brain tumor located in the left frontal lobe. The nurse would expect the patient to exhibit

(1) Unilateral hearing loss

(2) Personality changes

(3) Visual impairments

(4) Ataxia

210. A woman is diagnosed with endolymphatic hydrops (Ménière's disease). The nurse would expect the woman to exhibit

(1) Discharge from the ear and ear pain

(2) Vertigo and tinnitus

(3) Fever and headache

(4) Enlarged lymph nodes and draining sinuses

211. To assess an infant's pulse during cardiopulmonary resuscitation (CPR), the nurse should palpate the

(1) Femoral pulse

(2) Pedal pulse

(3) Carotid pulse

(4) Brachial pulse

212. A patient is admitted to the hospital with a diagnosis of Addison's disease and hyponatremia. Which of the following signs and symptoms would the nurse expect this patient to exhibit?

(1) Muscle cramps, fatigue, and hypotension

(2) Shortness of breath, pallor, and hirsutism

(3) Rales, maculopapular rash, and weight loss

(4) Hypertension, peripheral edema, and petechiae

GO ON TO NEXT PAGE

213. The nurse assesses a patient who has a chest tube and a three-chamber water-seal drainage system (Pleur-evac) connected to suction. Which occurrence would require an intervention by the nurse?

(1) There is continuous bubbling in the suction control chamber.

(2) The fluid in the water seal chamber fluctuates with the patient's respirations.

(3) The collection container contains 100 ml of serosanguinous fluid.

(4) There is continuous bubbling in the water-seal chamber.

214. A woman has had a cerebral infarct on the right side. The nurse should expect the patient to exhibit

(1) Weakness of her right arm

(2) Hyperactive reflexes on the left side

(3) Sluggish reflexes in both eyes

(4) Inability to distinguish words and letters

215. The nurse is caring for a patient 24 hours after a cast application to the right leg from the groin to the foot. Which findings would require an immediate intervention by the nurse?

(1) The patient's capillary refill of the right toes is one second.

(2) The patient's right toes are warm and dry to the touch.

(3) The patient can move her right toes.

(4) The patient states that her right toes are burning and tingling.

216. The nurse is counseling a patient with systemic lupus erythematosus (SLE) who is learning self-care management. The nurse should advise the client to avoid which of the following to help prevent an exacerbation?

(1) Nonsteroidal anti-inflammatory drugs (NSAIDs)

(2) Stress

(3) Citrus fruits

(4) Pets

217. A man has been diagnosed with hepatitis A. The man's wife asks the nurse how to avoid hepatitis spreading throughout the family. Which of the following statements is the most appropriate response by the nurse?

(1) "Do not eat any shellfish and seafood in restaurants."

(2) "Your husband should stay in a separate room from the family."

(3) "Keep your home well-ventilated."

(4) "Have the family use good hand-washing technique."

218. The nurse is caring for a patient who has just had a cardiac catheterization using the right femoral artery. Which of the following findings would require immediate intervention by the nurse?

(1) The right extremity is cooler to touch and paler than the left extremity.

(2) There is a quarter-sized amount of serosanguinous drainage on the femoral dressing.

(3) The patient's IV infusion is 30 minutes behind schedule.

(4) The patient is complaining of pain at the femoral insertion site.

219. A woman who has Bell's palsy comes to the clinic for a follow-up visit. During the visit, the woman tells the nurse, "I can't stand the way I look. I don't even want to go to work." The nurse's best response is

(1) "Your condition will last about a week."

(2) "I'll call a social worker to see you today."

(3) "You seem upset. Tell me how you feel."

(4) "If you wear dark glasses, your condition won't be as noticeable."

220. The clinic nurse is assessing a patient with multiple sclerosis. Which of the following findings would the nurse expect the client to exhibit? Select all that apply.

❑ (1) Bladder and bowel disturbances, including in urgency, frequency, retention, and incontinence

❑ (2) Blurred vision

❑ (3) Dyspnea

❑ (4) Ataxia and vertigo

❑ (5) Dysphasia

221. A nurse is advising a patient who has multiple sclerosis about how to manage her activities of daily living. Of these suggestions, which is correct?

(1) "Try to group many of your activities in the early part of the day."

(2) "Take a hot bath or shower to help you relax your body."

(3) "Limit fluids to avoid the interruptions of frequent voiding."

(4) "Stick to a strict, vigorous program of aerobic exercise."

222. A patient who has had a cerebrovascular accident (CVA) is diagnosed with receptive aphasia. This means that the patient

(1) Has difficulty understanding what is being said to him

(2) Has difficulty using language to express himself

(3) Does not recognize a number drawn on his hand

(4) Does not recognize a previously familiar household object

223. A nurse in the emergency department is triaging a group of patients. Which patient should be seen first?

(1) A 49-year-old male with a complex fracture of his right leg due to a motor vehicle accident who is complaining of severe pain

(2) An 11-year-old male who is holding his thumb with a bloody towel and who reports that he cut it on an old tin can

(3) A 78-year-old female who is complaining of difficulty speaking, left-sided weakness, and headache for the past two hours

(4) A 14-year-old female who has epilepsy and who had a grand mal seizure an hour ago at the beach

224. A patient is recovering from a brain contusion and a hairline skull fracture. The nurse should intervene if it is observed that the

(1) Head of the patient's bed is at 30 degrees

(2) Patient's intracranial pressure is 16 mm hg

(3) Patient has had a vest restraint applied

(4) Glasgow coma scale is unchanged at 12

GO ON TO NEXT PAGE

225. A nursing student is teaching a 120-pound patient about how to prevent urinary tract infections (UTIs). Which of these statements would the supervising nurse have to correct?

(1) "Avoid caffeine, alcohol, and spicy foods."

(2) "Your fluid intake should be about 2,500 ml per day."

(3) "Drink pure cranberry juice or take cranberry tablets each day."

(4) "After using the toilet, clean the perineal area from back to front."

226. A patient who has inquired about changing his diet shows that he has adequate information about nutrition if he makes all of the following statements except

(1) "Avoid foods high in fat content."

(2) "Eat one adequate meal per day."

(3) "Consume foods high in fiber."

(4) "Eat more than one meal per day containing foods from the major food groups."

227. A nurse is counseling a 63-year-old patient who has osteoporosis. Which of these measures should the nurse recommend to the patient to stimulate bone formation?

(1) Taking 300 mg of calcium daily

(2) Taking aluminum-based antacids

(3) Establishing a high protein intake

(4) Walking and swimming

228. A nurse is conducting an initial assessment for a newly admitted 83-year-old female patient. The nurse documents that the patient demonstrates "aphasia." The nursing student should know that this means that the patient

(1) Demonstrates mild hemiplegia when walking

(2) Has an inability to speak

(3) Will need a wheelchair for mobility

(4) Will be incontinent of urine

229. A nurse is teaching a group of older adults about normal changes in the eye related to aging. Which of these statements about eye changes and aging, if made by the nurse, is true?

(1) "There is increased peripheral vision with advancing age."

(2) "The pupil of the eye dilates more quickly in low light."

(3) "Depth perception decreases."

(4) "There is increased color perception."

230. A nurse is caring for a patient who has had major abdominal surgery. During the immediate postoperative period, what is the most important assessment parameter the nurse should monitor?

(1) Blood saturation of the dressings

(2) Rigidity of the abdomen

(3) Mobility of the patient from bed to chair

(4) Psychological impact of the surgery

231. A nurse is counseling a patient who has been told he has a high cholesterol level. The nurse should advise him to avoid

(1) Oatmeal

(2) Skim milk

(3) Sliced bologna

(4) Egg yolks

232. A new diet is being planned for an older patient in a nursing home who is becoming progressively confused. To preserve the patient's ability to feed herself, which of these foods should the nurse suggest may be best for this patient?

(1) Hamburger on a bun

(2) Beef stew

(3) Chicken fingers

(4) Tuna fish casserole

233. A nurse is advising a patient who is on a low-residue diet about which fruits to avoid eating due to their high fiber content. Which food is high in fiber?

(1) Pineapple

(2) Red cherries

(3) Apples

(4) Bananas

234. A nurse is caring for a patient who practices Orthodox Judaism. In helping the patient order his meals, the nurse should remember that according to dietary laws, an appropriate food tray would contain

(1) Pasta with shrimp and tomato sauce

(2) English muffins and cream cheese

(3) Chicken soup with bread and butter

(4) A ham and cheese sandwich

235. A patient who weighs 250 pounds asks the nurse why she has not lost weight even though she has stopped eating ice cream. The nurse's best response is that the reason for obesity and the lack of weight loss is directly related to

(1) The patient's low basal metabolic rate (BMR)

(2) A low level of hormonal activity

(3) Higher calorie intake than the energy used

(4) The patient's psychological responses to food

236. A nurse is counseling the parents of a 15-year-old girl who is strictly adhering to a vegan diet. Which of these foods would be most acceptable to the daughter while providing a complete protein per portion?

(1) Blueberries and vanilla yogurt

(2) Eggplant with legumes and rice

(3) A peanut butter and grape jelly sandwich

(4) Whole-wheat crackers and cheddar cheese

237. A woman who has osteoporosis has been advised to increase her intake of vitamin D. Which of these foods should the nurse advise the woman to eat?

(1) Liver

(2) Dark green, leafy vegetables

(3) Fortified milk

(4) Shredded wheat

238. A patient has been told that he has a low serum protein level. The nurse should know that which of these laboratory test results would confirm this finding?

(1) High hematocrit

(2) Low blood urea nitrogen

(3) High serum creatinine

(4) Low serum albumin

239. Following surgery, a patient has been placed on a clear liquid diet. Which of these fluids would be acceptable for the patient to eat?

(1) Clear chicken broth

(2) Soy milk

(3) Vegetable juice

(4) Vanilla custard

240. A nurse is assessing a patient's fluid and electrolyte balance. The nurse should know that the patient is at high risk for developing hyperkalemia if the patient

(1) Is experiencing two hours of profuse diaphoresis

(2) Has been vomiting for over 48 hours

(3) Is two hours post-deep partial thickness burns to trunk and arms

(4) Has had diarrhea for the past 72 hours

GO ON TO NEXT PAGE

241. The nurse is assisting during a paracentesis being performed on a patient who has ascites. During the procedure, 1,400 ml of fluid is removed. Which of these actions is most important for the nurse to take immediately after the procedure?

(1) Weigh the patient.

(2) Check the patient's blood pressure.

(3) Medicate the patient for pain.

(4) Measure the patient's abdominal girth.

242. A young woman is being assessed in the emergency department following her report of being raped by a neighbor in her home. The patient states, "I shouldn't have opened the door; my parents will kill me." The nurse's best response is

(1) "You should never open the door when you're home alone."

(2) "Don't worry, you're parents will have to understand."

(3) "This must be very difficult for you."

(4) "You shouldn't worry about this now."

243. A patient who is experiencing alcohol withdrawal calls the nurse and shouts, "Get those spiders out of my room right now!" The nurse's best response is

(1) "Tell me what the spiders look like and what are they doing."

(2) "Don't be concerned; the spiders won't hurt you."

(3) "There are no spiders in here; go back to sleep."

(4) "You are going through withdrawal and may see things that aren't real."

244. A nurse working in the community suspects that a child seen on a home visit is being physically abused. What is the most appropriate action for the nurse to take?

(1) Ask two colleagues to join the visit to the home the following week to confirm the suspicions.

(2) Discuss the concerns with the child's parents and grandparents who live in the home.

(3) Document the concerns and wait to see whether the situation improves by the next visit.

(4) Report the case as suspected child abuse to the nurse's superior and to the designated city, county, or state agency.

245. On entering a patient's room, the nurse sees flames and smoke spreading on the other side of the room. What is the first action the nurse should take?

(1) Run to the hall and pull the fire alarm.

(2) Remove the patient from the room.

(3) Throw water and blankets on the fire.

(4) Close the patient's door and call for help.

246. A nurse is visiting a patient in her home following discharge from the hospital to determine the patient's need for home health services. What is the most important assessment the nurse must make for this patient?

(1) The ability and willingness of family members to help the patient

(2) How much mobility the patient has in her home

(3) How safe the home environment is for the patient

(4) How fully the patient can contribute to the plan of care

247. When caring for a patient who is receiving total parenteral nutrition (TPN), what should the nurse do to prevent infection in the patient?

(1) Encourage the patient to take fluids by mouth each day.

(2) Monitor the serum blood urea nitrogen and blood sugar daily.

(3) Maintain strict intake and output records.

(4) Use strict aseptic (sterile) technique when caring for the IV site.

248. A nurse who is providing a secondary health-care service would be

(1) Helping a patient learn how to use assistive devices following a CVA

(2) Administering immunizations in a pediatric clinic

(3) Conducting cholesterol screenings at a health fair

(4) Teaching a group of second graders about hand-washing

249. A patient has been diagnosed with a vitamin K deficiency. What would the nurse expect to see on assessing this patient?

(1) Soft tissue bruising

(2) Night blindness

(3) Muscle weakness

(4) Bone loss

250. Following a craniotomy for a brain tumor, the nurse notes that the dressing is becoming saturated with a clear fluid. What action should the nurse take?

(1) Reinforce the dressing with sterile gauze.

(2) Mark the saturation pattern with a pen.

(3) Call the surgeon.

(4) Place the patient in a semi-Fowler's position.

STOP

Chapter 14

The Answers to All Your Questions (and Explanations to Boot)

This chapter contains the answers to every question on the practice exam in Chapter 13 along with explanations. I encourage you to read through each of the explanations, especially for any questions you missed, to help you reinforce the concepts tested. However, you can also find an answers-only key at the end of this chapter if you prefer.

Answers and Explanations

1. **2, 3, and 5.** The patient is an older adult at 75, which is a risk factor. He has a history of diabetes and hypertension — both risk factors. He's had an infection or sepsis and just finished the antibiotic for it, which puts him at risk for acute kidney injury. He has the signs and symptoms of acute kidney injury already: dyspnea, peripheral edema, fatigue, and decreased urine output over the past 24 hours. The diagnostics test for acute kidney injury would be the UA, UA culture and sensitivity, and a CT scan of the kidneys.

2. **3.** Choices (1), (2), and (4) are all within normal limits. The normal range for serum potassium is 3.5 to 5.5 mEq/L. Values above this range are abnormal and may indicate renal failure.

3. **1.** Oxybutynin chloride is an anti-cholinergic, antispasmodic used for an overactive bladder or urge incontinence. The other statements — Choices (2), (3), and (4) — have nothing to do with overactive bladder.

4. **1.** Painful muscle cramps are a common side effect of hemodialysis and result from the rapid removal of sodium and water from the extracellular space; cramps may also involve neuro-muscular sensitivity. Cramps aren't related to glucose metabolism or perfusion issues. Serum sodium and potassium don't rise during dialysis, but they may decrease.

5. **3.** Spinal anesthesia may induce a headache post-procedure due to leakage of the CSF at the injection site. Regional anesthesia doesn't require intubation, ventilatory assistance, and unconsciousness. Regional anesthesia causes immobility below the level of the injection site, but for a TURP, regional anesthesia doesn't involve levels that impact the arms or the diaphragm.

6. **2.** Renal failure caused by ischemia or toxins is characterized by the presence of tubular RBC and WBC casts. Casts are formed from mucoprotein impressions of the necrotic epithelial cells that slough into the tubules. Choices (1), (3) and (4) describe a kidney that is functioning normally.

7. **3 and 5.** Tight-fitting clothing can limit air to the area, increasing perspiration and the growth of bacteria in the perineal area. Wearing cotton underwear helps with increasing the air flow and decreasing the growth of bacteria. Choices (1) and (2) are incorrect, and Choice (4) is unrelated to the problem.

8. **4.** Pain relief is one of the first steps the nurse should take to help reduce the severity of pain and anxiety. Catheterization usually isn't indicated, and teaching would be done after the problem's resolved. Forcing fluids is avoided because it hasn't been shown to assist in excreting the stone and may exacerbate the colic of this condition.

9. **1, 2, 3, and 4.** If a client is experiencing a fat embolus, the nurse needs to notify the health-care provider, give IV fluids as prescribed, provide oxygen, and document the event and the actions taken. The nurse wouldn't place the client in Trendelenburg because the patient needs to increase venilation in the lungs. Placing in Trendelenburg would make breathing more difficult. Prone is the correct position for a patient with a fat emboli because this position increases lung expansion.

10. **1.** Chest pain indicates a pulmonary embolus, likely due to fat emboli post-long bone fracture. The other options aren't indicative of fat emboli and have nothing to do with the injury.

11. **3.** After hip surgery, the patient should be placed on the nonoperative side with legs abducted. Adducting the legs can result in dislocation.

12. **2.** Skin traction can cause pressure on the skin, leading to skin breakdown. Buck's traction doesn't use pins and doesn't cause arthritis or a rise in ICP.

13. **1, 2, 4, and 5.** Pain that gets better after rest and worsens after exercise, pain that gets worse in the cold or with changes in humidity, Heberden's nodes, and difficulty getting up after sitting for prolonged time are all signs of osteoarthritis. Swollen, hot joints with pain on movement, Choice (3), are a symptom of rheumatoid arthritis.

14. **1.** The most important parameter to monitor in the immediate postoperative period is vascular status; monitoring involves controlling bleeding to prevent blood loss and hypovolemic shock. The other issues are secondary considerations and will be cared for after control of bleeding and breathing.

15. **3.** Fatigue and impaired joint function (usually bilaterally) are characteristic of RA. Unilateral pain in a weight-bearing joint is normally related to osteoarthritis, as are Heberden's nodes on finger joints. ESR may increase with exacerbations of RA.

16. **2.** Three-point gait is where the patient advances both crutches and the foot of the affected leg together followed by the other foot. Choice (1) is the four-point gate, Choice (3) is the swing-through gait, and Choice (4) is the swing-to gait.

17. **1, 2, 4, and 5.** Interventions for lumbar disc herniation are to apply heat to decrease the muscle spasms, apply ice to decrease inflammation and swelling, apply pelvic traction as prescribed, and begin progressive ambulation as the inflammation, edema, and pain decrease. Skeletal traction isn't used with a lumbar disc herniation.

18. **4.** Drooling and inability to swallow indicate impairment of innervation, probably due to trauma and edema related to surgery. The other findings are normal postsurgery.

19. **3.** Profound headache is characteristic of a spinal cord injury at level C-5 with autonomic hyperreflexia, as are hypertension, bradycardia, nasal congestion, and sweating above C-5. The other options are incorrect.

20. **1.** Brown-Sequard syndrome results from damage to one half of the spinal cord. It involves loss of motor function, position, vibratory sense, and vasomotor paralysis on the same side as the lesion as well as loss of pain and temperature on the opposite side below the injury level. The other options are incorrect.

21. **1.** The patient can't feel pressure points due to complete transection and is at risk for skin breakdown or trauma with braces applied and not monitored. With a complete transection, the patient isn't able to perform active ROM or ambulate without help. Massage doesn't help with leg brace application and monitoring.

22. **4.** Following spinal cord injury, monitoring for signs of extending injury above and below the level of the trauma is critical. In the absence of head injury, the patient isn't at risk for seizures, and the patient isn't able to perform active ROM following a spinal cord injury. Skin breakdown is an issue but not a priority in the crisis period.

23. **3.** Injury from C-1 to C-4 requires wheelchair control using the muscles of the mouth or chin. The patient is completely paralyzed in a quadriplegic state and therefore can't use hand controls, transfer him or herself or ambulate, sit balanced without support, or feed himself or herself.

24. 1. In neurogenic shock, the patient will experience hypotension and bradycardia. Flacid paralysis of the skeletal muscles below the level of injury, hyperactive bowel sounds, and urinary urgency and frequency aren't symptoms of neurogenic shock. Massive vasodilation happens with neurogenic shock, which leads to blood vessels filling with pooling blood and hypoperfusion of tissue. This condition would impair cellular metabolism.

25. 2. Kyphosis is curvature of the spine with the curve in the posterior direction, which occurs secondary to microfractures as a result of arthritis and osteoporosis, with poor posture as contributing factor. Hemiplegia and urinary incontinence are unrelated, and patients with kyphosis don't lose mobility due to the kyphosis alone.

26. 3. With rising ICP, the patient's head should be in midline position with the head of the bed at 30 degrees. Having the lights and the TV on increases stimulation, and this patient needs decreased stimulation. Providing a sedative to promote rest isn't appropriate; the nurse can't assess responsiveness and level of consciousness. The patient should be NPO; the nurse shouldn't provide a regular diet.

27. 4. An atonic seizure is when the patient has a drop attack. They're sometimes associated with myoclonic seizures. A brief cessation of motor activity and blank stare, Choice (1), is absent seizure. Choice (2), alternating contraction and relaxation of extremity muscles and hyperventilation, is tonic-clonic activity, and Choice (3), motor activity that spreads sequentially to adjacent parts, fingers to arm, doesn't describe an atonic seizure.

28. 2. The nurse must first help prevent the patient from hurting herself. You should never attempt to force a bite stick in the patient's mouth. The other options are secondary to preventing harm.

29. 1. The only answer choice that accurately reflects information from the question scenario is Choice (1). The patient did have alternating stiffening/rigidity and relaxing of the muscles of the arms and legs. The seizure lasted for a minute (not two or five) minutes, and the patient fell asleep two minutes (not immediately) after opening his eyes.

30. 4. Cognitive functioning is best assessed by asking the patient for personal and current information that addresses memory, general knowledge, and orientation to place, person, and situation. Choice (1) addresses mood and affect, Choice (2) checks only long-term memory, and Choice (3) addresses only general appearance and behavior, not cognitive functioning.

31. 1. Increase in temperature can exacerbate intracranial pressure. The other readings are still within normal limits for vital signs.

32. 4. Before the first meal is attempted, the nurse should check the patient's gag reflex and ability to swallow. The other options aren't the most important actions and should be done only after making sure that the patient won't choke.

33. 1, 2, and 4. EEG is used to get a recording of electrical activity of the cerebral cortex. This test is used for head injuries, sleep disorders, and seizures. An EEG isn't necessary for myocardial infarction and deep vein thrombosis.

34. 3. The patient is subject to seizure activity with inflammation and infection of the meninges. Intake and output is important but not the priority. Vest restraints are contraindicated because their use can increase ICP. CSF wouldn't be leaking due to meningitis.

35. 3. In severe cases of cerebral edema, creating bilateral bone flaps (craniotomy) is most effective in decreasing ICP. Carbon dioxide levels can be decreased through mechanical ventilation. Most clients with Reye's syndrome recover without any resulting brain injury. Continuous monitoring of ICP is implemented through intraventricular catheter into the brain.

36. 4. Each patient's condition can contribute to skin breakdown, but the least likely risk is the lowered mental status. Choices (1), (2), and (3) identify physiological conditions that are risk priorities.

37. 4. Cyclobenzaprine is used only for short-term therapy — two to three weeks. Cyclobenzaprine isn't given with MAOIs and has an anti-cholinergic effect, not cholinergic. It's a skeletal muscle relaxant, not an antigout medication.

38. 3. A side effect of Solu-Medrol is hyperglycemia. Solu-Medrol normally doesn't affect level of consciousness, precipitate renal dysfunction, or cause dehydration.

39. 1. Mannitol is an osmotic diuretic that reduces ICP through renal diuresis. An increase in urinary output indicates the efficacy of the medication. Mannitol shouldn't increase diastolic BP, and it isn't directly responsible for reducing nausea or pain.

40. 3. Kayexalate (sodium polystyrene sulfonate) is a cation-exchange resin used to reduce blood serum potassium levels by exchanging potassium for sodium in the bowel. It removes 1 mEq of potassium per gram of the medication. It doesn't directly affect serum ammonia, RBC count, or arterial blood pH.

41. 1. Carbachol's action is to increase the outflow of aqueous humor by stimulating the iris sphincter to contract, causing miosis and the opening of the trabecular meshwork. Carbachol doesn't cause mydriasis, increase lens accommodation, or anesthetize eye muscles.

42. 4. Open-angle glaucoma has few early symptoms. The other options describe other eye problems; Choice (1) indicates infection, Choice (2) indicates closed-angle glaucoma, and Choice (3) indicates macular degeneration.

43. 4. The initial action of the nurse giving eyedrops is to ask the patient to tilt her head back slightly and have her look up. The other three options are tasks that come later in the process.

44. 4. In macular degeneration, the macula has degenerated, which leads to the loss of central vision. Choice (1) describes retinal detachment, Choice (2) describes cataracts, and Choice (3) describes glaucoma.

45. 2, 4, and 5. Interventions for Ménière's disease are to instruct the client to stop smoking; have the client lie down in a quiet, dark room during peak exacerbation; and give the prescription nicotinic acid for its vasodilatory effect. Choices (1) and (3) don't help a client manage the symptoms of Ménière's disease.

46. 3. Presbyopia is a normal process of aging that causes farsightedness. It's due to inelasticity of the lens, which means that the lens can't accommodate for near vision (which includes reading). Presbyopia is corrected through convex lenses. The other symptoms are unrelated to presbyopia and are related to other eye disorders.

47. **1, 3, and 4.** The tests used for glaucoma are tonometry, which tells the intraocular pressure; peripheral vision test; and complete eye exam. A CT scan and corneal staining aren't required.

48. **3.** The Amsler Grid is used to identify extending areas of visual distortion typical of macular degeneration. Choices (1), (2), and (4) relate to other visual problems.

49. **2.** Homonymous hemianopia is the loss of the same visual field in both eyes. The other options are unrelated to the symptoms of the disease.

50. **1, 2, and 5.** Furosemide, aspirin, and amikacin can be ototoxic and may damage the patient's hearing. The other two options have no effect on hearing.

51. **1.** A statement made by the patient indicating suicidal thoughts must be followed up first. The other measures are important and can be instituted, but they don't take first priority.

52. **2.** Codependence occurs when a partner subsumes his or her needs to meet the perceived needs of the partner, regardless of whether the choices necessary to meet the needs are sound. The term describes behaviors exhibited by family members or significant others that enable and protect the addicted individual so that addiction may continue at the expense of the family. Neither admission of inability to meet another's needs nor concurrence on mutually met needs is an indication of codependence.

53. **4.** Patients experiencing mania need fewer stimuli and shouldn't be given opportunities to act out unacceptable behaviors through group activities or discussion groups. Interacting one-on-one is more therapeutic than following the patient around the unit to discipline behaviors.

54. **3.** Giving away possessions may be an indication of preparation for suicide. Ritualistic behavior relates to obsessive-compulsive disorder, somatic complaints are made by anxious patients with hypochondriac tendencies, and expressions of hostility and anger don't indicate suicidal ideation.

55. **3.** Reflecting the feeling tone of the patient's remarks is the most therapeutic approach. The other options reinforce the patient's delusion. The nurse should try to understand what the delusion means to the patient without entering into the delusion.

56. **4.** Patients with borderline personality disorder have difficulties with interpersonal relationships. Giving the patient structure and realistic standards for behavior is a therapeutic approach. In contrast, offering recreational choices and leadership responsibilities gives the patient more freedom to manipulate other patients and staff. Isolating the patient for requesting special favors would be perceived as punishment by the patient and isn't therapeutic.

57. **3.** The patient's trying to deflect attention onto the nurse, so the nurse should help him refocus on himself. The other measures are too confrontational for an initial assessment and may close communication channels between the nurse and the patient.

58. **2.** Evaluating affect means that the nurse is making a judgment about the patient's overall expression of mood. Asking how the patient feels can elicit an expression of mood. The other options require yes/no answers or concrete information.

59. **1.** Depression may render the patient incapable of motivating himself or herself to participate in activities or make decisions. Allowing the patient to self-isolate encourages withdrawal, and forcing the patient to sit in the day room doesn't encourage the patient to participate in selected activities involving both solitary and group work.

60. **4.** Patients with antisocial personality disorder disregard the rights of others. They're focused on their own needs and will use manipulation or violence to obtain what they want. The other choices describe behaviors associated with other psychiatric disorders.

61. **1.** If untreated, common conditions in the early stages of alcohol withdrawal include anxiety, tremors, tachycardia, anorexia, insomnia, agitation, hypertension, nausea, and vomiting. These are followed by acute hallucinations, and then 24 to 72 hours post drink, the patient becomes disoriented, delusional, and agitated with tachycardia, fever, perspiration, and possible seizures. Depression, bradycardia, dyspnea, flat affect, drowsiness, and coma aren't commonly associated with withdrawal.

62. **4.** Narcotics stimulate endorphin receptors, producing a wide variety of changes in the nervous system, including a sense of comfort and pleasure, slowed bodily functions, rapid dependence on the drug, and an increase in pain threshold with diminished perception of pain.

63. **3.** Domestic violence doesn't occur primarily in low-income families; rather, it cuts across all socioeconomic groups. The other options are true.

64. **4.** The nurse is reflecting the feeling tone of the patient's statement without arguing with the patient, rationalizing the patient's refusal to eat, or using her own experiences to deal with the patient.

65. **4.** Calling a physician who can arrange for the patient to be medically evaluated is important. The patient's behavior may reflect a delirium that could be due to dehydration, drug interactions or toxicities, infection, hypoxia, or blood glucose abnormalities. This type of behavior change is fairly rapid and isn't likely dementia. Alcohol intoxication is unlikely, the patient won't be able to do a diet recall, and coughing and deep breathing aren't the most important actions to take.

66. **3.** Neuroleptic malignant syndrome is a rare but life-threatening complication of neuroleptic medications. Manifestations include high fever, confusion, decreased level of consciousness, rigidity, and akinesia. Dystonia is a common side effect of haloperidol. Tardive dyskinesia is a movement disorder that can occur after long-term use of neuroleptics, and aphasia is a speech disorder due to neurological damage sustained by a cerebral damage.

67. **1, 2, 4, and 5.** Haloperidol's side effects are rigidity, drooling, dysphasia, and Parkinsonism. You do need to monitor the vitals, but hypotension isn't a specific side effect of haloperidol.

68. **2.** Moderate toxicity is mild to moderate ataxia and incoordination. Nystagmus and the serum lithium level of 1.5 represent mild toxicity. Tonic-clonic seizures or a coma are signs of severe toxicity.

69. **3.** The patient may be developing dystonia, sustained involuntary muscle spasms that occur in the head and neck due to adverse effects of chlorpromazine. The other options don't provide for further patient assessment, which is important prior to notifying the physician.

70. **1.** This medication is an MAOI inhibitor and requires the patient to avoid foods that have tyramine in them because tyramine can cause a hypertensive crisis. Bananas, eggplant, papaya, and sauerkraut all have tyramine. All the other responses have nothing to do with an MAOI inhibitor.

71. **4.** Paracentesis removes fluid from the peritoneal cavity, which reduces pressure on the diaphragm and allows for improved lung expansion. A thoracentesis and Sengstaken-Blakemore tube aren't indicated for fluid removal from the peritoneal cavity. A Kayexalate enema is used to remove potassium from the bowel in order to reduce serum potassium in renal failure.

72. **1.** Changes in mental status such as confusion, agitation, or lethargy indicate increasing serum ammonia levels and impending hepatic coma. Change in abdominal girth yields information about increasing ascites. Urine specific gravity gives information about the concentration of urine, H&H doesn't signal impending hepatic coma but rather gives information about circulating red blood cells and iron levels.

73. **1.** Bleeding esophageal varices are treated with the Sengstaken-Blakemore tube. The other tubes have nothing to do with this condition. A Salem Sump/double lumen tube is used to decompress the gastrointestinal track, and the Miller-Abbott is also used to drain the GI system. The cantor tube is for draining the GI track.

74. **3.** Lifting and straining place stress on the varices through the Valsalva maneuver. Observing the neck and shoulders doesn't yield information or prevent bleeding varices, and excessive coughing and deep breathing may place stress on the varices. Aspirin has anticoagulant properties and facilitates the tendency to bleed.

75. **3.** After the weighted enteric tube is placed, the nurse should position the client on the right side. The left side is the side that would be used to give an enema or do a colonoscopy. Placing the client supine or with the head of the bed elevated at 30 degrees creates a risk for aspiration.

76. **3.** Adequate nutrition is essential for recovery from hepatitis C infection. Disposable dinnerware, fluid limitations, and HAV vaccine administration aren't related to recovery from hepatitis C.

77. **2.** Dark urine, light stools, and jaundice indicate entering the icteric phase. The other options are present in both the preicteric and icteric phases.

78. **4.** Spironolactone is a potassium-sparing diuretic, which means that hyperkalemia may result from this medication. Symptoms of hyperkalemia are nausea, diarrhea, abdominal cramps, tachycardia, peaked T waves, and oliguria.

79. **2.** When given to a patient with cirrhosis of the liver, lactulose decreases the ammonia level via fecal excretion. Choices (1), (3), and (4) have nothing to do with expected outcomes of cirrhosis of the liver.

80. **4.** Vasopressin is used to control bleeding episodes. Cyclosporine is an immunosuppressant used to reduce organ rejection after transplantation. Omeprazole reduces gastric acid production, and pancreatin is a pancreatic enzyme replacement.

81. **1.** This patient has tachycardia, which may be an early sign of sepsis. The other values are within normal limits.

82. **4.** Securing an airway is the first consideration following trauma. The other options are important but secondary to breathing.

83. **3.** Confusion is the only answer choice that's a symptom of moderate carbon monoxide poisoning. Other manifestations of moderate CO poisoning include pale to reddish-purple skin, decrease blood pressure, increased and irregular heart rate, decreased ST segment on the electrocardiogram, headache nausea and vomiting, drowsiness, tendonitis, and vertigo. The other options aren't related to carbon monoxide poisoning.

84. **3.** Loss of the pedal pulse after a full-thickness burn injury indicates that the circulation has become impaired due to edema and ischemia. Because the pulse was previously present, preexisting conditions wouldn't cause loss of the pedal pulse. The idea that pulses are never palpable after a severe burn isn't true.

85. **4.** After the burn injury, capillary permeability increases and water, sodium, and plasma proteins (albumin) are lost into the interstitial spaces. Hematocrit increases due to fluid loss, and renal blood flow and blood pressure decreases with hypovolemic shock.

86. **4.** Synthroid therapy will gradually improve the hypothyroid condition of the patient. Weight loss is more likely than weight gain. The medication is a lifelong therapy and shouldn't be stopped due to appetite changes or without talking to the physician.

87. **4.** Insomnia is a manifestation of hyperthyroidism. The other options are related to hypothyroidism.

88. **2.** Graves' disease results from a combination of genetic and environmental factors. It's not a bacterial infection, nor does it result from heavy metal poisoning or diabetes mellitus.

89. **1.** For a patient with hypoparathyroidism, calcium supplements are required as lifelong maintenance. Diets high in foods containing oxalic acid and phosphorus reduce calcium absorption, and large amounts of fluid intake are advised in hyperparathyroidism.

90. **3.** Hormonal influences due to manipulation of glandular tissue during surgery may cause fluctuations in fluid and electrolyte balance. Assessment for signs of infection, prevention of skin breakdown, and keeping the patient calm are important but not the primary concern in the immediate postoperative period.

91. **2.** The defibrillator pads are placed on the patient's chest just prior to discharging the defibrillator. The synchronizer switch is turned off, and the "all clear" warning is given after the paddles are placed on the patient's chest.

92. **4.** Pink, frothy sputum is characteristic of pulmonary edema due to leakage of fluid from pulmonary capillaries into the alveoli. Knife-like chest pain, hyperthermia, and sleepiness aren't characteristic of pulmonary edema.

93. **1, 2, 3, and 5.** Right-sided heart failure is evidenced by dependent edema, jugular vein distention, abdominal distention, and weight gain, along with anorexia, nausea, nocturnal diuresis, swelling of the fingers and hands, increased blood pressure, and potentially hepatomegaly and splenomegaly. Choice (4) is a symptom of left-sided heart failure.

94. **1.** Symptoms of cardiac tamponade are neck vein distention, narrowing pulse pressure, tachycardia, and tachypnea.

95. 3. The nurse should position the patient for respiratory and cardiac assessment and possible cardiopulmonary resuscitation. The other measures shouldn't be taken until the patient is assessed, and the nurse shouldn't leave the room to get help.

96. 2. Complaints of numbness and tingling are a sign that circulation has been lost. All the other answers are signs that the leg is perfusing well. Diarrhea has nothing to do with post-PTCA condition.

97. 1. Nitroglycerine dilates coronary arteries and is used in conjunction with dopamine to raise blood pressure. Nitroglycerine isn't used for electrolyte imbalance, doesn't prevent acidosis, and doesn't prevent dysrhythmias.

98. 3. Checking warmth and color of extremities is a way of checking circulation, especially in the leg into which the catheter is placed. The head of the bed (HOB) should be less than 45 degrees. The patient is on strict bed rest, and antihypertensives shouldn't be used because the patient is hypotensive.

99. 3. The patient's head should be elevated as high as is comfortable to improve tidal volume, drain lung lobes, and decrease venous return. The nurse shouldn't elevate the patient's legs because that position increases venous return and adds to the work of the heart.

100. 2. Epinephrine makes the heart muscle more responsive to defibrillation. Atropine is used to treat bradycardia, dopamine is used to raise blood pressure, and nitroglycerine dilates coronary arteries.

101. 3. Warfarin sodium interacts with vitamin K in that a diet high in vitamin K makes it difficult to maintain the INR (international normalized ratio — the standardized system of reporting PT) within a range necessary for those taking warfarin sodium. Foods high in vitamin K include green, leafy vegetables; broccoli, cabbage; Brussels sprouts; green tea; dairy products; and meat. Eggs and sweet potatoes contain negligible amounts of vitamin K. Chocolate cake contains small amounts of vitamin K.

102. 3. Parallel play is the characteristic play of toddlers, when they play independently but are among other children. Playing softball and an interactive board game are examples of cooperative play, which is organized play with children playing in a group that has a goal. One child watching a videotape and another sleeping are examples of children taking part in solitary activities. Parallel play is when children play next to each other, which is the case with the two children making towers in the sandbox side-by-side. The other activities are done by themselves.

103. 3. School-age children (ages 6 to 10) begin to develop "chumships" with children in their age groups. These friendships take on great importance but don't yet totally eclipse the importance the children place on their relationships with parents, on whom they're still dependent for emotional well-being. School-age children usually are neither completely self-focused nor involved in intimate relationships with others. Adolescents struggle to find out what they believe and value and where they fit in among their peers and in the wider world. They're also involved with establishing intimate relationships that take on more and more importance as adolescence progresses.

104. 1. Developing fears regarding strangers and separation is a normal developmental characteristic for the infant over 6 months of age. The nurse can mitigate this response by speaking softly at the infant's eye level, maintaining a safe distance from the infant, and avoiding sudden intrusive gestures. A weight gain of 6 pounds since birth is too little at age 8 months; most infants double their birth weight by 6 months and triple birth weight by 12 months.

The Moro reflex (abducting extremities and fanning fingers when startled) should dissipate by age 3 to 6 months. At age 8 months, most infants can sit without support, bear weight on legs when supported, and may stand holding onto furniture.

105. **3.** A school-age child is capable of understanding reasons that cooperation is needed, so an honest, simple explanation is the best approach with this age group. Equating medication with candy is inappropriate because it may lead to the child seeking other medications that taste like candy, and bribing the child is also inappropriate because it teaches the child that acceptable behavior can be bought with special rewards. The child shouldn't be coerced into cooperating with a therapeutic regimen through the use of threats.

106. **2.** During the diagnostic period, the parents should report any instances of forceful vomiting and the actions that may have precipitated them. A 2-month-old infant shouldn't be fed cereal thickened with formula because it crowds out the nutrition that the infant should be receiving from breast milk or formula. The infant who may have pyloric stenosis should be positioned in a semi-sitting position to feed, and the parents shouldn't decrease or stop feedings until the immediate preoperative period.

107. **1.** Management of pain during sickle cell crisis is extremely important. Crisis pain is usually severe and often requires opioids. The nurse needs to administer opioids around the clock to help alleviate pain. Hydration is necessary to both prevent sickling and to mitigate crisis through adequate hemodilution; if necessary, an IV will be started to help with hydration during a crisis. During crisis, the child should be encouraged to rest in order to reduce the cellular metabolism that increases tissue hypoxia but not to put their extremities dependent. Daily oxygen isn't required as a preventive measure to avoid crisis, but the child shouldn't be in an environment that has low oxygen concentrations, such as areas of high altitude or nonpressurized aircraft.

108. **3.** Crush injuries can result in serum potassium excess (hyperkalemia with K+ over 5.5 mEq/L), which can result in ventricular fibrillation and cardiac arrest. Laryngospasm isn't directly related to a crush injury of the right leg, and tetany is a manifestation of hypocalcemia. Hyperthermia isn't related to a crush injury involving an extremity, but it may be related to an injury to the CNS.

109. **3.** Excessive oral drooling indicates an inability to swallow that may herald progressive airway obstruction, hypoxia, hypercapnia, and acidosis. The sound related to acute epiglottitis is a frog-like croaking sound on inspiration. Endotracheal intubation may be required to protect the airway. Inspiratory crackles over both lungs may indicate pulmonary infection but isn't as emergent a finding as excessive drooling. Purulent nasal secretions may indicate a bacterial infection but also isn't an emergent finding. A barking cough is associated with acute laryngotracheobronchitis.

110. **2.** Fruity breath is a symptom of hyperglycemia and ketoacidosis, not hypoglycemia. The other options correctly describe symptoms of hypoglycemia.

111. **4.** Weight loss is a classic sign of chronic renal failure. Reddish-brown urine is significant and could indicate an acute urinary tract infection or a side effect of a medication, but it isn't a sign of chronic renal failure. A yellowish cast to the palate and conjunctiva is indicative of a liver problem, such as hepatitis. Trouble initiating a urine stream indicates an obstructive problem in the bladder.

112. **2.** Buck's traction is skin traction, so the nurse needs to assess the skin for pressure. Site and pin care and prevention of infection have to do with skeletal traction. Choice (4) is also unrelated to Buck's traction.

113. **4.** The most serious complication of Guillain-Barré syndrome is respiratory failure, which occurs when paralysis progresses to the thoracic nerves. The other choices are major problems but aren't immediately life threatening.

114. **3.** Clubbed fingers is a thickening and flattening of the tips of the fingers and toes due to chronic tissue hypoxemia. Clubbing is commonly seen in infants and children who haven't been surgically treated for tetralogy of Fallot. Clubbing is due to decreased pulmonary blood flow to the lungs with a reduced amount of oxygenated blood returning to the left side of the heart and to the peripheral arterial circulation. The condition isn't a result of delayed physical growth, but delayed growth can result from the effects of the cardiac defect on the body. Clubbing also isn't a result of iron-deficiency anemia or an altered immune response.

115. **4.** Passage of a normal brown stool after diagnosis is established usually indicates that the intussusception has reduced itself. The patient should immediately report the passage to the healthcare provider who determines alterations in the medical regimen. Twenty-four hours without colicky pain doesn't indicate resolution of the condition because there may be periods when the child is comfortable but the intussusception is still present. Raisin-sized, jelly-like stools are a classic symptom that occurs later in the disease, and long, ribbon-like stools indicate an obstructive area beyond which the stool can't normally progress. Neither indicates resolution of the disease.

116. **2.** Hand-washing is the single most effective and critical measure in the prevention and control of hepatitis in any setting, including the home. Standard precautions are followed in the hospital, and children aren't placed in isolation unless they're fecally incontinent or their toys and other items are likely to be contaminated by feces. Standard precautions may include the use of gowns, goggles, gloves, and masks to prevent contamination from blood and/or all body fluids (excluding sweat), nonintact skin, and mucous membranes. The necessity of this equipment depends on judgment; for example, it isn't necessary for the nurse to wear a mask when caring for this child.

Testing all the children on the unit would not be necessary if standard precautions are maintained. The contagious period is for two weeks prior and one week after jaundice appears. Immunizing all children on the unit with HAV is unnecessary because the mode of transmission of hepatitis is the fecal-oral route, so other children would have to be in close contact with the infected child or his possessions in order to be infected.

117. **2.** Fat embolism is the greatest threat to an adolescent with a long bone fracture. Fat droplets from the marrow move to the circulation system, where they can go to the lungs or brain. This type of embolism generally occurs within first 24 hours postinjury. Malunion of bone isn't an issue in the first 24 to 72 hours. Avascular necrosis, which is cell death due to lack of circulation to an area, is usually seen after 72 hours and often occurs near joints. Osteomyelitis is a bone infection that can occur after a fracture. However, it generally develops after the first two to three days postinjury.

118. **3.** Ataxia is a sign of cerebellar malfunction. Periorbital edema isn't related to cerebellar brain tumor but may be seen in children who are in renal failure, or have other conditions such as brain infections/brain abcesses. Homonymous hemianopia is sometimes seen in post-CVA patients or patients with disorders affecting the occipital lobe of the brain. High-pitched cry isn't related to cerebellar brain tumor but is sometimes seen in infants with other neurological disorders.

119. **3.** Restraints should be avoided in patients who have head injuries with potential for increasing intracranial pressure because straining against restraints can increase ICP further. A GCS of 13 is within normal limits. HOB at 30 degrees is acceptable, and ICP at 12 is also within normal limits.

120. **2.** The lab values indicate respiratory acidosis. The oxygen saturation is only 87%, so oxygen isn't being adequately exchanged or distributed throughout the body. Carbonic acid is high, the pH is abnormally low, and bicarbonate is normal. In respiratory acidosis, bicarbonate is usually in normal range until the renal compensatory mechanism begins to operate. The patient doesn't have metabolic acidosis because there's no bicarbonate deficit. The compensatory response to metabolic acidosis is to increase carbon dioxide excretion by the lungs so that carbon dioxide is normal (uncompensated) or low (partially compensated). Excessive ingestion of antacids results in metabolic alkalosis, which produces a high bicarbonate value, a normal carbonic acid value (uncompensated), and a high carbonic acid (partially compensated). If the patient were in respiratory alkalosis, he would likely be hyperventilating, and the carbon dioxide value would be abnormally low. Because the carbon dioxide (carbonic acid) value is abnormally high, the patient has respiratory acidosis.

121. **4.** An electroencephalogram (EEG) records the electrical activity of the brain to evaluate seizure disorders, cerebral disease and CNS effects of systemic diseases, and brain death. EEG isn't used to diagnose myasthenia gravis disease, and it isn't the primary method of assessing pituitary tumors or diagnosing meningitis.

122. **2.** The high pressure alarm generally indicates a resistance in the system, usually related to a buildup of secretions. The nurse should oxygenate the patient and then suction. Alarms should never be reset or turned off without checking the nature of the problem. Loose connections are indicated by a low pressure alarm. The high pressure alarm doesn't indicate that arterial blood gases need to be drawn but rather that the system needs to be cleared of obstructive material.

123. **4.** Decreased urination is a sign of dehydration. Decreased blood pressure, tachycardia, and depressed anterior fontanel in an infant are also signs of dehydration.

124. **2.** Singed hair and a smoke-covered face or smoky breath indicates possible smoke inhalation with the potential for upper airway edema. The first priority is to establish and maintain an airway. Establishing an IV line and fluid replacement is the next priority. The need for administering tetanus prophylaxis must be evaluated by the care provider, and obtaining baseline laboratory studies should be done shortly after.

125. **2.** The lab that shows glomerulonephritis is the lab that shows recent streptococcal infection. All the other answers don't confirm the diagnosis.

126. **3.** Lyme disease isn't characterized by a fine rash on palms, soles, and extremities. It typically appears as a skin lesion occurring at the deer tick bite site. The red macule or papule expands to form a larger lesion with a red border and central clearing. Viral symptoms, headache, stiff neck, swollen lymph nodes, and muscle pain may also occur. Lyme disease can be prevented by avoiding heavily wooded areas where the infected deer tick may live and by using insect repellent. Deer ticks feed on mice, dogs, horses, deer, and humans. If not treated, Lyme disease can cause severe neurologic problems, facial paralysis, poor motor coordination, arthritis, and cardiac abnormalities.

127. **3, 4, 2, 1, and then 5.** The nurse should explain the procedure to the patient first. Suctioning is the next step to clear the airways. The cuff should be deflated before the patient is extubated, and oxygen should be ready for administering immediately after extubation.

128. **2.** The lab values indicate impaired gas exchange. The oxygen saturation is only 88%, so oxygen isn't being adequately exchanged or distributed throughout the body, indicating COPD. Carbonic acid is high, and the pH is abnormally low. The serum bicarbonate usually remains at normal levels until the renal compensatory mechanism begins to operate. If the

patient were hyperventilating, the carbon dioxide value would be abnormally low. Because the carbon dioxide (carbonic acid) value is abnormally high, the patient has respiratory acidosis. The patient also doesn't have a metabolic acidosis, which results in bicarbonate deficit. In addition, with metabolic acidosis, carbon dioxide is normal (uncompensated) or low (partially compensated). The compensatory response to metabolic acidosis is to increase carbon dioxide excretion by the lungs. Excessive ingestion of antacids would result in metabolic alkalosis, which would result in a high bicarbonate value, a normal carbonic acid value (uncompensated), or a high carbonic acid (partially compensated).

129. **3.** The high pressure alarm generally indicates a resistance in the system, usually related to a buildup of secretions. The nurse should oxygenate the patient and then suction. Alarms should never be turned off, and sighing the patient doesn't address the high pressure in the system. The nurse shouldn't waste time looking for the last set of lab values until a solution for the immediate problem is attempted. Asking the respiratory therapist to see the patient due to a high pressure alarm is unnecessary unless the nurse can't resolve the issue by suctioning the patient.

130. **4.** Of the options, the most important is establishing a communication system with the patient. Doing so helps to reduce patient anxiety and improves the management of the patient on a ventilator. Condensed moisture that has pooled in the tubing should never be drained toward the patient at the risk of causing water aspiration and potentially introducing microorganisms into the patient's respiratory tract. An increase in IV fluids may be ordered for the patient, depending on the patient's condition, but in this scenario, whether the patient is at risk for hypotension is unknown. Morphine isn't given when a patient is moving from a controlled mode to an SIMV mode on the ventilator. CMV takes over for the patient so that the patient has respirations without any initiation. SIMV also assists patients who can't breathe on their own.

131. **2.** Maintenance on ventilatory support can result in complications. Gastrointestinal ulcers are one common complication. Ventilator support in and of itself wouldn't cause the BUN and the creatinine to rise or cause PVCs or focal seizures.

132. **3.** The nurse should immediately obtain a pulse oximetry reading to determine oxygen saturation. Increasing the IV rate may be done after respiratory assessment is complete. Increasing the IV rate without the assessment could exacerbate conditions such as pulmonary edema. Increasing the oxygen rate must be discussed with the physician because an oxygen rate that's too high could exacerbate respiratory failure in a patient with chronic obstructive pulmonary disease. Checking the peripheral and other pulses doesn't address the issue.

133. **3.** The low pressure alarm signals a break somewhere in the ventilator-patient system. The first action the nurse should take is to check the integrity of the system, including the endotracheal tube cuff and all connections. The patient's blood pressure doesn't affect the low pressure alarm. If the patient needed to be suctioned, the high pressure alarm would sound. The level of humidification isn't related to low pressure in the system.

134. **1.** The correct method for using an inhaler is to exhale completely, insert the inhaler, and inhale the medication while dispensing the cartridge. The other options are ineffective and incorrect.

135. **3.** Stridor, or a crowing sound, is a sign that respirations are difficult for the patient. A respiratory rate of 20 is within the normal range. Hearing crackles bilaterally in the lungs is a sign of pneumonia or fluid overload. The of blood pressure of 130/88 is slightly elevated but not related to the airway being removed.

136. **4.** The first action the nurse should take when a patient complains of shortness of breath is to listen to the patient's breath sounds to ascertain the presence of abnormal sounds such as rhonchi, rales, or expiratory wheezing. After listening to breath sounds, the nurse should do further assessment, which includes vital signs, use of accessory muscles, retractions, and color of mucous membranes.

137. **1.** CD4+ T cell counts are an important tool to monitor the progression of HIV infection. As AIDS progresses, a decrease in the number of CD4+ T cells is a marker for decreased immune function. First, the EIA or ELISA tests are done to detect serum antibodies that bind to HIV antigens. If these tests are positive, then the Western blot (WB) test or immunofluoresecence assay (IFA) may be completed to validate a positive HIV diagnosis. Western blot uses purified HIV antigens electrophoresed on gels and incubated with serum samples from the patient. If antibody in the serum is present, this method detects it. IFA is used to identify HIV in infected cells. Blood is treated with a fluorescent antibody against p17 or p24 antigen and examined by fluorescent microscope. The EIA or ELISA, Western blot, and p24 aren't used to determine progression of HIV.

138. **3.** An exacerbation of rheumatoid arthritis (RA) includes fatigue and general limited joint function, usually occurring bilaterally. A unilaterally swollen weight-bearing joint is more characteristic of osteoarthritis. RA doesn't cause the erythrocyte sedimentation rate (ESR) to decrease; often the ESR is elevated, demonstrating an inflammatory response. Heberden's nodes on distal finger joints are indicative of osteoarthritis of the hands.

139. **4.** *Cryptosporidium muris* is an opportunistic illness that affects the GI tract of immune-suppressed patients, including those with HIV, causing watery diarrhea, abdominal pain, weight loss, and nausea. HIV patients are susceptible to conditions that can cause the other symptoms listed, however those symptoms aren't related to Cryptosporidium muris. For example, partial blindness may be caused by *cytomegalovirus* retinitis (CMV retinitis), herpes virus type I (HSV1), or varicella zoster virus (VZV) affecting the eye. Mental status changes may be caused by *Toxoplasma gondii*, JC papovirus, cryptococcal meningitis, CNS lymphomas, and AIDS-dementia complex (ADC). Productive cough may be caused by *Pneumocystis carinii*, *Histoplasma capsulatum*, *Mycobacterium tuberculosis*, *Coccidioides immitis*, or Kaposi's sarcoma.

140. **1.** Triggers of systemic lupus erythematosis (SLE) include fatigue, overexposure to the sun, emotional stress, infection, medications, and surgery. Vitamins, a high-protein diet, and mild exercise not leading to fatigue don't trigger exacerbation of SLE and may be protective.

141. **2.** *Mycobacterium avium* complex (MAC) is an opportunistic illness that affects the GI tract, causing watery diarrhea and weight loss. This organism can be found anywhere in the environment and in food and water. MAC affects immune-suppressed individuals. It's not found in birds, cat litter, or respiratory infections in children.

142. **4.** The person least likely to contract HIV is the 9-year-old child whose best friend is HIV positive. HIV infection isn't contracted through casual contact but rather is spread through infected body fluids that ultimately spread through the healthy person's vascular system. Examples of such fluids are breast milk, semen, blood, and blood products. The 4-month-old born to an HIV-infected mother is at high risk, as is the 17-year-old who has been receiving long-term treatment for hemophilia with blood products. The 16-year-old sexually active woman is also at high risk. Because she seeks to become a mother, she is not using birth control such as condoms, which are protective against the spread of HIV.

143. **3.** Bilaterally swollen joints that are painful on movement indicate an exacerbation of rheumatoid arthritis (RA). Accelerated pedal pulses and a normal heart rate are incorrect and unlikely. RA doesn't cause the erythrocyte sedimentation rate (ESR) to decrease; often, the ESR is elevated. Unilateral hip and groin pain lasting more than two hours may indicate a fractured or dislocated hip.

144. **1.** Fevers greater than 104 degrees Fahrenheit can cause delirium and seizures. The first action the nurse should take is to administer antipyretics to prevent acute elevation or swings in temperature. Exposing the skin to the air is a secondary measure that may follow medication. A sponge bath with iced water induces shivering and isn't therapeutic because shivering is a compensatory mechanism to restore body heat. Water used to induce evaporative heat loss and a hypothermia blanket may be helpful but should be given after administering the antipyretic.

145. **2.** The most important nursing diagnosis is related to the risk of bleeding due to thrombocytopenia. Fatigue, stomatitis, and body image are also related to the diagnosis of ALL and its therapies, but bleeding is the highest priority because of its effect on circulation, cardiovascular integrity, and oxygen-carrying hemoglobin.

146. **4.** Cyclosporine is an immunosuppressant used to prevent rejection of a transplanted organ while maintaining enough immunity to prevent infection. Zidovudine is used for treatment of HIV, and ceftriaxone is an antibiotic used for a variety of serious bacterial infections, including meningitis. Hydroxyzine is a medication with antihistamine properties used for mild sedation and to control nausea and vomiting.

147. **4.** Shortness of breath may indicate an allergic reaction, congestive heart failure, or cardiotoxicity. The other options are expected side effects of cancer chemotherapy.

148. **1, 2, 3, and 5.** Syndrome of inappropriate antidiuretic hormone, spinal cord compression, a calcium level of 12.5, and periorbital edema in the morning are all manifestations of oncological emergencies. The only listed choice that isn't one is diabetes insipidus, Choice (4).

149. **1.** Deep vein thrombosis is a serious side effect of tamoxifen, a medication used as a chemotherapeutic agent for breast cancer. None of the other choices are related to this medication.

150. **1, 4, 5.** Aphasia, headache, and blindness are symptoms related to cerebral tumors. The other answers are not related to cerebral tumors.

151. **4.** Sentinel node mapping is a procedure that helps track movement of cancer cells into lymph nodes using a blue dye. The other modalities don't represent node mapping; it isn't hormonal therapy, radiation seed treatment, or genetic testing.

152. **4.** Platelet count of 50,000/mm3 (or μl) indicates that the count is low due to the side effects of the bone marrow suppression caused by 5FU cancer chemotherapy. A low platelet count indicates the potential for bleeding. Hematocrit of 55% is high and may indicate dehydration, but that count isn't related to the medication. Agnosia and hypertension aren't related to the effects of 5FU.

153. **1.** A loose cotton bra prevents irritation in a patient who has undergone a lumpectomy and radiation. The patient should only use soaps and lotions that are permitted by the surgeon. Exposure to the sun should be avoided due to the effects of the radiation therapy, and the skin shouldn't be exposed to any extremes of hot or cold.

154. **4.** Stomatitis, or mouth ulcerations, is an early side effect of chemotherapy. The nurse should assess the client's mouth twice a day and give mouth care frequently. The client should use a soft toothbrush and avoid extremely hot or cold foods, spices, and all citrus juices. The weight loss and malnutrition associated with chemotherapy are long-term effects resulting from anorexia, nausea, and vomiting. Skin ulcerations aren't an early effect of chemotherapy.

155. **2.** A testicular self-exam should be performed once a month. Testicular cancer affects mostly young men between the ages of 15 and 34. Annual exams aren't performed often enough, and the exam should be done routinely, not just when discomfort is felt.

156. **3.** Allopurinol and vigorous hydration are part of the patient's treatment plan prior to vincristine therapy. The treatment plan reduces the risk of uric acid neuropathy because vincristine can be neurotoxic. Allopurinol doesn't change the effectiveness of vincristine. Chemotherapeutic medications help destroy rapidly multiplying cells, but allopurinol isn't an antineoplastic or chemotherapeutic agent and doesn't suppress the bone marrow.

157. **2.** A glycosylated hemoglobin level would provide information about the average blood glucose level over a two- to three-month period. Keeping a written record doesn't provide a reliable source of information on compliance over a two-month period. A postprandial blood glucose only gives information about blood sugar levels after one meal. A shopping receipt doesn't provide information about compliance over a two-month period.

158. **2.** Putting a large drop of blood on the test strip is necessary for proper interaction with chemicals on strip; the patient shouldn't smear the drop or allow his or her finger to touch the strip. Elevating the hand above the level of the heart before the procedure decreases blood flow to the fingers, soaking hands in cold water before the procedure causes vasoconstriction, and sticking the center of the phalanx is too painful.

159. **2.** Checking the blood glucose level frequently will indicate if the patient is hyperglycemic or hypoglycemic. Signs and symptoms of hyperglycemia (DKA) include dehydration, tachycardia, lethargy and weakness, confusion, abdominal pain, anorexia, nausea, and vomiting. Emotional and physical stress can increase blood glucose level, resulting in hyperglycemia. Even minor illnesses can cause hyperglycemia. Patients with hyperglycemia should continue with their regular meal plans if possible and increase the intake of noncaloric foods such as broth or water. If the illness causes the patient to eat less than normal, the patient should continue to take insulin or oral hypoglycemic medications as prescribed with carbohydrate-containing fluids. Insulin shouldn't be withheld automatically during times of illness, and physical activity shouldn't be increased with signs of illness or impending DKA. Eating foods high in simple sugars worsens the hyperglycemia. Symptoms of hypoglycemia (insulin reaction) include irritability, confusion, tremors, diaphoresis, hunger, weakness, and visual disturbances.

160. **3.** Sudden unconsciousness is usually related to hypoglycemia. In the event that the blood glucose can't be obtained immediately, the safest course of action is to inject glucagons to prevent cellular death. Administering glucagon reverses hypoglycemia and usually produces a quick improvement in the patient's level of consciousness. The family shouldn't inject regular insulin because the sliding scale isn't applicable unless the blood glucose is known and because doing so further compromises the patient if he's hypoglycemic. Fluids by mouth can't be given to an unconscious patient. The family should call 911 rather than take the patient to the hospital themselves.

161. **2.** The patient is hypoglycemic because peak for NPH is 4 p.m., between the client's meals. The onset of NPH insulin is 1 to 2 hours, peak is 4 to 12 hours, and duration is 8 to 18 hours (usually 12 hours). The patient's walk and nap aren't significant, and her breakfast food and the evening glass of wine don't impact her symptoms at 4 p.m. The fact that the patient takes her medication at 11 a.m. also isn't important.

162. **2.** A symptom of peripheral artery disease (PAD) is paresthesia of the lower extremity, especially the foot. The patient with numbness is unable to feel sharp and dull pressure. The leg appears pale and may be cool unless it's dangled, in which case the leg may become red. Pain relief generally isn't obtained by elevating the legs. Dangling the legs may be more effective, especially at night. Swelling of the foot is unrelated to PAD.

163. **3.** Symptoms of a vein thrombosis include a palpable, firm, subcutaneous cord-like vein, tenderness, redness, warmth, inflammation, induration, and venous distention. Pale, cold skin around the area indicates an arterial, not a venous, obstruction. Erratic, bounding pulse; tingling; and numbness are unrelated to a vein thrombosis.

164. **1.** The nurse should intervene if the student nurse places a pillow under the knee because this action increases the risk of clot formation in the affected extremity. Providing thigh-high or knee-high TED hose, administering continuous warm moist compresses, and measuring the circumference of the thigh in calves and recording it in the chart are all appropriate actions by the student nurse.

165. **2.** Rest pain occurs most often at night because cardiac output drops during sleep and the legs are at heart level. The patient may try to achieve partial pain relief by dangling the leg over the side of the bed to allow gravity to improve blood flow. Elevating the legs on a pillow actually reduces blood flow to the legs. Blankets aren't necessarily contraindicated, but keeping the legs warm doesn't improve circulation enough to reduce pain.

166. **3.** *Malpractice* is professional negligence compared to the actions of another professional in a similar situation. Malpractice is characterized by four elements: duty (professional relationship); failure to meet standard of care (breach of duty); harm, injury, or damage to the patient (harm); and harm that is a direct result of the nurse's failure to follow the standards of care (causation). *Battery* is the willful touching of a person that may or may not cause harm, *assault* is a threat or attempt to touch another person unjustly, and *libel* is false communication about another person by print, pictures, or the written word.

167. **2.** Consent for surgery must be signed before the patient receives any medication that depresses the central nervous system (CNS), thus impacting judgment and decision making. The other measures listed may be taken but don't need to be performed before administration of the sedating medication.

168. **4.** *Slander* is a false, spoken statement resulting in damage to a person's character or reputation. The nurse's action isn't a breach of duty because the action doesn't involve a standard of care, nor is it libel, which involves the written word. The action also isn't a violation of patient confidentiality because the nurse didn't share patient information.

169. **4.** Checking the apical pulse of a patient following a detected irregularity in the radial pulse is a complex task that requires the assessment skills of an RN. Checking the apical pulse may require problem-solving and intervention on a higher level. Transferring a patient isn't a complex task; it requires basic knowledge of how to use the mechanical lift and simple problem-solving skills. Although patient transfer has the potential to harm the patient if not done properly, this task is within the scope of practice for an unlicensed assistive personnel. Changing the bed sheets for a patient with an altered level of consciousness isn't a complex

task; although this action has the potential to cause harm if the assistant doesn't maintain ventilator connections, it's within the assistant's scope of practice and doesn't require complex decision making. Taking the temperature of a patient with TB is also within the unlicensed assistive personnel's scope of practice. Being in a negative pressure room requires basic knowledge of isolation precautions and isn't a complex task.

170. **3.** Demonstration with explanation is the safest way to assess the LPN's readiness to perform the task. The RN delegating care is responsible for the actions of the LPN and for ensuring the staff member's competency. Assigning the procedure to another staff member doesn't explore the LPN's knowledge deficit or concern about doing the procedure. This procedure is within the scope of practice for an LPN. Having the LPN read the procedure manual before performing the task doesn't ensure competency or safety for the patient and therefore is unsafe. A unlicensed assistive personnel shouldn't be asked to help the LPN because this task isn't within the unlicensed assistive personnel's scope of practice, and the assistant shouldn't be held responsible for the outcome of the task.

171. **1 and 4.** An unlicensed assistive personnel (UAP) can empty catheter bags of urine and ambulate a postoperative patient for the second day post-op. A UAP shouldn't be explaining what a myocardial infarction is, and starting IV fluids after the IV has been inserted isn't within this person's scope of practice, period.

172. **2.** A patient with an open wound or an incision shouldn't be in a room with a patient who has an infection. Putting a postsurgical patient with one who has an FUO is taking an unnecessary risk because the source of the fever is yet unknown and may negatively impact the health of the surgery patient. It's not important that roommates communicate. A surgical patient rooming with a ventilated patient or with a patient with a CVA isn't contra-indicated because the communicability of a disease isn't an issue. Bone cancer also isn't a communicable issue. Many patients are depressed, so rooming with a depressed or emotion-ally stressed patient isn't contraindicated unless the patient is a danger to himself/herself or others.

173. **3.** A myocardial infarction patient who's receiving alteplase for a clot to break-up is a priority. A heart failure patient who has furosemide ordered for 9 a.m. is not a priority. The atrial fib patient isn't high-risk enough to warrant the medication, so a call to the MD is required, and this patient isn't currently a priority. Cough is a normal side effect of captopril and doesn't constitute a priority in this case.

174. **1.** Addressing the behavior quickly and conducting a counseling session confidentially and in private with the employee are important responses by the manager. Ignoring lateness or absenteeism isn't prudent because they may be symptomatic of other issues and can nega-tively affect other employees. Other inappropriate actions include humiliating the employee with a remark intended to highlight the lateness and waiting for a yearly evaluation when steps can be taken much earlier to resolve the situation.

175. **3.** This patient should be assigned to a private room because contact precautions may need to be taken to protect susceptible patients in the semiprivate rooms from possible environmen-tal contact with body fluids infected with hepatitis A. An Alzheimer's patient may not be able to keep the bathroom environment clean or may not do a thorough hand-washing before touching environmental surfaces. The remaining patients, whether they're cancer patients, preoperative patients, or patients with minor infections who are bedfast, may be assigned to semiprivate rooms because their conditions carry no evidence of droplet, airborne, or contact issues requiring precautions.

176. **3.** Full, bounding pulses signal fluid volume excess; thready pulses indicate dehydration or fluid volume deficit. An excess in fluid volume causes tachycardia, not bradycardia, because the heart tries to keep up with the increasing volume. Pulse pressure (the difference between systolic and diastolic pressures) increases with fluid volume excess and decreases with fluid volume deficit. Paralytic ileus is unrelated to the signs of fluid volume excess.

177. **2.** Enteric formulas are usually hypertonic, which pulls fluid into the GI tract, resulting in intestinal cramping and diarrhea. The patient's high Fowler's position, vitamin and mineral intake from the formula, and the intermittent nature of the feeding aren't causative factors for diarrhea.

178. **3.** Type O Rh− blood can be used for all other blood types and is called the universal donor. The Rh negative factor matches the patient's blood. Blood type B and Rh+ aren't compatible with A−. Blood type B isn't compatible with A, and Rh+ isn't compatible with Rh−.

179. **1.** Distended neck veins and moist crackles are signs of fluid volume excess, whereas the other options aren't. Hypotension, dry skin, decreased urinary output, and thirst may indicate fluid volume deficit.

180. **4.** The lettuce salad with tofu, salmon, and milk contains more calcium than the other three choices. The milk and salmon are both calcium sources, and the tofu can be depending on how the manufacturer prepares it. In Choice (1), the only good source of calcium is the yogurt; in Choices (2) and (3), it's the rhubarb in the pie and the cheese in the sandwich, respectively.

181. **1.** Fluid volume deficit yields an increased pulse rate with a thready quality, decreased BP, and an increased rate and depth of respirations. It can be associated with fever. Dyspnea; pale, cool skin; pitting edema; headache; and changes in level of consciousness are related to fluid volume overload.

182. **3.** Placing the client in left side-lying position with the head lower than the feet is a position of safety. It would also help prevent an air embolism from traveling farther into the heart. Checking the tubing connections is something you do in this situation, but after you place the client in the proper position. Obtaining a blood glucose level would be a third priority, and reassuring the client that nothing is wrong is an inappropriate reaction to this situation.

183. **2.** Preferred areas for assessing turgor in the older patient are the forehead and the sternum because these areas don't have the normal decreases in skin elasticity that can mask skin turgor changes. The forearm is a preferred site for other age groups. The ankle and cheek aren't used for checking skin turgor because the ankle may accumulate fluid in the older adult and may not be a reliable source of information about turgor, and the cheek is subject to loss of elasticity due to exposure to the elements and aging.

184. **3.** Phosphate intake is restricted to less than 900 mg/day. Dairy products contain large amounts of phosphate and calcium. Therefore, dairy products should be restricted and replaced with other sources of calcium. The patient may take calcium supplements as well as phosphate-binders such as sevelamer, which doesn't contain calcium or aluminum. Calcium-based phosphate-binders such as calcium carbonate and calcium acetate are also used to bind phosphate, which is then excreted in the stool.

185. To take a carotid pulse, your fingers go on the side of the neck over the carotid artery.

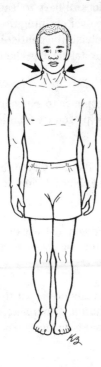

186. **1.** These symptoms indicate that ruptured membranes may be the cause. Lightening is when the fetal head has dropped into the true pelvis. Lightening occurs between the 36th and 40th week and indicates that the uterus has settled into the pelvis. Typical symptoms of lightening include urinary frequency and lower abdominal pressure. Ruptured membranes result in fluid being expelled. The fluid isn't always expelled quickly; it can be a slow leak. Urinary frequency isn't a usual symptom of ruptured membranes. Quickening occurs in the second trimester and occurs when fetal movements are detected. The patient's frequent urination doesn't indicate effacement, which is the thinning of the cervix and is a slow process that occurs in the last part of pregnancy into early labor. Effacement doesn't cause bladder pressure.

187. **4.** The newborn in Choice (4) has an Apgar score of 2, and a score between 0 and 3 requires full resuscitation and rescore at later intervals. The other choices have scores high enough not to require full intervention, though you would stimulate or rub the back of and administer oxygen to the newborn in Choice (2) because it scores a 4.

188. **2.** Shifting the woman to her left side takes pressure off the umbilical cord, which improves oxygenation to the fetus. Cesarean section isn't indicated for one episode of variable decelerations. Increasing the IV flow rate helps only if the mother is dehydrated and decreased cardiac output is causing fetal distress. Decelerations are due to hypoxia, and waiting for several hours can cause significant oxygen deprivation to the fetus.

189. **4.** The patient has developed uterine hypertonicity that has resulted in fetal distress. The oxytocin should be stopped. Putting oxygen on at 8 to 10 liters, obtaining vitals and the fetal heart rate, and documenting the signs and symptoms observed all come later.

190. **1, 2, 3, and 4.** Being a woman under the age of 19 is a predisposing condition for preeclampsia, as is having diabetic mellitus, a family history of gestational hypertension, and/or chronic renal disease. Epilepsy isn't related.

191. **1.** Folic acid should be increased prior to conception to lower the risk of neural tube defects, and prenatal vitamins help supplement the diet. The cat doesn't have to leave the home, but after the pregnancy is established, the partner should take over cleaning the litter box to avoid possible exposure to toxoplasmosis. The best time to visit the dentist is before a pregnancy, and a shield should be worn if dental X-rays are taken. The client should stop drinking alcohol immediately.

192. **4.** RhoGAM suppresses maternal antibodies produced in response to exposure to Rh+ red blood cells. RhoGAM doesn't affect iron studies, doesn't help produce fetal antibodies, and doesn't decrease maternal hemoglobin.

193. **3.** Orange juice enhances the absorption of iron, whereas milk of any type can inhibit the absorption of iron. Tea, even if decaffeinated, isn't the best choice. Water, although acceptable, isn't the best choice either.

194. **4.** A nonstress test is a measure of fetal well-being. A reactive nonstress test doesn't indicate potential complications, nor is it inconclusive. The fetal neurological system isn't measured by a nonstress test.

195. **3.** Ovulation can occur before menstrual periods return, usually no earlier than 27 days after delivery. This means that ovulation can occur before involution is complete, which is at about six weeks postdelivery and therefore may begin before four months postdelivery. Breastfeeding doesn't protect against conception.

196. **2.** Gentle pressure on the head prevents damage due to the change of pressure as it emerges. The patient's pushing at this point increases the potential for a traumatic birth; rapid expulsion of the infant could result in dural or subdural newborn tears and maternal lacerations. Pushing the baby's head back is contraindicated and may cause harm to the baby. Having the woman squat hastens a precipitous delivery and is contraindicated.

197. **2.** Naegele's rule is to determine the first day of the last normal menstrual period, count back three months, and add seven days plus one year. This calculation assumes that most women have a 28-day cycle and ovulate on the 14th day. February 11 is too early, and the April dates are too late.

198. **3.** The nurse's first action is to cause the uterus to contract and slow the bleeding. Manual massage should be initiated while help is arriving. In an emergency, the nurse should remain with the patient and call for help because the patient's safety is of highest priority. High Fowler's position doesn't slow postpartum hemorrhage and may contribute to hypotension. Oxygen is recommended, but it isn't the first priority. Urinary catheterization and increasing fluid rate may also be initiated but aren't top priority.

199. **1.** Bloody show may be present just before or during labor, not several days before labor begins. Backache often becomes more severe and continuous with labor. A weight loss of 0.5 to 1.5 kilograms occurs during labor due to electrolyte shifts and water loss, not prior to delivery. The mucous plug is often lost in the days before labor begins.

200. **1.** Chlamydia infections are destructive and can recur with exposure, so the partner must be treated to avoid reinfection. Younger clients are at greater risk than older clients, and chlamydia is usually asymptomatic in women.

201. **2.** Timing contractions from the beginning of one contraction to the beginning of the next indicates how many minutes apart they're occurring. Timing from the end of one contraction to the end of the next contraction doesn't yield information about how often contractions are occurring. Timing from the end of one contraction to the beginning of the next gives information about how long the uterus is in a relaxed state. Timing the length of a contraction is simply a measure of how long a contraction lasts.

202. **1.** After establishing respirations, warming the newborn to regulate thermoregulation is most critical to the newborn's survival. Monitoring the newborn's sensory functions is the nurse's next priority, and that's done as part of the newborn assessment in the nursery. The blood glucose level isn't routinely checked immediately after delivery. The newborn may be wiped off but shouldn't be washed right after delivery because vernix is protective.

203. **1.** The infant is getting enough milk if there are at least six to eight wet diapers per day. Newborns should have eight feedings per day and feed every four hours at night. Crying may or may not be related to adequacy of milk intake.

204. **4.** Explaining that the woman's outburst is an expected behavior takes the pressure off both the woman and her partner. Threatening the husband is unproductive and can lead to further problems. The coaching partner shouldn't leave while the patient is going through transition. Transition isn't an appropriate time to tell the patient that she's out of control; it's normal for women in transition to feel out of control briefly.

205. **3.** The fetus's heart rate should be immediately monitored after amniotomy. Determining pain level after amniotomy is unnecessary because the procedure doesn't normally cause pain. Vital signs aren't immediately required after the procedure. Although rupture of membranes can improve the labor process, the frequency of uterine contractions doesn't have to be monitored immediately after amniotomy.

206. **4.** The quantitative sweat chloride test is diagnostic for cystic fibrosis. Normal sweat chloride content is 30-59 mEq/L, and 60 mEq/L or greater is diagnostic of cystic fibrosis. Bone marrow aspiration isn't used to diagnose cystic fibrosis but rather to examine bone marrow for hematological abnormalities. Doctors use a lung scan to examine abnormalities in the lungs and a renal biopsy to diagnose abnormalities in the kidneys and ureters.

207. **3.** With an ileal conduit, the possible complications are pyelonephritis, as well as leakage at the anastomosis site, hydronephrosis, calculi, skin irritation and ulceration, and stomach defects. Being embarrassed about the appearance of the abdomen isn't a complication. Having a bowel movement in two to three days is normal for after having an ileal conduit surgery. Patients with ileal conduits don't self-catheterize; that happens with a Kock pouch.

208. **3.** A pneumothorax patient could have a tracheal deviation to one side. She would have absent breath sounds on the affected side and be hypotensive (not hypertensive) and tachycardic (not bradycardic).

209. **2.** The frontal lobe controls voluntary activity, concentration, motivation, ability to plan and problem solve, and aspects of personality. The temporal lobe controls hearing, the occipital lobe controls vision, and the cerebellum controls balance and gait.

210. **2.** Vertigo and tinnitus are symptoms of Ménière's disease. Discharge and ear pain are symptoms of acute otitis media, which is an acute infection of the middle ear. Fever isn't related to Ménière's disease, although the disease may cause headache. Enlarged lymph nodes and draining sinuses are indicative of sinusitis.

211. **4.** During infant CPR, the nurse uses the brachial pulse to assess for a pulse on an infant. The femoral pulse is used to assess circulation of the leg and may be used only if other pulses aren't palpable during cardiac arrest. The apical pulse or PMI is used for auscultation of heart sounds. The carotid pulse is used to assess the pulse of an adult during CPR. A child would have the pulse checked at the carotid or femoral during CPR.

212. **1.** Muscle cramps, fatigue, and hypotension are seen with hyponatremia in Addison's disease. Shortness of breath, pallor, hirsutism, rales, and maculopapular rash aren't characteristic of Addison's disease and hyponatremia. Hypertension, peripheral edema, and petechiae aren't indicative of Addison's disease.

213. **4.** Continuous bubbling in the water seal chamber indicates a leak in the drainage system that should be reported immediately. Continuous bubbling in the suction chamber is expected. Fluid fluctuating in the water seal chamber with the patient's respirations indicates that the drainage system is patent; absence of fluctuation indicates that the tubing is obstructed, a dependent loop has developed, the suction isn't working, or the lung has reexpanded. Serosanguinous drainage is expected after surgery; immediately post-op, more than 100 cc/hour of drainage is expected.

214. **2.** A cerebral infarct on the right side affects motor responses on the left side. The initial reflex response is hyporeflexia, which progresses to hyperreflexia. Right-sided weakness isn't seen because a lesion on one side of the brain affects motor function on the opposite (contralateral) side of the brain. Unequal pupils occur after an infarct; both pupils responding sluggishly indicate a central nervous system disorder or systemic effect of substances. Inability to distinguish words and letters is a symptoms of left sided cerebral infarct.

215. **4.** Burning and tingling may be the first sign of impaired circulation to the leg and foot and requires immediate follow-up. All other options are normal findings.

216. **2.** Fatigue, stress, or sudden exertion can bring about a relapse of SLE symptoms. NSAIDs may be prescribed for the treatment of pain or inflammation associated with lupus erythematosus. Citrus fruits and exposure to pets don't affect SLE.

217. **4.** Hepatitis A is spread via the oral-fecal route, not the airborne route; good hand-washing is critical to prevent the spread of the disease. It's spread by contaminated food and water, not by eating seafood. Isolating the patient doesn't prevent hepatitis A. This disease isn't spread by casual contact.

218. **1.** Coolness or blanching may indicate arterial obstruction. Pain at the insertion site and a small amount of drainage is expected after a cardiac catheterization using the right femoral artery. An IV that's 30 minutes behind isn't a high priority compared to the assessment finding.

219. **3.** This response by the nurse allows the patient to express her feelings and temporarily reduces stress. The effects of Bell's palsy can last several weeks to several months. Calling in a social worker passes responsibility on to another professional when the nurse can handle the issue. Advising the patient to wear dark glasses doesn't address her emotional distress.

220. **1, 2, 4, and 5.** Multiple sclerosis patients have bladder and bowel disturbances that include urgency frequency, retention, and incontinence. They experience blurred vision. Other symptoms are ataxia, vertigo, and dysphasia. Dyspnea isn't a symptom.

221. **1.** Patients with multiple sclerosis should cluster activities early in the day when their energy levels are higher and muscle fatigue is at a minimum. Later in the day, their energy levels are lower, and fatigue is more marked.

222. **1.** Patients who have difficulty understanding what's being said to them have receptive aphasia. Patients who have difficulty expressing themselves have expressive aphasia. If a patient doesn't recognize a number drawn on his hand, he has agraphesthesia. Agnosia is the inability to recognize common objects.

223. **3.** This patient is demonstrating signs of an evolving cerebrovascular accident (CVA). Timing is important in this case because she's only had symptoms for two hours. This patient may benefit from the administration of recombinant tissue plasminogen (tPA), which can lyse a thrombotic clot, thus preventing cell death in brain tissue. However, for maximum effect, this medication must be given within three hours of onset of symptoms. The other patients are in need of attention, especially the patient with the complex fracture, but the patient with the potential evolving CVA takes priority.

224. **3.** The nurse should intervene if a vest restraint has been applied because the patient can raise his intracranial pressure by resisting or straining against the restraint. The head of the bed may be at 30 degrees. An ICP of 16 mmHg is slightly elevated but not imminently a problem, and a GCS of 12 indicates possible moderate injury, but is unchanging.

225. **4.** The nurse should correct the statement that to prevent further urinary tract infections, the patient should wipe or clean herself from back to front. This information is incorrect because of the high risk of fecal contamination. All other measures are correct preventive measures for urinary tract infections (UTI).

226. **2.** If the client eats only one adequate meal each day, he will have a deficit of essential nutrients. Avoiding foods high in fat content and consuming large portions of foods containing fiber indicate that the client has good knowledge about nutrition. The client would need to eat three meals a day to get the right number of servings of all the food groups, not just more than one meal.

227. **4.** Weight-bearing exercise such as walking or swimming stimulates bone formation, and swimming also improves coordination, balance, and stamina. Taking a calcium dose of 300 milligrams is too little for a postmenopausal woman, who should have 1,200 milligrams daily. Aluminum-containing antacids interfere with bone formation, and high protein intake isn't directly related to bone formation.

228. **2.** Expressive aphasia occurs after a stroke or other compromising event and is an inability to speak. Expressive aphasia isn't related to hemiplegia (paralysis on one side of the body). Expressive aphasia doesn't necessarily result in a patient becoming wheelchair-bound, nor is it related to urinary incontinence.

229. **3.** Aging is related to a decrease in depth perception. Aging isn't related to an increase in peripheral vision or color perception. The pupil of the eye dilates more slowly in low light as a person ages.

230. **2.** The most important assessment the nurse should make after major abdominal surgery is the rigidity of the abdomen. A rigid abdomen can be a sign of internal bleeding. Blood saturation of the dressings, mobility issues, and the psychological impact of the surgery are important but secondary to monitoring for potential hemorrhage.

231. **4.** Each egg yolk contains about 184 milligrams of cholesterol. Oatmeal contains little or no cholesterol. One cup of skim milk contains about 4 milligrams of cholesterol, and two slices of bologna contain about 31 milligrams of cholesterol.

232. **3.** Chicken fingers facilitate feeding oneself because they're easy to handle and manipulate. A hamburger on a bun may be too difficult for the patient to eat effectively unless it's cut into smaller pieces. A patient who's confused may have difficulty using utensils; therefore, beef stew and tuna casserole may be harder for the patient to eat than foods that are easily moved from hand to mouth. Patients who feel overwhelmed by the task of eating may refuse to eat.

233. **4.** A medium raw apple with skin has 2.4 g of fiber per 100 g of edible portion. Raw pineapple has 1.4 g of fiber per 100 g of edible portion. Red cherries have 1.6 g of fiber. Bananas win with 2.6 g of fiber per 100 g of edible portion.

234. **2.** An English muffin with cream cheese constitutes part of an acceptable breakfast because Orthodox Jewish dietary law prohibits milk products and meat combined in the same meal. If the meal contains meat, milk products may be eaten before but not with the meal. Fish is allowed only if it has scales and fins. Shellfish isn't permitted, so the nurse shouldn't give the patient shrimp. Chicken soup may not be eaten with butter, and cheese can't be eaten with meat. Ham isn't permitted because it's derived from the pig, the consumption of which is prohibited.

235. **3.** The main reason for obesity is caloric intake that supersedes energy expenditure. The patient may have a low basal metabolic rate, hormonal influences, and psychological issues surrounding food, but these are factors that contribute to the inefficient use of calories or excessive intake of calories.

236. **2.** Each cup of legumes has about 8 grams of protein, 1 cup of cooked rice has about 5 grams of protein, and 1 cup of cooked eggplant has 1 gram of protein for a total of about 14 grams. People on a vegan diet don't eat any foods that originate with an animal or animal product. Although blueberries are acceptable, yogurt isn't because its source is the cow. One tablespoon of peanut butter has 5 grams of protein, two slices of bread have 4 to 6 grams of protein, and jelly has no protein, for a total of 11 grams of protein. Crackers are acceptable, but cheddar cheese isn't because of its animal origin.

237. **3.** Fortified milk contains 40 IUs (international units) of vitamin D per 100 grams of edible food. Beef liver contains 16 IUs. Green, leafy vegetables and shredded wheat don't contain measurable amounts of vitamin D.

238. **4.** Low serum protein may be detected through serum albumin testing. Normal range for albumin is 3.5 to 5.0 mg/dl. Serum albumin has limitations in that it lags behind actual protein changes by more than two weeks. Hematocrit is the ratio of red blood cells to plasma, and a normal range for a male is 40% to 54%. A high hematocrit may indicate dehydration. Blood urea nitrogen (BUN) is diagnostic of renal problems and indicates the concentration of urea in the blood and the kidneys' ability to clear the urea. Normal range for BUN is 10 to 30 mg/dl. Serum creatinine indicates efficacy of renal function by examining the kidneys' ability to clear the end products of muscle and protein metabolism; normal range is 0.5 to 1.5 mg/dl.

239. **1.** Clear chicken broth is considered a "clear" liquid because such diets are composed chiefly of water and carbohydrates. Vegetable juice, soy milk, and vanilla custard aren't clear fluids but rather are full fluids.

240. **3.** In the first 24 hours post-burn, serum potassium is elevated due to oliguria and tissue destruction. After the initial phase, during the diuretic phase, sodium shifts back from the interstitial compartment to the intravascular compartment, and the patient may develop hypokalemia. Profuse sweating causes hypokalemia in this situation because sweat contains water, potassium, sodium chloride, glucose, urea, and lactate. Gastrointestinal fluids are high in potassium, so vomiting and diarrhea also cause hypokalemia.

241. **2.** Complications of paracentesis include hypotension, tachycardia, and pallor due to hypovolemic shock from fluid shifts. Measuring weight and abdominal girth and assessing pain aren't immediate priorities.

242. **3.** This response by the nurse demonstrates empathy and reflects the patient's feelings; it opens channels of communication. Admonishing the woman about opening the door just reinforces guilt and negative feelings. Telling the woman not to worry offers reassurances that may not be real because the nurse has no way of knowing the parents' reactions. Telling the woman not to think about what happened dismisses the woman's anxiety and pain.

243. **4.** This response by the nurse offers an explanation and orients the patient to reality. Asking for a description encourages the hallucination, as does telling the patient that the spiders are harmless. Dismissing the hallucination doesn't offer the patient any reassurance about what's happening.

244. **4.** Reporting suspected child abuse immediately is state law. Waiting for validation from colleagues violates the law and wastes time. Documenting concerns but not reporting the case also violates state law. Discussing the suspicion with the people who may be participating in the abuse is inappropriate.

245. **2.** The nurse should remove the patient from the room immediately. The RACE acronym is rescue, alarm, contain, and extinguish; these actions should be done in that order. Running to pull the alarm, trying to extinguish the fire, and containing the fire aren't the first actions to take.

246. **3.** The most important assessment is the safety of the home environment. The patient's mobility, family support, and the ability to contribute to the care plan are issues secondary to safety. Adaptations may be made to address these secondary factors, but safety must be ascertained before all else.

247. **4.** When administering TPN, a nurse must use strict aseptic (sterile) technique to prevent infection at the IV catheter insertion site; infection could cause sepsis in a vulnerable patient. Taking fluids by mouth every day wouldn't prevent infection in the patient and may be contraindicated depending on the condition or illness of the child. Monitoring the BUN and blood sugar isn't a preventive measure against infection but provides useful information about the efficacy of the TPN formula. Maintaining strict intake and output records is necessary for the patient who's receiving TPN, but this monitoring also doesn't prevent infection.

248. **3.** Health screening is an example of a secondary healthcare service. Helping to restore function after a stroke is an example of tertiary care. Giving immunizations and teaching about hand-washing are examples of primary prevention and care.

249. **1.** Vitamin K plays an essential role in the production of clotting factors II, VII, IX, and X. Lack of this vitamin can lead to bleeding. Night blindness is a result of vitamin A deficiency, muscle weakness is related to a deficiency in thiamin, and bone loss may be related to calcium deficiency.

250. **3.** The nurse must notify the surgeon immediately because the clear fluid indicates that cerebrospinal fluid is leaking from the surgical site. This is a finding that must be assessed by the surgeon. Reinforcing the dressing, marking the saturation, and placing the patient in semi-Fowler's position don't stop the leakage of CSF and the potential hazards related to it.

Answer Key

1. 2, 3, 5	34. 3	67. 1, 2, 4, 5	100. 2
2. 3	35. 3	68. 2	101. 3
3. 1	36. 4	69. 3	102. 3
4. 1	37. 4	70. 1	103. 3
5. 3	38. 3	71. 4	104. 1
6. 2	39. 1	72. 1	105. 3
7. 3, 5	40. 3	73. 1	106. 2
8. 4	41. 1	74. 3	107. 1
9. 1, 2, 3, 4	42. 4	75. 3	108. 3
10. 1	43. 4	76. 3	109. 3
11. 3	44. 4	77. 2	110. 2
12. 2	45. 2, 4, 5	78. 4	111. 4
13. 1, 2, 4, 5	46. 3	79. 2	112. 2
14. 1	47. 1, 3, 4	80. 4	113. 4
15. 3	48. 3	81. 1	114. 3
16. 2	49. 2	82. 4	115. 4
17. 1, 2, 4, 5	50. 1, 2, 5	83. 3	116. 2
18. 4	51. 1	84. 3	117. 2
19. 3	52. 2	85. 4	118. 3
20. 1	53. 4	86. 4	119. 3
21. 1	54. 3	87. 4	120. 2
22. 4	55. 3	88. 2	121. 4
23. 3	56. 4	89. 1	122. 2
24. 1	57. 3	90. 3	123. 4
25. 2	58. 2	91. 2	124. 2
26. 3	59. 1	92. 4	125. 2
27. 4	60. 4	93. 1, 2, 3, 5	126. 3
28. 2	61. 1	94. 1	127. 3, 4, 2, 1, 5
29. 1	62. 4	95. 3	128. 2
30. 4	63. 3	96. 2	129. 3
31. 1	64. 4	97. 1	130. 4
32. 4	65. 4	98. 3	131. 2
33. 1, 2, 4	66. 3	99. 3	132. 3

133. 3	163. 3	191. 1	221. 1
134. 1	164. 1	192. 4	222. 1
135. 3	165. 2	193. 3	223. 3
136. 4	166. 3	194. 4	224. 3
137. 1	167. 2	195. 3	225. 4
138. 3	168. 4	196. 2	226. 2
139. 4	169. 4	197. 2	227. 4
140. 1	170. 3	198. 3	228. 2
141. 2	171. 1, 4	199. 1	229. 3
142. 4	172. 2	200. 1	230. 2
143. 3	173. 3	201. 2	231. 4
144. 1	174. 1	202. 1	232. 3
145. 2	175. 3	203. 1	233. 4
146. 4	176. 3	204. 4	234. 2
147. 4	177. 2	205. 3	235. 3
148. 1, 2, 3, 5	178. 3	206. 4	236. 2
149. 1	179. 1	207. 3	237. 3
150. 1, 4, 5	180. 4	208. 3	238. 4
151. 4	181. 1	209. 2	239. 1
152. 4	182. 3	210. 2	240. 3
153. 1	183. 2	211. 4	241. 2
154. 4	184. 3	212. 1	242. 3
155. 2	185. **See answer explanation earlier in this chapter.**	213. 4	243. 4
156. 3		214. 2	244. 4
157. 2		215. 4	245. 2
158. 2	186. 1	216. 2	246. 3
159. 2	187. 4	217. 4	247. 4
160. 3	188. 2	218. 1	248. 3
161. 2	189. 4	219. 3	249. 1
162. 2	190. 1, 2, 3, 4	220. 1, 2, 4, 5	250. 3

4

The Part of Tens

Chapter **15**

Ten Myths about the NCLEX-RN

D id you hear that more people pass the NCLEX-RN on Thursdays than on Fridays? Did you know that you don't stand a chance of passing if your name has an *R* in it? These are just a few of the wild — and false — rumors and myths that surround the NCLEX-RN. In this chapter, I tell you the whole truth and nothing but the truth about some of the rumors you're sure to hear about the exam.

Length Matters

More people agonize over when the test "shuts off" than any other topic concerning the NCLEX-RN. Rumor says that if your test stops at 75 questions, you've passed, and if you get 265 questions, you've failed. (You may also hear the reverse — fewer questions equal failure and more questions equal passing.)

The truth is that the length of your test has nothing to do with whether you pass or fail. The number of questions you get is based on how you answer the questions. If you answered correctly, a harder question is given to you. If you answer incorrectly, an easier question is given to you.

The NCLEX-RN uses a program called Computer Adaptive Testing (CAT), which assesses a test taker's abilities (as in whether you can answer difficult questions correctly or only simple ones) based on his or her answers to exam questions and searches its bank of test questions for questions that are equal to the test taker's abilities. The fact that the NCLEX-RN uses CAT means that, depending on your performance, you may answer fewer questions than you'd have to answer on other types of tests that determine your knowledge of safe and effective nursing care.

Although the exam doesn't have a time limit for each question, keep a steady pace and try to spend about one minute on each question.

Every Question Counts

This point may sound like a reasonable assumption for any exam, but for the NCLEX-RN, it's false. The NCLEX-RN uses you as a guinea pig to try out new questions that aren't yet part of the scored test. Each candidate's exam contains up to 15 experimental questions, but, tricky devils that they are, the exam folks don't tell you which ones are the experimental items. So despite the myth, treat every question as if it counts, even though it really may not, to be on the safe side.

Computer Savvy Is Essential

You don't have to be a computer whiz to take the NCLEX-RN. When you show up for the exam, the test administrator conducts an orientation, and you work through a tutorial that explains how to use the keys and how to record your answers. (When taking the exam, you only use two keys: the space bar to move the cursor and the Enter key to highlight and lock in your answer.) The tutorial also covers how to respond to questions that may use a format other than multiple choice. (See Chapter 3 for more about the different types of questions on the exam.)

REMEMBER

You're allowed to ask the test administrator for help if you have trouble with the computer during the test.

You Can't Stop 'til You're Done

After you sit down at the computer to take the NCLEX-RN, two breaks are prescheduled. The first break comes after 2 hours of testing, and the second break comes after 3.5 hours of testing. (You have up to 6 hours to take the test, though most test takers finish in 2.) The computer even tells you when you can take a break, so all you have to do is focus on the test.

TIP

Taking a break at prearranged times or at times you choose, counts against your testing time, so don't overdo it. But if you need a quick breath of fresh air and a stretch, a few minutes away from the test may be worth it. Clearing your head and relaxing your body may be just what you need to keep your momentum going, your brain sharp, and your anxiety at bay.

You take breaks outside the testing room, and the test administrator makes sure you follow all the rules and get back to your test without any problems.

The Test Plays Off Your Weakness

The NCLEX-RN isn't out to get you. When you answer a question incorrectly, the computer automatically chooses an easier question for you to answer. If you answer that question correctly, it chooses a slightly more difficult question. Throughout the exam, the computer gives you questions based on your answer to a previous question's difficulty level. What the computer is trying to establish is your competence level, or ability to correctly answer approximately 50 percent of the questions you're given, which means you need to be above the passing standard consistently to show competency. The computer is able to establish your competence level after a minimum number of questions. It then compares your competence level to the passing standard competence level and makes one of the following assessments:

» You're above the passing standard. You pass, and the test ends.

» You're below the passing standard. You fail, and the test ends.

» You're close to the passing standard, but it's still not clear whether you should pass or fail. You continue answering questions until either the computer can make the determination of whether you should pass or fail or the time runs out.

The NCLEX-RN tries to give you every opportunity to demonstrate that you have the knowledge, judgment, and skill to get that license. This type of testing actually improves your chances of demonstrating a passing score.

You Have to Wait Eons to Retake a Failed Test

The waiting period for retesting is 45 days. This period gives you enough time to continue studying and reviewing, but you don't have to wait so long that the knowledge you have becomes obsolete.

If you fail the exam at any point, the state's board of nursing sends you a Candidate Performance Report (CPR). This report summarizes your strengths and weaknesses based on the NCLEX-RN test plan, breaking down whether you were above, near, or below passing standard in a given area. (The preceding section explains what these standards mean.) This information is very helpful because it lets you know exactly what you need to study so that you don't waste precious time studying what you already can demonstrate knowledge of.

Your First Instinct Is Probably Wrong

The NCLEX-RN doesn't allow you to go back and review the questions you've already answered. When you submit an answer, it's gone forever. The ability to only move forward prevents that pitfall of reconsidering and changing your answers and, in the process, losing precious time.

The questions are presented one at a time, and you can review each one for as long as you want before you submit your answer. You must confirm your submission before you can go on to the next question, so you can be sure of your choice.

REMEMBER

You can change your answer before you submit it, but keep in mind that you're most likely to choose the correct answer right off the bat because you make the choice calmly and rationally. When you change your answers, you're second-guessing yourself, which leads to uncertainty and doubt that just balloons until you aren't sure about anything anymore. That's definitely not a good way to make a correct decision. So read the question, find your keywords (see Chapter 4), analyze your answers, and then choose your answer based on what you see in the question and know about the content being tested. If you're having a "could-be" or "might-be" conversation with yourself, move on and leave your first answer as it is.

The Same Question Popped Up Twice

The NCLEX-RN doesn't contain repeat questions, so you won't see the same question more than once. You may receive a question that contains similar symptoms or diseases to another question but actually addresses a different area of the nursing process.

Don't assume that you receive a similar question because you answered a previous question incorrectly. As I note in the earlier section "Every Question Counts," some items on the test are trial questions. Seeing two similar questions may (or may not) indicate you've gotten one of those experimental items. Always choose the best answer for each question; don't select an answer based on information you may have seen in a previous question.

Your Test Schedule Chooses You

You can choose not only your test date but also the time you want to take your test. This control gives you the upper hand in scheduling yourself for success. After you receive your Authorization to Test (ATT) from the board of nursing in the state in which you're taking your exam, you can schedule your test date and time. Don't wait to schedule, though, because the longer you wait, the less likely you are to get the schedule you want.

If you're a first-time test taker, you're offered an appointment within 30 days; if you're a repeat test taker, you will be offered an appointment after 45 days. You may choose to make an appointment later than what you're offered, but make sure you stay within your ATT time frame when you schedule. Otherwise, you lose that attempt. By choosing your own test schedule, you ensure that the day of your test doesn't conflict with anything else you may have scheduled.

REMEMBER

Schedule your test so that you have a six-hour window. Keep in mind that the NCLEX-RN session can last up to six hours (including orientation).

Choice (3) Is the Magic Answer, and Other Multiple-Choice Fails

Conventional wisdom claims that multiple-choice tests use Choice (C) as a correct answer more than any other answer choice. In the language of the NCLEX-RN, Choice (C) translates to Choice (3), but the fact remains that the correct answers don't follow any particular pattern. The chance of the correct answer to any NCLEX-RN question being Choice (3) is no better than the correct answer being Choice (1), Choice (2), or Choice (4).

Another trap: When test takers don't know the answer to a question, they tend to choose the answer option that they know nothing about. They assume that if they don't know what it is, it must be the right answer. Nothing could be more incorrect. If you can't determine the correct answer, your best option is to choose an answer option that you know something about. When you're unsure of the correct choice, choosing something you know is an educated guess, and it may be correct.

Chapter **16**

Ten Common Phrases Found in NCLEX-RN Questions

This book is full of techniques to help you do your best on the NCLEX-RN. One of the best ways to prepare for the test is to answer as many questions as you can; that's why I include so many sample questions throughout this book. Whether you work your way through this entire book or just pop in and out, you'll probably notice that the test has a language all its own. Understanding the language will make you much more successful on the test. In this chapter, I help you speak NCLEX by reviewing ten phrases most likely to appear in NCLEX-RN questions. I tell you how to find the real question behind the question and provide example questions with answers and explanations.

As with many exams, answering NCLEX-RN questions correctly isn't always as easy as it seems. Sometimes figuring out exactly what the question is asking can be difficult, which is why the first step is to find the keywords as I discuss in Chapter 4. Keeping an eye out for certain phrases that alert you to the keywords of a question can help you identify how to answer it successfully. These phrases usually relate to one of the five steps of the nursing process. In this chapter, I cover all the steps and describe common uses of the phrases that you'll see on the test. (Chapter 4 also has details on the nursing process.)

Assessment and Priority

The first stage of the nursing process is always assessment. Common questions related to the assessment phase of the nursing process may require you to set priorities when performing patient assessments. Questions may ask which assessment is most important, has the highest priority, or is the priority for a particular client. These kinds of questions are likely to start with or include the phrases *Which priority assessment* or *Who would the RN see first.* The latter is a priority assessment of which client is in the most life-threatening condition.

EXAMPLE

A nurse is caring for a client who has just had elective nasal surgery for a deviated septum. Immediately after the surgery, the nurse performs which priority assessment?

(1) Measuring intake and output

(2) Determining the client's pain level

(3) Checking for impaired swallowing

(4) Assessing respiratory status

The correct answer is Choice (4). The biggest keywords here are *nasal surgery, highest priority,* and *immediately after surgery.* When answering questions about priority assessments, remember that more than one answer option may be correct. In this question, all the options are assessments that should be performed immediately post-op nasal surgery. But the question asks which assessment assumes the highest priority, and for priorities you need to remember that life-threatening issues are the priority in every case. As a result of the nasal packing and edema of the airway, the nurse should carefully assess for signs of respiratory compromise. Nasal packing may also dislodge, resulting in obstruction of the airway.

EXAMPLE

A client with an acute gastrointestinal bleed is receiving an intravenous infusion of packed red blood cells and normal saline solution. Which nursing assessment would assume the highest priority?

(1) Level of consciousness

(2) Fluid balance/intake and output

(3) Signs of anaphylactic reaction

(4) Pain assessment

The correct answer is Choice (3). Again, focus on the phrase *highest priority* as a keyword. It tells you that more than one option is probably correct. Ask yourself

>> What's the key concept of the question?

>> What's the most life-threatening problem I'm assessing the patient for?

During a blood transfusion, a transfusion reaction can be life threatening. Therefore, the priority assessment is to check for signs and symptoms of an allergic/anaphylactic reaction, which may include pruritis (itching), urticaria (hives), facial edema or edema of the epiglottis, fever, chills, low back pain, dyspnea, and shock. If a reaction occurs, the nurse must immediately stop the transfusion, leave the intravenous line intact, and notify the physician. Although it's a concern during a blood transfusion, fluid balance isn't as immediately life threatening as an anaphylactic reaction. Level of consciousness should be assessed in any patient with a gastrointestinal bleed because a change may indicate the development of shock. However, it doesn't directly relate to a blood transfusion. Pain assessment isn't a concern for this client.

Diagnosis

Questions relating to the nursing diagnosis step of the nursing process usually present information about a patient situation and ask you to identify an appropriate nursing diagnosis or the priority diagnosis. In order to make any kind of diagnosis, you need to

» Organize the data that you're given

» Analyze the data

» Determine what you feel is the highest priority in terms of nursing care

These kinds of questions are likely to ask *Which nursing diagnosis is the most appropriate?*

EXAMPLE

A client with a newly created colostomy has verbalized to the nurse that he thinks the opening in his abdomen is disgusting and he doesn't want to look at it. Which nursing diagnosis would be most appropriate?

(1) Knowledge deficit related to the care of a stoma

(2) Disturbed personal identity related to change in appearance

(3) Disturbed body image related to colon surgery

(4) Hopelessness related to irreversible changes in body functioning

The correct answer is Choice (3). Organize the data (new colostomy, client's feelings about the stoma, refusal to look at it) in the keywords. Then analyze that information and determine what the priority concern is. In this case, the primary concern is that the patient has verbalized negative feelings about his stoma in terms of how it looks. Therefore, the priority nursing diagnosis is disturbed body image. The client's feelings aren't related to a knowledge deficit but rather to a permanent change in physical appearance. Hopelessness may be an issue, but the question contains no data to support this diagnosis. Disturbed personal identity relates to a client's inability to distinguish between self and nonself.

Planning and Assigning Care

Many exam questions address your ability to plan patient care that meets all the patient's needs. Common questions pertaining to the planning step of the nursing process may address one of the following topics:

» Planning for delegation of tasks

» Developing patient teaching plans

» Formulating patient outcomes/goals

Questions on planning for delegation of tasks may include phrases such as *The nurse is assigning care, The patient understands teaching by,* or *A goal for this patient is.*

EXAMPLE

A nurse is assigning the care of a patient with a modified radical mastectomy to a unlicensed assistive personnel (UAP). Which intervention can't be delegated to the UAP?

(1) Collecting a clean catch urine specimen and sending it to the lab

(2) Emptying the patient's Foley catheter and recording output

(3) Assisting the patient out of bed and into the chair on the first day post-op

(4) Assessing the operative site for drainage

The correct answer is Choice (4). When answering questions about delegating care, first look at who the care is being delegated to and consider what that person is qualified to do. The Nurse Practice Act and individual hospital policy define and limit the scope of nursing practice, but generally, unlicensed personnel aren't permitted to perform patient assessments, administer medications, or perform medical treatments. Unlicensed assistive personnel can perform activities such as ambulation, positioning of patients, bathing, hygiene measures, and collection of some urine and stool specimens. In this question, assessment of the operative site for drainage is a nursing responsibility and therefore can't be delegated. The other activities can safely be performed by the UAP, but the nurse is accountable for the assistant's activities.

The Teaching Plan

Nurses are teachers; making sure that patients understand their care is an important part of nursing. Questions pertaining to patient teaching may be worded something like *Which instructions would the nurse include in the teaching plan?*

EXAMPLE

The nurse is preparing for the discharge of a toddler admitted with nephrotic syndrome. Which instructions would the nurse include in the teaching plan for the parents?

(1) "Call the physician if the child has an increase in urine output."

(2) "Keep the child away from others with infections."

(3) "Administer antipyretic medication as ordered."

(4) "Assess urine specific gravity every day."

The correct answer is Choice (2). Find who the client is, the condition, and what the question is wanting, in this case teaching plans. When answering questions about teaching plans, think about what you know about the patient's condition and incorporate this information into the teaching plan. The child recovering from nephrotic syndrome should be protected from infection. The physician should be notified if the child has a decrease, not an increase, in urine output. Specific gravity assessments aren't appropriate for a child being discharged to home, and antipyretic medication isn't indicated.

Outcomes and Goals

As a nurse, you need to know why you perform specific nursing interventions. In other words, what are you expecting to happen when you do certain things? These expectations are called *expected outcomes and goals.* NCLEX-RN questions on planning patient outcomes and formulating goals may contain the phrase *Which would be an expected outcome.* An easy way to understand this concept is to think about the expected outcome of taking, say, cold medication. If you take one of those fizzy tablets, for example, you probably expect not to have a cold anymore, or be able to breathe freely.

EXAMPLE

The nurse is planning care for a patient admitted with bacterial pneumonia. Which would be an appropriate expected outcome for the patient?

(1) The patient performs activities of daily living without dyspnea.

(2) The patient expectorates a moderate amount of yellow sputum.

(3) The patient's white blood count (WBC) is 14,000 cells/mm³.

(4) The patient's urine output is greater than 30 ml/hr.

The correct answer is Choice (1). When formulating outcomes, first consider the patient and his or her condition. Figure out what the nursing or medical diagnosis is, and then ask yourself, "How will I know the patient is getting better?" An appropriate expected outcome

>> Is observable and measurable

>> Specifically addresses the patient's nursing or medical diagnosis

In this question, it's evident that a patient with bacterial pneumonia is getting better when he or she can ambulate and perform activities of daily living without being short of breath. This activity is an observable, measurable goal that specifically addresses the patient's condition. Expectorating a moderate amount of yellow sputum indicates that the disease process isn't resolving. A white blood count of 14,000 is elevated (normal is 4,500 to 11,000 cells/mm³) and indicates an infection. Although a urine output of greater than 30 ml/hr is within normal limits, it doesn't specifically address the patient's pneumonia.

Best Response

The implementation step of the nursing process refers to how the nurse carries out nursing actions. Common questions pertaining to the implementation step of the nursing process may ask you to

>> Identify the nurse's best or most therapeutic response in a certain situation

>> Identify the nurse's immediate or priority action

>> Identify the appropriate nursing interventions for a specific disease or condition

Implementation questions may employ the phrase *Which would be the nurse's best response?*

EXAMPLE

A client who has been hospitalized frequently for major depression tells the nurse, "I don't understand why I get so depressed." Which would be the nurse's best response?

(1) "I'm sure you'll improve with the right medication."

(2) "Would you like to talk about the reasons you're depressed?"

(3) "This must be very upsetting to you."

(4) "Your depression is most likely caused by a chemical imbalance in the brain."

The correct answer is Choice (4). In answering implementation questions, carefully consider all the responses to determine which one contains accurate information and is therapeutic for the client. In this situation, the best response acknowledges that depression has a biochemical basis. Stating that the client will improve with medication or is upset doesn't address the client's immediate concern about the cause of his depression. "Asking about whether or not the client wants to talk is a closed-ended question, and does not respond appropriately to the client's concern."

REMEMBER

This situation is where you want the client to talk about his feelings or emotions. When you see this type of question, use therapeutic communication techniques such as

>> **Reflecting:** Directing the client's question back to client

>> **Restating:** Repeating what the client has said

>> **Using silence:** Allowing time for formulating thoughts

>> **Focusing:** Keeping the conversation focused on the topic.

Nontherapeutic communication techniques include

>> **Asking closed ended questions:** These questions elicit only a yes or no response.

>> **Giving advice:** "You really shouldn't . . ."

>> **Minimizing the client's feelings:** "Cheer up."

>> **Making a value judgment:** "I don't think that's good."

Check out Chapter 8 for more on therapeutic communication.

Priority Action

Nursing care actions need to be performed in a certain order. Some actions are always more essential than others, and you need to know what to do first.

Exam questions relating to priority action are likely to be worded "What should the nurse's priority action be?" or use the phrases *initial action* or *immediate action*.

EXAMPLE

A client with chronic immune thrombocytopenic purpura undergoes a splenectomy. Upon receiving the patient in the PACU (postanesthesia care unit), the nurse immediately assesses the client's airway and vital signs. What should the nurse's next priority action be?

(1) Checking the patient's Foley catheter for urinary output

(2) Administering pain medication as ordered

(3) Checking the patient's dressing for excessive bleeding and drainage

(4) Administering platelets as ordered

The correct answer is Choice (3). To determine priority action, first consider the patient and his or her condition. Next, determine what the essential nursing interventions are for the condition and determine which condition is the most life threatening for the client. In this case, chronic immune thrombocytopenic purpura (ITP) is an immune-mediated disorder of platelet destruction. A client undergoing a splenectomy with a history of ITP is at high risk for hemorrhage, and therefore the priority assessment is to check the dressing for signs of bleeding. Although the nurse should check the urine output and pain level, these conditions aren't immediately life threatening.

Interventions

Nursing requires you to anticipate what may happen with your patient given his disease process. Thinking ahead in this manner allows you to watch for signs of problems and intervene as quickly as possible. To determine whether you know the appropriate nursing interventions for a particular disease or condition, exam questions on this topic usually ask "The nurse can anticipate which intervention?"

EXAMPLE

A client has developed hepatic encephalopathy as a result of liver disease. Which intervention can the nurse anticipate incorporating into the plan of care?

(1) Restricting fluid to 1,000 ml/day

(2) Inserting a nasogastric tube

(3) Administering intravenous salt poor albumin

(4) Implementing a low-protein diet

The correct answer is Choice (4). From the way the question is worded, you know that only one of the interventions listed is a priority in this situation. When hepatic encephalopathy develops as a result of liver disease, one of the treatment goals is to reduce the production of ammonia. One of the by-products of protein breakdown is ammonia, so protein should be limited in the patient's diet. Fluid restriction and salt poor albumin are used to treat ascites (a complication of liver failure). A nasogastric tube may be inserted as the disease progresses, but it isn't the best answer here.

Further Teaching

The last step of the nursing process is evaluation. Common phrases in these types of questions pertain to determining whether patient goals have been achieved and interventions have been successful. For example, questions may include the phrases *Further teaching is necessary when*, *Interventions have been effective when*, or *Intervene when*.

EXAMPLE

The nurse is caring for a client receiving subcutaneous injections of enoxaparin sodium (Lovenox) for a pulmonary embolism. Which statement made by the patient indicates that further teaching about the medication is needed?

(1) "I'll watch for signs of bleeding and notify my physician immediately if I notice anything."

(2) "I'll avoid medication that contains aspirin."

(3) "My doctor will be checking my platelet count regularly."

(4) "I'll need to have my coagulation levels checked daily."

The correct answer is Choice (4). *Needs more teaching* means you're looking for the incorrect statement. When you see this type of question, rephrasing the question in your mind is often helpful to figure out what it's really asking. In this case, you can rephrase the question to be "Which is an incorrect statement made by the patient?" Choice (4) is incorrect and is therefore the right choice. Enoxaparin sodium (Lovenox) is a low molecular weight heparin used to prevent deep vein thrombosis; it's also given to patients with pulmonary edema. As for the other options, patients with normal coagulation who are receiving enoxaparin don't require regular monitoring of coagulation levels. The patient needs to watch for signs of bleeding and to avoid aspirin. Platelet levels are checked periodically because thrombocytopenia is a potential side effect of the drug.

EXAMPLE

A client with a history of chronic obstructive pulmonary disease (COPD) is admitted with a diagnosis of respiratory failure and hypercarbia. The nurse knows that nursing interventions have been effective when the client exhibits

(1) An improvement in level of consciousness

(2) A decrease in respiratory rate and depth

(3) An increase in CO_2 levels

(4) A decrease in breath sounds

The correct answer is Choice (1). Rephrasing these types of questions may make it easier for you to pick the correct answer. You can rephrase this question to read, "For a COPD patient with respiratory failure and high pCO_2 levels (hypercarbia), how would I know my interventions have been successful?" High CO_2 levels may cause an alteration in mental status; therefore, improvement in level of consciousness may indicate that levels are beginning to decrease. A decrease in respiratory rate, depth, and breath sounds may be a sign of further deterioration and CO_2 retention. An increase in CO_2 levels is a sign that interventions have been ineffective.

Chapter **17**

Ten Rules to Remember When Prepping for the NCLEX-RN

E very test has rules, and the NCLEX-RN is no exception. The ten rules that make up this chapter don't come from a rule book, however. They come from years of experience with the NCLEX-RN, and I chose them specifically to help you focus on what can really help you succeed on the exam. Follow these ten rules as you get ready for and take the exam, and you'll be well on your way to putting "RN" after your name!

Read Each Question in Its Entirety

When you read a question, you may identify a keyword or phrase right away and think you know the answer. You check out your four answer options; see the answer that you came up with; say to yourself, "That was easy"; and choose that perfect answer. But if you were to read the question more carefully, you may see that your perfect answer doesn't really answer the question — it just seems like it does. Sometimes all the answers are right and you must choose the best one. Speed-reading questions and jumping to answers isn't an effective way of identifying the real problem the question is presenting and often leads you to an incorrect answer.

TIP

The best approach is to read the entire question at least once before reading the answers. Take the opportunity to think about what the question is asking before you rush to the answers. Part of the skill required for success on this exam is reading comprehension, so read carefully and thoroughly. And make sure you read all of the answer, too, checking carefully for any bits that are wrong.

Don't Read into the Question

Many students fall victim to the pitfall of thinking too deeply about a question and inserting bits and pieces that aren't actually in the question (see Chapter 4 for more). Adding information to a question — from words to responsibilities and situations — is deadly. It almost always encourages you to choose an incorrect answer because your mind is already heading in one direction. Instead of reading into a question, take the information in the question and choose an answer that best reflects the stated problem. Keywords, which I also discuss in Chapter 4, can help you stay on track.

For example, you may read a question that asks a nurse to complete a very time-consuming task. You may ask yourself, "How could I possibly have time to complete that task when I have six other patients to care for?" Well, the question never presented any other patients in the scenario. If the question asks you about one patient and doesn't tell you that you're responsible for any others, don't assume that you have that responsibility — just answer the question.

Answer Questions with the Ideal Situation in Mind

One tried-and-true characteristic of the NCLEX-RN is that all the questions reflect nursing practice in a perfect world, which is majorly different from the NCLEX-RN world. On the day of the test, remember that the real world doesn't belong on the NCLEX-RN. When you read a question and its answer options, ask yourself, "If all conditions were optimal, what would I choose to do?" Follow all the steps you learned in nursing school regardless of how time-consuming or laborious they may seem. The exam is testing your knowledge of how you'd provide care for a patient under the most optimal circumstances.

Many students choose an incorrect answer even though they've identified a better and safer choice; they say to themselves, "I saw a nurse do that in clinical, and if an experienced nurse does it that way, then how could I know better?" The truth is, most new graduates practice safer nursing care because they follow all the steps in the process and don't take shortcuts. Don't use what you see other nurses do at work. The people who write the exam are aware of how many nurses in practice may take shortcuts to save time but also may put the patient at risk. Therefore, they test to make sure you aren't taking any shortcuts. Always choose an answer that includes all the steps in a process in the correct sequence.

Avoid Changing Your Answers

Most students change their answer to a question only to find out that they changed a correct answer to an incorrect answer. Second-guessing yourself is probably one of the most dangerous things you can do on a test. Students change answers because they don't trust their judgment or knowledge about a subject. As a new nurse, you probably don't have much experience to draw on, so when faced with a situation in which making a choice confirms your decision about how to handle a particular situation, you may feel that you aren't "qualified" to make that decision.

You couldn't be more wrong. By virtue of your graduation from nursing school, you're qualified to make the decisions that new graduate nurses are allowed to make. The exam asks only questions that are within the scope of practice of a new graduate, not of an experienced ICU nurse. Nursing schools are very careful about making sure that all graduates are able to safely and competently make the decisions necessary to care for patients.

REMEMBER

Your first choice is usually well thought out and rational; changing your answer indicates doubt and insecurity. Be confident in your instincts!

Don't Call the Doctor until You're Sure You Need To

Calling the patient's doctor is always a tempting choice because, after all, who better to make patient care decisions than the doctor? However, the NCLEX-RN examiners have prepared this test as a *nursing practice* test and are testing you on what a nurse would do in a particular situation, not what a doctor would do. Doctors have their own tests!

Besides, anytime you call a doctor, he or she asks questions about the patient, such as what vital signs and symptoms you've observed and what actions you've taken to address the problem. Always think about what appropriate nursing actions would be important to implement before calling the doctor, and you have your answer.

Also remember to consider what you can do to help this patient prior to calling the doctor. The doctor won't magically appear when called; getting there takes time. Can you do something in the meantime? Both scenarios help you find your answer.

Avoid Answers That Make You Choose All or Nothing

Very few things happen either all the time or none of the time. Life's just not like that. Even if you want things to be black and white, they never are. So avoid choosing answers that include specific, finite words like *all, every, always, none,* and *never.* These words should be a red flag that the answer has some flaw. Rarely can you describe a situation in such concrete terms. Even if the rest of the answer seems possible and only that one little word gives you doubt, the fact that the situation is presented in an all-or-nothing way makes it very unlikely to be correct.

REMEMBER

Nurses must be prepared to function in an ever-changing environment, so answers with words that indicate the flexibility of a situation are more likely to be correct.

Don't Memorize Facts, Questions, or Other Useless Trivia

Memorizing a lot of factoids, questions, and other information is a lot of work and very time-consuming. It exhausts you and takes up time that you could spend studying the really important stuff. Anyway, questions in books like this one or in online testing for the NCLEX-RN never show up word for word. Memorizing them isn't worth your time. You may see a question with the same content, but it's likely to be asking something completely different than the question you memorized.

Knowledge and understanding of content is a much more successful path to take; believe it or not, actually learning the information doesn't take any longer than memorizing it. The main difference is that the information you learn and understand stays in your head much, much longer than what you memorize by rote. And you can apply learned information to many different situations, which enables you to answer so many more questions correctly. A little knowledge can go a long way.

Don't Think You Can Be Ready without Hard Work

Many new graduates and NCLEX-RN candidates are accustomed to cramming for exams. In nursing school, you may have only had a few weeks to prepare for a test in a particular course because the next test was just around the corner. Well, cram no more — you can take more time to prepare for the NCLEX-RN than any other test you took in nursing school. This is *the* test — the last test you need to take prior to receiving your nursing license — so you can spend all your study time preparing for only this test.

I recommend that you begin to study as soon as you graduate. Continue to review your notes and study your textbooks every day until you actually take the test. Don't leave long gaps in your study schedule. As time goes on, most people tend to forget more, not remember more; continuous review and practice keeps much of that precious nursing knowledge in your head until the big day.

Know Your Strengths and Weaknesses

As you prepare yourself for the NCLEX-RN, you should take as many practice tests as you can. Practice tests reveal two things:

>> Content areas that you need to spend more time reviewing

>> Test-taking strategies that you need to brush up on

Going over your answers and understanding the rationales for the correct answers helps you identify your weak areas content-wise, and identifying areas that you're good at relieves you from studying what you already know. You free up your study time to focus on things that need the most work.

TIP

Write down the content you missed on practice tests, and any other content on that topic you don't know. Review this content at least daily to limit the number of times you look up a specific subject. "One and done" is my motto.

Be Kind to Yourself

For many, taking the NCLEX-RN is so overwhelming that it seems more like a punishment than a reward. Remember, taking the NCLEX-RN is a reward for successfully completing nursing school. Therefore, you should treat yourself extra well during the time you spend preparing for this exam. Many people lock themselves away from family and friends and just study day and night. But that approach may not be as beneficial as you think. Having the support of those who are closest to you and care most about you makes the triumph of passing much sweeter.

Taking good care of yourself during preparation time ensures that you have maximum energy and can get the most out of the hard work you put in. Continue all your regular healthy habits, like exercising, eating right, sleeping well, and, most of all, taking some time to relax. (If you lost those habits during nursing school, get them back!) Pick family outings or events and go spend time with the people who are important to you. People who are successful in what they do know how to take good care of themselves.

5
Appendixes

IN THIS PART . . .

Review information about state boards of nursing, their general NCLEX-RN fees and requirements, their contact information, and testing centers that offer the NCLEX-RN.

Take on the exam as an aspiring nurse from outside the United States. Find out about registration and certification information. Understand how particulars of American culture factor into nursing practice in the United States.

Tackle important terminology to strengthen your nursing vocabulary.

Appendix A

Additional Info about Exam and Licensing Logistics

Getting and maintaining a nursing license isn't as easy in the United States as it may be in other countries because each state and territory has its own regulations for nursing licensure. If you were born in one place and plan to stay there until you die, you are less likely to have a problem with licensure. But the United States is a nation of nomads; the average resident moves 11 times during his or her lifetime! So your New York license won't get you hired in Nebraska; you'll need to obtain a license in your new state as well. Fortunately, you only have to know your own state's requirements, unless you're a real nomad — or a traveling nurse!

Suppose one day your significant other comes home and says, "Guess what? I've been transferred to Alaska!" Your first thought is, "But I don't have a nursing license for Alaska!" You know that you don't have to retake the NCLEX-RN, but that doesn't mean that you can simply show up in Alaska, flash your Idaho license, and snag a job. You need to contact the Alaska board of nursing (using the info provided later in this appendix) to find out what the state requirements are. You don't have to give up your Idaho license when you move; you're allowed to hold multiple state licenses at once. In fact, if you live in an area where several states come together and job opportunities are available in all of them, holding multiple licenses is a good idea in case you want or need to make a quick job change.

To make things even more complicated, a nursing license is like a driver's license: You have to renew it on a regular basis, even if you remain in the state in which you earned the license for the rest of your life. In this appendix, I stress the importance of keeping your license current and give you advice about renewal. I also list each individual state's licensure requirements and tell you how to make transferring your license as painless as possible.

TIP

Some good news is that as of 2000 you can get a compact state license, which allows you to work in any state that's part of the compact. The two compacts are the Enhanced Nurse Licensure Compact (eNLC) and the Original Nurse Licensure Compact (NLC). I cover compact licensing in more detail in Chapter 2. Throughout this appendix, I note whether a given state/territory participates in compact licensing as of this writing. Remember the compact state license gives you the ability to work in those states, but you have your main nursing license in your state of residence — where you actually live and work and where your driver's license is from. You have to change this license any time your main job, residence, or driver's license changes states.

Identifying Individual State and Territory Licensing Requirements

The nursing school you graduated from most likely has helped you file to take the NCLEX-RN in the state where you plan to work — even if that's not the state you currently live in. For instance, if you live in New Jersey but are sure you're going to work in New York, you can take the test in New York. However, you'd be wise to also obtain a New Jersey license after you pass the test in case you decide to work closer to home at some point. (As of this writing, New Jersey isn't a compact state.) If you want to get your license in more than one state and a compact license isn't an option, just have your current state of licensure send a letter of endorsement to the state where you're looking to become licensed.

TIP

A temporary permit allows you to work in some states before you take the NCLEX-RN. Back in the old days when the NCLEX-RN was given twice a year, graduate nurses (GNs) were allowed to work before taking the boards. Some states still allow this practice; others don't. (If you decide that you don't want to work until you pass your boards, that's okay, too.)

Your license is good for a limited time (expiration varies from state to state). Like a driver's license, you can renew your nursing license without taking the test again. You get one — and only one — notice that your license needs to be renewed. Don't expect the state to nag you about this; you're responsible for knowing when your license is about to expire. If you don't get a renewal notice in the mail, notify the state board of nursing a month or more before your license expires. State boards of nursing, like most bureaucratic agencies, aren't always quick to do things.

WARNING

Whatever else you do, don't let your license expire; if your license expires, you can't work. Hospitals keep track of nursing licenses, and legally they can't afford to let nurses work without valid and current licenses.

Some, but not all, states require continuing education units (CEUs) to renew your license. Make sure you know where your state stands on this point because cramming all your CEU credits into the last month before your license expires is nearly impossible. Work on CEUs throughout the year, and you'll have no problem.

Testing and Licensing Information Arranged by State and U.S. Territory

This section provides the following information (to the extent that it's available) for each state:

>> State board contact info

>> State board fee: How much you have to pay

>> Background check: What clearance, if any, the state requires (such as fingerprinting), and cost information

>> Nurse Licensure Compact: Whether the state is a compact state

>> Temporary permit: Whether the state allows one and what it costs

>> Application: How you apply (online and/or on paper)

» Renewal: How often you have to re-up your license and how much doing so costs

» CEU: Whether the state requires continuing education units (CEUs) and, if so, the specifics

REMEMBER

The information in this section is up-to-date as of this printing. However, state licensing requirements, fees, and compact licensure arrangements may change, so you should contact the state licensing agency for updated information. For the five U.S. territories, I've provided contact information as it was available, but you need to contact those without information for specific NCLEX-RN details.

Alabama

Board of Nursing
770 Washington Ave., RSA Plaza, Ste. 250
Montgomery, AL 36104
Phone 334-293-5200 or 800-656-5318
Fax 334-293-5201
Website www.abn.alabama.gov/

» State board fee: $100

» Background check: Required; contact state for cost

» Nurse Licensure Compact: Yes (NCL effective January 1, 2020)

» Temporary permit: Allowed; $50

» Application: Online

» Renewal: $100. RN licenses are valid from January 1 of each odd-numbered year and expire December 31 of each even-numbered year.

» CEU: Alabama requires 24 contact hours every two years; for the first license renewal, the state requires four contact hours of Alabama board–provided continuing education related to Board functions, the Nurse Practice Act, regulations, professional conduct, and accountability.

Alaska

Board of Nursing
550 West Seventh Ave., Ste. 150
Anchorage, AK 99501-3567
Phone 907-269-8161
Fax 907-269-8196
Website www.commerce.alaska.gov/web/cbpl/ProfessionalLicensing/BoardofNursing.aspx

» State board fee: $100 nonrefundable; $200 license

» Background check: $75

» Nurse Licensure Compact: No

» Temporary permit: $100

» Application: Online or paper

» Renewal: November 30 of even years

>> CEU: Before a license can be renewed, registered and practical nurse licensees must complete two of the following:

- 30 contact hours of continuing education prescribed under 12 AAC 44.610 (certified by ANCC, ANA, AMA, a nurse practitioner or nurse anesthetist certifying body, or approved by another board of nursing)

- 60 hours of participation in uncompensated professional activities prescribed under 12 AAC 44.620

- 320 hours of employment as an RN prescribed under 12 AAC 44.630

American Samoa

American Samoa Health Services Regulatory Board
Department of Health
Pago Pago, AS 96799
Phone 684-633-1222
Fax 684-633-1869
Website N/A
Nurse Licensure Compact: No

Arizona

Board of Nursing
1740 West Adams, Ste. 2000
Phoenix, AZ 85007
Phone 602-771-7800
Fax 602-771-7888
Website www.azbn.gov/

>> State board fee: $300 application fee

>> Background check: $50 for fingerprints

>> Nurse Licensure Compact: Yes (eNLC)

>> Temporary permit: Allowed; 48-hour emergency temporary licenses must be completed in person at the board offices with all supporting documents at the time of application.

>> Application: Online only

>> Renewal: Arizona requires 960 hours of practice (equivalent to 24 weeks full time) every 5 years to renew. Renewal occurs every four years; the date varies by when each license was issued.

>> CEU: N/A

Arkansas

Board of Nursing
University Tower Bldg., 1123 S. University, Ste. 800
Little Rock, AR 72204-1619
Phone 501-686-2700
Fax 501-686-2714
Website www.arsbn.org/

- » State board fee: $100

- » Background check: $36.25

- » Nurse Licensure Compact: Yes (eNLC)

- » Temporary permit: Allowed; $30

- » Application: Online

- » Renewal: $100

- » CEU: 15 contact hours every two years, or certification or recertification during the renewal period by a national certifying body, or completion of a recognized academic course in nursing or a related field.

California

Board of Nursing
1747 North Market Blvd., Ste. 150
Sacramento, CA 95834
Phone 916-322-3350
Fax 916-574-8637
Website www.rn.ca.gov/

- » State board fee: California-educated, $300; other, $350

- » Background check: $49

- » Nurse Licensure Compact: No

- » Temporary permit: Allowed; $100

- » Application: Online or paper

- » Renewal: $190

- » CEU: 30 hours of continuing education

Colorado

Board of Nursing
Division of Professions and Occupations, 1560 Broadway, Ste. 1350
Denver, CO 80202
Phone 303-894-2430
Fax 303-894-2821
Website www.colorado.gov/pacific/dora/Nursing

- » State board fee: $200; maximum of three attempts allowed

- » Background check: Fingerprinting

- » Nurse Licensure Compact: Yes (eNLC)

- » Temporary permit: Allowed. Four months with no extension if an individual has an active license in another state or U.S. territory; fee included in application fee

- » Application: Online; $88

- » Renewal: By September 30 every two years

- » CEU: N/A

Connecticut

Board of Nursing
Dept. of Public Health, 410 Capitol Ave., MS# 13PHO
Hartford, CT 06106
Phone 860-509-7603
Fax 860-509-7553
Website portal.ct.gov/DPH/Public-Health-Hearing-Office/Board-of-Examiners-for-Nursing/Board-of-Examiners-for-Nursing

>> State board fee: $180

>> Background check: Background check and drug testing required, $25; fingerprint check, $5

>> Nurse Licensure Compact: No

>> Temporary permit: Allowed; 120-day nonrenewable permit

>> Application: Online only

>> Renewal: $100 every year and by email only

>> CEU: N/A

Delaware

Board of Nursing
861 Silver Lake Blvd., Cannon Building, Ste. 203
Dover, DE 19904
Phone 302-744-4500
Fax 302-739-2711
Website dpr.delaware.gov/boards/nursing/

>> State board fee: $110

>> Background check: Fingerprinting

>> Nurse Licensure Compact: Yes (eNLC)

>> Temporary permit: Allowed; $40

>> Application: Online, $156. If 24 months or more have elapsed since graduation, you're required to submit evidence of completing an NCLEX-RN review course within the previous six months. The course must include a test(s) and provide either a certificate or letter from the provider as proof of completion.

>> Renewal: Online, $110; must have completed the required continuing education and have practiced nursing at least 1,000 hours in the past five years or 400 hours in the past two years. Depending on the original license issue, licenses expire on February 28, May 31, or September 30 of odd years. All newly issued RN licenses expire on September 30 of odd years.

>> CEU: 30 contact hours every two years, 3 of which must be in substance abuse

District of Columbia

Board of Nursing
Department of Health
Health Professional Licensing Administration
899 North Capitol St., NE
Washington, DC 20002
Phone 877-672-2174
Fax 202-727-8241
Website dchealth.dc.gov/service/health-professionals

- » State board fee: $200 exam fee

- » Background check: Fingerprinting, $50

- » Nurse Licensure Compact: No

- » Temporary permit: Allowed; $187

- » Application: Online or paper, $187 application fee

- » Renewal: Online, $145. Renewal occurs every two years (in even years) on June 30.

- » CEU: 24 hours of continuing education; RNs are required 24 contact hours every two years, 3 of which must be in HIV/AIDS and are required to complete 2 hours of instruction in cultural competency focusing on patients who identify as LGBTQ.

Florida

Board of Nursing
4042 Bald Cypress Way, Bin C02
Tallahassee, FL 32399
Phone 850-245-4125
Fax 850-617-6460
Website floridasnursing.gov/

- » State board fee: $110; includes fees for both application and board licensing

- » Background check: Electronic fingerprinting

- » Nurse Licensure Compact: Yes (eNLC)

- » Temporary permit: Not allowed

- » Application: Online; fee included in state board fee. An additional $200 is also owed to Pearson VUE, the vendor of the testing site.

- » Renewal: $75 every two years on April 30 or July 31, depending on licensing group date

- » CEU: 27 hours every two years: 16 general hours, 2 hours on prevention of medical errors, 2 hours on Florida laws and rules, 2 hours on recognizing impairment in the workplace, 2 hours on human trafficking, 2 hours on domestic violence, and 1 hour on HIV/AIDS training

Georgia

Board of Nursing
237 Coliseum Dr.
Macon, GA 31217-3858
Phone 844-753-7825
Fax 877-371-5712
Website sos.ga.gov/index.php/licensing/plb/45

- ›› State board fee: $200 exam fee
- ›› Background check: Electronic fingerprinting
- ›› Nurse Licensure Compact: Yes (eNLC)
- ›› Temporary permit: Allowed; $75
- ›› Application: Online; $40; by endorsement, $60
- ›› Renewal: $65
- ›› CEU: 30 contact hours every two years by license renewal

Guam

Board of Nursing
P.O. Box 2816
Hagatna, Guam 96932
Phone 671-735-7407
Fax 671-735-7413
Website dphss.guam.gov/guam-board-of-nurse-examiners-2/

- ›› State board fee: $100 exam fee
- ›› Background check: Police and local court clearance dated within two months of the date of the application
- ›› Nurse Licensure Compact: No
- ›› Temporary permit: Allowed; $25
- ›› Application: Online and paper, $150
- ›› Renewal: Online, $80 biennially (odd years) by September 30
- ›› CEU: 30 contact hours every two years by license renewal

Hawaii

Board of Nursing
King Kalakaua Bldg.
P.O. Box 3469
335 Merchant St., 3rd Floor
Honolulu, HI 96813
Phone 808-586-3000
Fax 808-586-2689
Website cca.hawaii.gov/pvl/boards/nursing/

- » State board fee: $200

- » Background check: Fingerprinting, starts at $52.50

- » Nurse Licensure Compact: No

- » Temporary permit: Allowed; $50, must be currently employed

- » Application: Online (paper by request), $40

- » Renewal: Online, $166, due by June 30 every odd year or July 1 every even year. Fingerprints must also be submitted at each renewal.

- » CEU: 30 contact hours every two years by license renewal

Idaho

Board of Nursing
280 N. 8th St., Ste. 210
Boise, ID 83702
Phone 208-577-2476
Fax 208-334-3262
Website https://ibn.idaho.gov

- » State board fee: $110

- » Background check: $25

- » Nurse Licensure Compact: Yes (NLC)

- » Temporary permit: Allowed; $25, good for 120 days

- » Application: Online only

- » Renewal: $90 in odd years

- » CEU: To renew an RN license, a licensee needs to accomplish at least two of any of the learning activities (in the Practice, Education, or Professional engagement sections) within the 2-year renewal period, from the date of renewal to the following expiration date.

Illinois

Board of Nursing
IDFPR/Nursing Unit
320 W. Washington St., 3rd Floor
Springfield, IL 62786
Phone 800-560-6420
Fax N/A
Website www.idfpr.com/profs/Nursing.asp

- » State board fee: $60

- » Background check: Fingerprinting, cost varies by vendor

- » Nurse Licensure Compact: No

- » Temporary permit: Allowed; $75

- » Application: Online or paper, $91

>> Renewal: $60 every two years

>> CEU: Complete 20 hours of approved continuing education per 2-year license renewal cycle. All CE must be completed in the 24 months preceding expiration of the license.

Indiana

Board of Nursing
Professional Licensing Agency
402 W. Washington St.
Indianapolis, IN 46204
Phone 317-234-2043
Fax 317-233-4236
Website www.in.gov/pla/nursing.htm

>> State board fee: $50

>> Background check: Fingerprinting, $35.95+

>> Nurse Licensure Compact: Yes (eNLC as of July 2020)

>> Temporary permit: Allowed; $10

>> Application: Online or paper

>> Renewal: $50

>> CEU: N/A

Iowa

Board of Nursing
RiverPoint Business Park
400 S.W. 8th St., Ste. B
Des Moines, IA 50309-4685
Phone 515-281-3255
Fax 515-281-4825
Website https://nursing.iowa.gov/

>> State board fee: $200

>> Background check: Fingerprinting, $50 (included in application fee)

>> Nurse Licensure Compact: Yes (eNLC)

>> Temporary permit: Allowed; granted for 30 days, fee is included in the application

>> Application: Online by exam, $143 (includes the $93 application fee and the $50 fee for the criminal history background check); by endorsement, $169 (includes the $119 application fee and the $50 fee for the criminal history background check)

>> Renewal: $99 every three years, due 30 days prior to the 15th of the licensee's birth month

>> CEU: 36 contact hours every three years

Kansas

Board of Nursing
Landon State Office Bldg.
900 S.W. Jackson, Ste. 1051
Topeka, KS 66612
Phone 785-296-4929
Fax 785-296-4939
Website https://ksbn.kansas.gov/

>> State board fee: $125

>> Background check: Fingerprinting, $48

>> Nurse Licensure Compact: Yes (NLC)

>> Temporary permit: Allowed; $150

>> Application: Online; $50 by exam (exam fee $200), $125 by endorsement

>> Renewal: $85

>> CEU: 30 contact hours every two years

Kentucky

Board of Nursing
312 Whittington Pkwy., Ste. 300
Louisville, KY 40222
Phone 502-429-3300
Fax 502-429-3311
Website https://kbn.ky.gov/

>> State board fee: $110

>> Background check: Fingerprinting, $13.25

>> Nurse Licensure Compact: Yes (eNLC)

>> Temporary permit: Allowed; one-time, six-month temporary permit given, fee included in endorsement application

>> Application: Online; by endorsement, $165, by exam, $125

>> Renewal: Online, $65 (paper application available for additional $40 charge); by October 31

>> CEU: 14 contact hours, including 3 hours on domestic violence and 1.5 hours on pediatric head abuse trauma within three years of Kentucky licensure

Louisiana

Board of Nursing
17373 Perkins Road
Baton Rouge, LA 70810
Phone 225-755-7500
Fax 225-755-7584
Website www.lsbn.state.la.us/

>> State board fee: $100

>> Background check: $39.25

>> Nurse Licensure Compact: Yes (NLC)

>> Temporary permit: Allowed; a temporary permit good for 90 days is included in the cost of application and background check

>> Application: Online only

>> Renewal: Annually for the first year and then every two years

>> CEU: The annual CEU requirements for renewing Louisiana nurses vary according to the time spent practicing nursing throughout the year:

- Nurses who've practiced nursing at least 1,600 hours within the calendar year: Minimum of 5 contact hours of ANCC or State BON accredited nursing continuing education required annually for license renewal

- Nurses who've practiced nursing between 160 hours and 1,600 hours: Minimum of 10 contact hours of ANCC or State BON accredited nursing continuing education required annually for license renewal

- Nurses who've practiced nursing less than 160 hours during the calendar year: Minimum of 15 contact hours of ANCC or State BON accredited nursing continuing education required annually for license renewal

Maine

Board of Nursing
161 Capital St.
Augusta, ME 04333
Phone 207-287-1133
Fax 207-287-1149
Website www.maine.gov/boardofnursing/

>> State board fee: $75

>> Background check: $52; if you've been out of school more than two years, you need another certificate of completion from a school of nursing

>> Nurse Licensure Compact: Yes (NLC)

>> Temporary permit: None noted on website

- >> Application: Online

- >> Renewal: Every two years after initial renewal; renew on or before birthday

- >> CEU: N/A

Maryland

Board of Nursing
4140 Patterson Ave.
Baltimore, MD 21215
Phone 810-585-1900
Fax 410-358-3530
Website https://mbon.maryland.gov/Pages/default.aspx

- >> State board fee: $100

- >> Background check: $57.25

- >> Nurse Licensure Compact: Yes (NLC)

- >> Temporary permit: Allowed; $40

- >> Application: Online

- >> Renewal: $13

- >> CEU: N/A

Massachusetts

Board of Nursing
239 Causeway St., Ste. 500, 5th Floor
Boston, MA 02114
Phone 877-877-9727
Fax 617-973-0984
Website www.mass.gov/orgs/board-of-registration-in-nursing

- >> State board fee: $230

- >> Background check: Not required

- >> Nurse Licensure Compact: No

- >> Temporary permit: Not allowed

- >> Application: Online

- >> Renewal: $120 on your birthday in even years

- >> CEU: 15 contact hours

Michigan

Board of Nursing
Department of Licensing and Regulatory Affairs
Bureau of Professional Licensing
611 W. Ottawa
P.O. Box 30670
Lansing, MI 48933
Phone 517-241-0199
Fax N/A
Website www.michigan.gov/lara/0,4601,7-154-89334_72600_72603_27529_27542---,00.html

>> State board fee: $54; application fee, $200

>> Background check: Fingerprinting

>> Nurse Licensure Compact: No

>> Temporary permit: Not allowed

>> Application: Online

>> Renewal: Every two years from date of issue, $128.50

>> CEU: 25 hours of continuing education (including at least 2 hours in pain and symptom management) every two years. If your Michigan license has been lapsed for less than 3 years and you hold a current and valid license in another state, you don't need to submit proof of Continuing Education.

Minnesota

Board of Nursing
1210 Northland Dr., Ste. 120
Mendota Heights, MN 55120
Phone 612-317-300
Fax 652-688-1841
Website https://mn.gov/boards/nursing/

>> State board fee: $138.25

>> Background check: $33.25 (included in fee for test)

>> Nurse Licensure Compact: No

>> Temporary permit: May apply with license application, good for 6 months

>> Application: Online or paper

>> Renewal: $85 every two years unless stated otherwise on license

>> CEU: 24 hours per 24 months

Mississippi

Board of Nursing
713 Pear Orchard Rd., 3rd Floor
Ridgeland, MS 39157
Phone 601-957-6300
Fax 601-957-6301

Website www.msbn.ms.gov/

>> State board fee: $100

>> Background check: Fingerprinting, $75

>> Nurse Licensure Compact: Yes (eNLC)

>> Temporary permit: Allowed; by endorsement, reorientation, or camp, $25

>> Application: Paper $100 by exam, $100 by endorsement

>> Renewal: $100; September 1 through December 31 in even numbered years

>> CEU: None for standard renewal. If the nurse hasn't practiced in the last 5 years, license reinstatement requires 20 hours of CEU.

Missouri

Board of Nursing
3605 Missouri Blvd.
P.O. Box 656
Jefferson City, MO 65102-0656
Phone 573-751-0681
Fax 573-751-0075
Website www.pr.mo.gov/nursing.asp

>> State board fee: $55

>> Background check: Fingerprinting, $44.80

>> Nurse Licensure Compact: Yes (eNLC)

>> Temporary permit: Allowed; issued for 6 months and fee included in endorsement application

>> Application: Online by exam, $45; online by endorsement, $55

>> Renewal: $60, every two years

>> CEU: N/A

Montana

Board of Nursing
301 S. Park Ave.
P.O. Box 200513
Helena, MT 59601-0513
Phone 406-841-2300
Fax 406-841-2305
Website http://boards.bsd.dli.mt.gov/nur

>> State board fee: $100 exam fee

>> Background check: Fingerprinting, $30

>> Nurse Licensure Compact: Yes (NLC)

- » Temporary permit: Allowed; 90 days by endorsement or exam, $25

- » Application: Online or paper

- » Renewal: $100 by December 31, every two years

- » CEU: 24 contact hours every two years due by the time of license renewal

Nebraska

Board of Nursing
Nebraska State Office Bldg.
301 Centennial Mall South, 1st Floor
14th & M Streets
Lincoln, NE 68508
Phone 402-471-4376
Fax 402-742-2360
Website http://dhhs.ne.gov/licensure/Pages/Nurse-Licensing.aspx

- » State board fee: $123

- » Background check: $42.25

- » Nurse Licensure Compact: Yes (NLC)

- » Temporary permit: Allowed; valid for 60 days

- » Application: Online

- » Renewal: $123, every 2 years on even years

- » CEU: Have practiced nursing for at least 500 hours during the past five years and have completed at least 20 contact hours of acceptable continuing education/in-service education within the past two years. Of the 20 hours, no more than 4 hours may be from CPR or BLS, and at least 10 hours must be peer reviewed. All of the required contact hours can be taken via home study or Internet courses.

Nevada

Board of Nursing
5011 Meadowood Mall #201
Reno, NV 89502-6547
Phone 775-687-7700
Fax 775-687-7007
Website https://nevadanursingboard.org/

- » State board fee: $100

- » Background check: $40 and make an appointment to be fingerprinted

- » Nurse Licensure Compact: No

- » Temporary permit: Allowed; one-time, six-month permit; contact state for fee

- » Application: Online

- » Renewal: $100

- » CEU: The Nevada Nurse Practice Act requires all renewing RNs and LPNs to complete 30 hours of nursing-related continuing education.

New Hampshire

Board of Nursing
121 S. Fruit St.
Concord, NH 03301
Phone 603-271-2323
Fax 603-271-6605
Website www.oplc.nh.gov/nursing/

» State board fee: $120

» Background check: $ 48.25

» Nurse Licensure Compact: Yes (eNLC)

» Temporary permit: Allowed for an extra $20

» Application: Paper only

» Renewal: $80

» CEU: Each applicant for licensure by endorsement, renewal, or reinstatement for an RN or LPN license must complete at least 30 contact hours of workshops, conferences, lectures, or in-service educational offerings that are designed to enhance nursing knowledge, judgment, and skills. Current national certification may be used to fulfill such continuing education requirements.

New Jersey

Board of Nursing
P.O. Box 45010
124 Halsey St., 6th Floor
Newark, NJ 07101
Phone 973-504-6430
Fax 973-648-3481
Website www.njconsumeraffairs.gov/nur/

» State board fee: $200 exam fee

» Background check: Fingerprinting, $70.25

» Nurse Licensure Compact: Partially, allowing nurses with compact state license to practice in New Jersey

» Temporary permit: Allowed; $140

» Application: Online, $80

» Renewal: $80, May 31 every two years

» CEU: 30 contact hours every two years by license renewal

New Mexico

Board of Nursing
6301 Indian School Road, NE, Ste. 710
Albuquerque, NM 87110
Phone 505-841-8340
Fax 505-841-8347
Website http://nmbon.sks.com/

- » State board fee: $200 exam fee

- » Background check: Fingerprinting, $44

- » Nurse Licensure Compact: Yes (eNLC)

- » Temporary permit: Allowed; $50 after cleared fingerprints are received

- » Application: Online, $110

- » Renewal: $110, every two years from date of issue

- » CEU: 30 contact hours every two years by license renewal; earned CEU hours proof must be uploaded online

New York

Board of Nursing
Education Bldg., 89 Washington Ave., 2nd Floor West Wing
Albany, NY 12234
Phone 518-474-3817, Ext. 120
Fax 518-474-3706
Website www.op.nysed.gov/prof/nurse/

- » State board fee: $143

- » Background check: N/A. Applicants must report all criminal convictions and disciplinary actions, regardless of whether they occurred in New York State or elsewhere.

- » Nurse Licensure Compact: No

- » Temporary permit: Allowed; valid for up to 90 days for new nursing graduates (can't obtain if NCLEX-RN has already been taken/attempted). Costs $35 unless submitted with examination; then application fee is included.

- » Application: Online, $143

- » Renewal: $73, every three years

- » CEU: 3 contact hours on infection control every three years. Two contact hours on child abuse are required only for initial licensure. New nursing graduates will not have to complete these requirements because they're fulfilled in their nursing school course work.

North Carolina

Board of Nursing
4516 Lake Boone Trail
Raleigh, NC 27607
Phone 919-782-3211
Fax 919-781-9461
Website www.ncbon.com/

>> State board fee: $75

>> Background check: Fingerprinting, $38

>> Nurse Licensure Compact: Yes (eNLC)

>> Temporary permit: Allowed; permit valid for 120 days or until the permanent license has been issued (whichever comes first). Fees are included in application.

>> Application: Online by exam, $75, by endorsement, $150

>> Renewal: $100, every two years during month of birth

>> CEU: 15 contact hours of continued education and 640 hours of active practice within previous 2 years, or 30 contact hours of continued education

North Dakota

Board of Nursing
919 South 7th St., Ste. 504
Bismarck, ND 58504
Phone 701-328-9777
Fax 701-328-9785
Website www.ndbon.org/

>> State board fee: $130

>> Background check: Fingerprinting, $41.25

>> Nurse Licensure Compact: Yes (eNLC)

>> Temporary permit: Allowed; valid for up to 90 days, fees included in application for endorsement

>> Application: Online by exam, $130, by endorsement, $160

>> Renewal: $120 by December 31 of expiration year

>> CEU: 400 hours within four years

Northern Mariana Islands

Board of Nursing
CDA Bldg., 2nd Floor
San Jose, Beach Road
Saipan, MP 96950
Phone 670 233 2263
Fax 670- 664-4823
Website https://nmibon.info/

- » State board fee: $150

- » Background check: Contact board of nursing for clarification

- » Nurse Licensure Compact: No

- » Temporary permit: Allowed; $60

- » Application: Paper

- » Renewal: $100 60 days prior to expiration; $120 30 days prior to expiration (considered late, incurs an additional $20 fee)

- » CEU: 30 contact hours. CE providers will be accepted from all nursing boards as well as accredited sources.

Ohio

Board of Nursing
17 South High St., Ste. 660
Columbus, OH 43215-3413
Phone 614-466-3947
Fax 614-466-0388
Website https://nursing.ohio.gov/

- » State board fee: $75

- » Background check: Fingerprinting

- » Nurse Licensure Compact: No

- » Temporary permit: Allowed; valid for up to 180 days, fee included in endorsement application

- » Application: Online by exam, $75, by endorsement, $75

- » Renewal: $65 July 1–September 15 in odd years; $115 September 16–October 31 in odd years

- » CEU: 24 contact hours that include at least one contact hour for each renewal. A nurse who has been licensed in Ohio by reciprocity for less than or equal to one year prior to the first Ohio license renewal must complete at least 12 contact hours rather than 24.

Oklahoma

Board of Nursing
2915 N. Classen Blvd., Ste. 524
Oklahoma City, OK 73106
Phone 405-962-1800
Fax 405-962-1821
Website http://nursing.ok.gov/

>> State board fee: $85

>> Background check: Applicants with a history of arrest or disciplinary action must provide documentation of incident and outcome

>> Nurse Licensure Compact State: Yes (eNLC)

>> Temporary permit: Allowed; licensure by endorsement for the U.S.–educated nurse (LPN/RN) with temporary license request, $95

>> Application: Paper or online ($3.50 online processing fee)

>> Renewal: $75 (additional $3.00 online processing fee). License must be renewed every two years by the end of your birth month. RNs renew in even years and LPNs renew in odd years.

>> CEU: N/A

Oregon

Board of Nursing
17938 SW Upper Boones Ferry Rd.
Portland, OR 97224
Phone 971-673-0685
Fax 971-673-0684
Website www.oregon.gov/osbn/Pages/apply-NCLEX.aspx

>> State board fee: $160 (plus $9 fee for Oregon Nursing Advancement Fund)

>> Background check: Fingerprinting, $64.50

>> Nurse Licensure Compact: No

>> Temporary permit: Not allowed; individual must have an active license before beginning orientation

>> Application: Online by exam, $160 (plus $9 fee for Oregon Nursing Advancement Fund), by endorsement, $195 (plus $9 fee for Oregon Nursing Advancement Fund)

>> Renewal: $145 every two years by licensee's birthday

>> CEU: 7 hours of pain management training; 1 hour must be from the Oregon Pain Management Commission module (doesn't have to be repeated for each renewal). The remaining 6 hours can be the licensee's choice of pain management topics and providers.

Pennsylvania

Board of Nursing
P.O. Box 2649
Harrisburg, PA 17105-2649
Phone 717-783-7142
Fax 717-783-0822
Website www.dos.pa.gov/ProfessionalLicensing/BoardsCommissions/Nursing/Pages/default.aspx#.VTEYxCFVhBd

>> State board fee: By exam, $95; by endorsement, $120

>> Background check: Criminal History Records Check (CHRC) from the state police or other state agency for every state in which you've lived, worked, or completed professional

training/studies for the past 10 years. The report(s) must be dated within 90 days of the date the application is submitted.

» Nurse Licensure Compact: No

» Temporary permit: Allowed; $70, extension fee $85

» Application: Online or paper, $95

» Renewal: $122 every two years prior to license expiration date

» CEU: 30 hours including 2 hours of approved training on child abuse recognition and reporting from an approved provider and 2 hours of opioid education if CRNP with prescriptive authority

Puerto Rico

Board of Nursing
Commonwealth of Puerto Rico Board of Nurse Examiners
800 Roberto H. Todd Ave., Room 202
Santurce, PR 00908
Phone 787-999-8989 or 787-705-8364
Fax not available
Website www.board-of-nursing.com/puerto-rico-board-of-nursing.php

Rhode Island

Board of Nursing
3 Capitol Hill
Providence, RI 02908
Phone 401-222-5960
Fax N/A
Website https://health.ri.gov/licenses/

» State board fee: $135

» Background: $35

» Nurse Licensure Compact: No

» Temporary permit: Allowed; $135 for 90 days

» Application: Online

» Renewal: $135

» CEU: Nurses seeking to renew a nursing license must complete 10 continuing education hours during every two-year licensing cycle; 2 of those hours must be about substance abuse.

South Carolina

Board of Nursing
Synergy Business Park
Kingstree Bldg.
110 Centerview Dr., Ste. 202
Columbia, SC 29210
Phone 803-896-4550
Fax 803-896-4515
Website https://llr.sc.gov/nurse/

- » State board fee: $90

- » Background check: Fingerprinting

- » Nurse Licensure Compact: Yes (eNLC)

- » Temporary permit: Allowed; $10

- » Application: Online by exam, $90, by endorsement, $100

- » Renewal: $75 by April 30 every other year

- » CEU: 30 contact hours during two years before renewal

South Dakota

Board of Nursing
4305 South Louise Ave., Ste. 201
Sioux Falls, SD 57106-3115
Phone 605-362-2760
Fax 605-362-2768
Website https://doh.sd.gov/boards/nursing/

- » State board fee: $100

- » Background check: Fingerprinting, $25

- » Nurse Licensure Compact: Yes (eNLC)

- » Temporary permit: Allowed; $25, good for 90 days

- » Application: Online by endorsement, $100, by exam, $100

- » Renewal: $115. Must have worked at least 140 hours in any 12-month period, or an accumulated total of at least 480 hours worked within the preceding 6 years.

- » CEU: Contact the state.

Tennessee

Board of Nursing
665 Mainstream Dr.
Nashville, TN 37243
Phone 615-532-5166
Fax 615-741-7899
Website www.tn.gov/health/health-program-areas/health-professional-boards/nursing-board/nursing-board/about.html

- » State board fee: None

- » Background check: Fingerprinting, $35.15

- » Nurse Licensure Compact: Yes (eNLC)

- » Temporary permit: Allowed. May only be issued to graduates of international medical schools for temporary clinical practice; nonrenewable.

- » Application: Online by exam, $0, by endorsement, $115.00

- » Renewal: $100 every two years

- » CEU: You must maintain proof for two items from the following list of options:

  - Copy of a satisfactory employer evaluation

  - Letter from a peer providing a satisfactory evaluation of your nursing performance

  - Letter from a patient or family member giving evidence of a satisfactory nurse/patient relationship

  - Copy of a contract of renewal or reappointment to a nursing position

  - Written self-evaluation based on the standards of competence listed in the rules

  - Evidence of current national certification

  - A document that identifies two nursing goals and how you met these goals

  - A letter from the agency where you volunteered as a nurse

  - Documentation from a school of nursing stating that you participated in the education of nursing students (RNs only)

  - Certificate/evidence of five contact hours of continuing education (for RNs/LPNs who aren't practicing, ten contact hours will fulfill the competency requirement)

  - Copy of a published article relevant to nursing you've written

  - Letter of satisfactory completion of a nursing refresher course

  - Letter of satisfactory completion of a comprehensive nursing orientation program

  - Official transcript (may be student issued) demonstrating two hours of nursing credit

  - Evidence of successfully retaken NCLEX

Texas

Board of Nursing
333 Guadalupe, Ste. 3-460
Austin, TX 78701
Phone 512-305-7400
Fax 512-305-7401
Website www.bon.state.tx.us/

- » State board fee: $186

- » Background check: Fingerprinting, $39.75 ($10.00 plus a $29.75 fee for the State and National Criminal History Record Information)

- » Nurse Licensure Compact: Yes (eNLC)

- » Temporary permit: Allowed; good for up to 120 days. Issued to nurses who haven't been a Licensed Vocational Nurse during the past four years. Are also used for completing a refresher program, extensive orientation, or a nursing program of study under an RN Instructor. Fee included in application.

- » Application: Online or on paper by exam, $100, by endorsement, $186

- » Renewal: $68 every two years

- » CEU: 20 contact hours

U.S. Virgin Islands

Board of Nursing
#3 Kongens Gade (Government Hill)
St. Thomas, Virgin Islands 00802
Phone 340-774-7477
Fax 340-777-4003
Website N/A

Utah

Board of Nursing
Heber M. Wells Bldg., 4th Floor
160 East 300 South
Salt Lake City, UT 84111
Phone 801-530-6628
Fax 801-530-6511
Website https://dopl.utah.gov/nurse/index.html

>> State board fee: $100 (includes $60 application fee and two background check fees)

>> Background check: Fingerprinting, $40 ($20 per fingerprinting card)

>> Nurse Licensure Compact: Yes (eNLC)

>> Temporary permit: Not allowed

>> Application: Online or paper; by exam, $95, by endorsement, $95

>> Renewal: $58, January 31 every odd year

>> CEU: Every 2 years, must have completed at least 400 hours licensed practice, at least 200 hours with 15 hours of approved continuing education, or 30 hours of approved continuing education

Vermont

Board of Nursing
Office of Professional Regulation
Board of Nursing
89 Main St., Floor 3
Montpelier, VT 05620-3402
Phone 802-828-2396
Fax 802-828-2484
Website https://sos.vermont.gov/nursing/

>> State board fee: $60

>> Background check: Not required

>> Nurse Licensure Compact: Yes (NLC)

>> Temporary permit: Allowed for 60 days

>> Application: Online

>> Renewal: Every 2 years, must have worked a minimum of 50 days (400 hours) in the last two years or 120 days (960 hours) in the last 5 years under that license

>> CEU: N/A

Virginia

Board of Nursing
9960 Maryland Dr., Ste. 300
Henrico, VA 23233
Phone 804-367-4515
Fax 804-527-4455
Website www.dhp.virginia.gov/Boards/Nursing/

>> State board fee: $190 first time

>> Background check: Fingerprinting, $35.95

>> Nurse Licensure Compact: Yes (eNLC)

>> Temporary permit: Allowed; valid up to 90 days, fees included in endorsement application

>> Application: Online or paper ($50 additional fee), $190 by exam or renewal

>> Renewal: $140 every two years

>> CEU: 30 contact hours of workshops, seminars, conferences, or courses relevant to the practice of nursing

Washington

Dept. of Health, Nursing Care Quality Assurance Commission
111 Israel Rd. S.E.
Tumwater, WA 98501
Phone 360-236-4703
Fax 360-236-4738
Website www.doh.wa.gov/LicensesPermitsandCertificates/NursingCommission

>> State board fee: $120

>> Background check: $34.25

>> Nurse Licensure Compact: No

>> Temporary permit: Not allowed

>> Application: Online

>> Renewal: $120 on birthday

>> CEU: Registered nurses (RN) and licensed practical nurses (LPN) are required to keep documentation of 531 hours of active practice and 45 clock hours of continuing education within a three-year cycle.

West Virginia

Board of Examiners for Registered Professional Nurses
101 Dee Dr.
Charleston, WV 25311
Phone 877-743-6877 or 304-558-3596
Fax 304-558-3666
Website https://wvrnboard.wv.gov/Pages/default.aspx

>> State board fee: $51.50

>> Background check: Required; contact state for cost

>> Nursing Licensure Compact: Yes

>> Temporary permit: Allowed; 90 days pending results of first exam; 90 days if by endorsement, $25

>> Application: Online $70

>> Renewal: $25 December 31 every year

>> CEU: 30 contact hours every odd year. If initial licensure occurs during the first half of any two-year reporting period, the nurse must complete 12 contact hours before end of that reporting period. If initial licensure occurs during the second half of any two-year reporting period, the nurse is exempt from CEU requirements for the entire reporting period.

Wisconsin

Board of Nursing
4822 Madison Yards Way
Madison, WI 53705
Phone 608-266-2112
Fax N/A
Website https://dsps.wi.gov/Pages/Professions/RN/Default.aspx

>> State board fee: $75

>> Background check: $45

>> Nurse Licensure Compact: Yes (NLC)

>> Temporary permit: Allowed; $10, good for three months

>> Application: Online or on paper depending on where you live

>> Renewal: $82

>> CEU: Survey required 8 weeks prior to renewal online or paper version

Wyoming

Board of Nursing
130 Hobbs Ave., Ste. B
Cheyenne, WY 82002
Phone 307-777-7601
Fax 307-777-3519
Website https://wsbn.wyo.gov/

» State board fee: $130

» Background check: $60

» Nurse Licensure Compact: Yes (eNLC)

» Temporary permit: Allowed; $25

» Application: Online

» Renewal: Online, $110

» CEU: Complete one of the following in the past 2 years (waived during first renewal period if you were licensed by exam): 400 hours of active nursing practice, 200 hours of active nursing practice and 15 hours of continuing education, or 30 hours of continuing education.

Appendix **B**

Information for International Nurses Moving to the United States

re you one of the many nurses from all over the world planning a move to the United States in search of a job? Given the shortage of nurses in the U.S., you can certainly benefit from a wealth of nursing opportunities, and hospitals in need of nurses welcome international folks as long as they have the necessary credentials. However, no matter what field you're in, moving to a foreign country isn't easy; cultural differences can make the practice of nursing in America very different from what it is at home. In this appendix, I tell you how to navigate the legal waters necessary to obtain the paperwork to practice nursing in the U.S. In addition, I give you a crash course in U.S. nursing practices you may not be familiar with, including NCLEX-RN practice questions on therapeutic communication, which is specific to the American language and culture.

Following the Two-Step Process for Becoming Eligible to Take the NCLEX-RN

Before an international nurse is eligible to take the NCLEX-RN, most states in the U.S. require that he or she receive certification from the Commission on Graduates of Foreign Nursing Schools (CGFNS) by completing a federal screening program. The screening program comprises two main steps:

1. Getting a VisaScreen certificate from the CGFNS
2. Getting a certificate from the CGFNS

After you complete both parts of the certification program, you receive a CGFNS CP certificate. If you don't have a CGFNS certificate, you may be granted eligibility to take the NCLEX-RN to provide proof of nursing knowledge (see "Getting the NCLEX-RN go-ahead without a certificate" later in this appendix). You can find out more about the CGFNS by visiting www.cgfns.org.

REMEMBER

A foreign-educated nurse who's licensed and practicing nursing in the United States is required to obtain a VisaScreen certificate (see the following section).

Getting a VisaScreen certificate

The first step of the screening process, getting a VisaScreen certificate, includes educational analysis, credential review, and license verification. The International Commission on Health Care Professions, a division of the CGFNS, completes these tasks. Here's what you have to do to get the VisaScreen certificate:

>> **Submit the following paperwork to the CGFNS:**

- Proof of completion of senior secondary school education, separate from any professional certification

- Proof of completion of a government-approved professional healthcare program of at least two years in length

- Documentation that you completed a minimum number of clock and/or credit hours in specific theoretical and clinical areas while in nursing school

>> **Get your license verified by the CGFNS:** You must present all current and past licensure for review.

For more on the VisaScreen, visit www.cgfns.org/services/certification/visascreen-visa-credentials-assessment/.

Securing a CGFNS certificate

Many state boards of nursing require internationally educated nurses to obtain a certificate from the CGFNS before applying for initial licensure as a registered nurse. Check with the state board where you want to be licensed before you even apply for the license. Appendix A has state board websites.

Obtaining a CGFNS certificate involves

» An assessment of proficiency in the English language

» An examination that tests nursing knowledge

The English proficiency exam and the CGFNS qualifying exam must be taken within two years of each other, and scores are valid for two years after you take the tests.

Showing your knowledge of English language

To get your CGFNS certificate, you must submit proof of a passing score on an English proficiency examination approved by the U.S. Department of Education and Health and Human Services. You have three exams to choose from:

» **Test of English as a Foreign Language (TOEFL):** If you take the pencil-and-paper exam, you need a score of 540 to pass. If you take it on a computer, you need a score of 207. The TOEFL has two additional components that carry their own passing scores:

  • **Test of Written English (TWE):** You need a score of 4 to pass.

  • **Test of Spoken English (TSE):** You need a score of 50 to pass.

» **Test of English for International Communication (TOEIC):** You need a score of 725 to pass.

» **International English Language Testing System (IELTS):** You need a score of 6.5 to pass.

The contact information for the testing organizations that administer the three proficiency tests is as follows:

» **To take the TOEFL,** contact the Educational Testing Service, P.O. Box 6151, Princeton, NJ 08541-6151; phone 443-751-4862 or 1-800-468-6335; online form www.ets.org/toefl/contact/test-takers/contact-forms; website www.toefl.org

» **To take the TOEIC,** contact the TOEIC Services America, 1425 Lower Ferry Road, Ewing, NJ 08618; phone 609-734-1560; email toeic@ets.org; website www.toeic.org

» **To take the IELTS,** contact www.ielts.org/en-us/info-pages/contact-us

TIP

If you graduated from a nursing program in an English-speaking country such as Australia, New Zealand, England, or Canada (except Quebec), you don't have to take the English proficiency exam.

Proving your nursing knowledge on the CGFNS exam

The CGFNS qualifying exam, which tests your nursing knowledge, is a one-day exam offered four times a year (typically in March, July, September, and November) at over 40 sites worldwide. The CGFNS assessment is the most important qualifying exam for nurses wanting to work in the United States. It ensures that foreign-educated healthcare professionals are eligible and qualified to meet licensure and other practice demands in the U.S. It also assures that they have the same level of understanding of nursing as recent graduates of schools in U.S.

Applications for the exam are free, and you can download them at www.cgfns.org. On the website, you can also find application deadlines, submit your application and educational and professional documentation, and pay all exam fees by credit card.

Getting the NCLEX-RN go-ahead without a certificate

If the state in which you intend to be licensed doesn't require CGFNS certification, it still may require submission of some of the same documents that the CGFNS requires. The state may require you to provide the following:

» Proof of citizenship or legal alien status

» Official transcripts of educational credentials sent directly to the board of nursing from the school of nursing

» Validation of theoretical instruction and clinical practice in a variety of nursing areas, including medical nursing, surgical nursing, pediatric nursing, maternity and newborn nursing, and mental health nursing

» A copy of your nursing license and/or your diploma

» Proof of proficiency in the English language

» A photo of yourself

» Application fees

Taking the NCLEX-RN Abroad

If you're a nurse abroad hoping to practice nursing in the United States, the amount of paperwork and testing necessary to make the switch may seem bewildering. Especially if you've been a nurse for many years, having to prove yourself as a nurse all over again may seem somewhat insulting. Take heart — all this testing is designed to make sure you can safely handle the language and cultural issues faced by anyone moving to a foreign country. It measures your clinical knowledge and critical thinking in caring for clients.

In the U.S. as in any country, patient safety comes first. The NCLEX-RN is designed to measure the competency of an RN in the U.S. You must demonstrate that you're a safe and effective nurse by answering an appropriate number of multiple-choice questions as well as some special questions that involve diagrams, fill-in-the-blanks, or putting options in order.

You may not be accustomed to the types of questions on tests like the NCLEX-RN. This type of test is common in the United States because

» It's easy to administer to large groups of people.

» It measures knowledge more objectively than other types of tests do.

In the area of licensing and credentials, the United States is anything but united. Each state has its own rules and requires you to become licensed in that state before you can practice. For example, a license from Idaho doesn't allow you to practice nursing in Oklahoma unless you have a compact state license, which I discuss in Chapter 2. Appendix A tells you which states are compact states. You may already know where you intend to live and practice nursing. If you don't, you need to decide now, before you take the NCLEX-RN, because you have to take the test in the state you intend to work in (with a few exceptions).

TIP

The first step to practicing nursing in America is to contact the board of nursing in the state where you want to practice. I've included contact information and websites for the individual state boards of nursing in Appendix A.

Your state board's website should list the requirements for international nurses, and through the site, you can request an application packet for initial licensure as a nurse who has been educated outside of the United States. Exams are usually good for two years, so plan accordingly to avoid having to retake it.

Previously, the NCLEX-RN could be taken only in the United States and its territories, but now it's administered internationally exclusively at Pearson VUE professional testing centers. (Remember, all current state licensure requirement processes still apply.) In addition to the U.S. sites, you can take the NCLEX-RN at Pearson professional centers in the following countries:

>> Australia

>> Brazil

>> Canada

>> England

>> Hong Kong

>> India

>> Japan

>> Korea

>> Mexico

>> South Africa

>> Taiwan

>> The Philippines

These international locations were selected because they rated highly in areas such as national security, examination security, and similarity with United States intellectual property and copyright laws and because they have Pearson locations with high-stakes testing. The examination given internationally is exactly the same as the exam given in the U.S. Before taking the test, you need to pass specific requirements of eligibility by a member board and any state or practice entity where you want to practice (see Appendix A for state board information). Also, regardless of where you take the exam, you must first apply for licensure with a U.S. state or territorial board of nursing to receive an Authorization to Test (ATT).

REMEMBER

On the National Council of State Boards of Nursing's website (www.ncsbn.org), you can register for the NCLEX-RN and access the candidate bulletin. This bulletin provides detailed information regarding all facets of the NCLEX-RN, including the examination fee, other initiation processes, and scheduling procedures for both international and domestic test centers.

The exam fee is $200 USD, and scheduling your exam at an international test center requires an additional international scheduling fee of $150 USD plus taxes, where applicable. If you already have an appointment at a test center in the United States, you may change your appointment to an international center for an additional $150 USD international scheduling fee. For further information regarding international testing, contact the National Council of State Boards of Nursing at 1-866-293-9600.

Navigating Nursing Roles in the U.S.

Whereas some international nurses find nursing in the U.S. very similar to the nursing that they've learned and experience in their home countries, others find it very different. The NCLEX-RN may ask you questions about procedures, communication skills, diet, and foods that are unfamiliar to you. In order to be successful on the NCLEX-RN, you must be able to correctly answer questions regarding nursing practice in the U.S.

You may be thinking, "How different can it be?" All countries have their own cultural norms that carry over into nursing practice and make it vary greatly from one country to the next. The following sections provide an overview of the skills nurses are expected to perform in the U.S.

Forming partnerships with clients

REMEMBER

Nurse-client relationships in the U.S. are partnerships in that both parties work together to improve the client's health. This partnership involves

>> Agreeing on goals for treatment

>> Giving information on how the goals can be reached

>> Designing a plan to achieve those goals

>> Working together toward the desired and expected outcome

Nurse-client relationships can forge powerful emotional bonds, but at all times the nurse must

>> Remain objective

>> Communicate therapeutically

>> Assist patients without being patronizing

>> Preserve clients' privacy

As a nurse in the U.S., you must also be able to put the clients' needs and concerns before your own and be proficient in the nursing skills required to safely deliver care to your clients. Accept clients' dependency on you while encouraging them to strive for independence and health and well-being.

Teaching and instructing

In some cultures, instruction may be the responsibility of doctors or families, but in the U.S., nurses are responsible for teaching patients and their families how to manage healthcare needs. Nurses are involved with disease prevention, health screening, and treatment of illness for people of all ages from birth to death. The nurse needs to be able to identify how to best teach each individual patient. For example, some clients may prefer to be shown with pictures or a model, and others may learn better from printed material. And when you teach matters, too. Clients in pain or severely anxious aren't going to be receptive to teaching because these are non-teachable circumstances.

Nurses also help patients understand the complex healthcare system of the United States and assist them in making decisions about their healthcare. They serve as patient advocates, talking to patients about their rights and treatment options. (Check out Chapter 5 for more about patient advocacy.)

Providing care

In the U.S., nurses provide hands-on nursing care for patients in the hospital setting. This arrangement may be very different from some cultures in which families provide care under the nurse's guidance and teaching. In the U.S., nurses are held legally accountable for their practice and are legally responsible for their actions. They must utilize a large base of nursing knowledge to provide the best possible nursing care, which often means mastering very high-tech equipment.

REMEMBER

The emphasis is on treating the whole person, not just the illness. A nurse's focus is the needs of the patient and how the patient is responding to his or her illness and treatment.

Working with other professionals

In the U.S., nurses and physicians share responsibility for patient care. Nurses must also communicate with all the members of the healthcare team, including other nurses, nursing assistants, housekeeping staff, physicians, dietitians, and social workers. Communication between healthcare workers is just as important as the technical adeptness of the nurse. Nurses should be assertive in asking questions of other healthcare professionals when necessary, including physicians. The nursing style of communication should be direct but also polite and collaborative. (To find out more about communicating and collaborating with the healthcare team, turn to Chapter 5.)

Getting Accustomed to U.S. Cultural Values

Every country has defining cultural values. In order to practice nursing effectively in the U.S., you need to understand the socio-cultural factors of this country, especially as they apply to healthcare. U.S. culture emphasizes the following values:

>> **It's a democratic society.** The principles, policies, and norms of democracy are emphasized by social equality and representation by the people, for the people. In healthcare, all clients must receive equal time and consideration.

>> **People in the U.S. expect to be in optimal health.** This expectation contrasts with societies in countries where health isn't a major concern and receives little financial, social, and political support.

>> **People in the U.S. relate cleanliness with optimal health.** Clients may be very outspoken about the cleanliness of the facilities they're in and the healthcare workers assisting them. Very few countries emphasize cleanliness as much as the United States does, and you may be shocked by the way people there order their lives around cleanliness and insist upon it.

>> **All individuals, rather than certain social or religious groups, receive primary consideration.** Human rights, dignity, and individualism are emphasized.

>> **Success is marked by hard work and achievement.** The cultural value of achievement means that self-worth is often tied to personal success. In contrast, many other cultures emphasize enjoying what you have without worrying about accumulating more.

>> **Time is very valuable to people in the U.S.** Considerable emphasis is placed on schedules. People carry various electronic devices just to keep up with their own schedules, and punctuality is very important.

>> **The United States is culturally diverse, especially in major metropolitan areas.** Nurses must be concerned with the cultural care and preservation of those that they care for, accommodating cultural needs and requirements. Also, they must be able to make accommodation and negotiate with families and other caregivers who may be involved in the care patterns for particular patients.

Communicating Therapeutically

In the United States, the development of therapeutic communication skills is essential to a successful nursing career. Therapeutic communication is conversational — you speak to patients in a way that encourages them to be comfortable and honest with you. Saying the wrong thing can shut down communication and make meeting patient needs more difficult. Many questions on the NCLEX-RN relate to therapeutic communication, so a strong understanding of this technique can help you pass the exam. (I also cover therapeutic communication in Chapter 8.)

Practicing therapeutic communication

Therapeutic communication helps you communicate not only with your patients but also with their family members and with other members of the healthcare team. Therapeutic communication requires active listening, which involves listening to what your patient tells you, decoding the information, and then verbalizing to the patient what you gathered from his or her remarks. Repeating patients' remarks indicates that you understand their concerns and helps clarify their needs. Interpreting what they say may change the meaning.

Nurses must convey respect, warmth, and genuineness through active listening. They must also demonstrate interest and empathy for the concerns of everyone involved in the care of the patient, thus creating an environment that allows them to comfortably communicate their concerns.

Conversation should be focused on clients' feelings and concerns. You need to validate clients' feelings and listen to what patients say both verbally and nonverbally in order to properly work with them to improve their health. You also must anticipate that clients may experience some difficulty as they learn new behaviors and ways of coping with their conditions.

You can approach therapeutic communication in many ways. Although nurses in the U.S. use therapeutic responses that are based on an assessment of what each client needs, some general guidelines apply.

>> **Be accepting.** Don't impose your values on the patient. Indicate a nonjudgmental attitude toward clients and their perceptions by nodding and following along with what they say.

>> **Clarify.** Encourage patients to state their feelings more explicitly, perhaps by asking, "Could you explain that to me?"

>> **Encourage description.** Ask patients to verbalize their perceptions of what's going on. You may ask, "What is happening to you right now?"

>> **Give recognition.** Acknowledge your patients, letting them know that you're aware of them and their behaviors. You may say, "Good evening, Mr. Jones. You look well tonight." Intervene when a client behaves inappropriately and respond directly to a client by reinforcing positive behaviors.

>> **Keep eye contact.** Maintain eye contact with patients, especially during conversations. Lean toward them and use facial expressions to indicate your feelings while you're listening. When speaking to a child, kneel down or squat so that you're on the child's level and able to look the child directly the eye when you're speaking. ***Note:*** However, some cultures don't accept direct eye contact, so this point is one of those areas where you need to keep the individual patient's background in mind.

>> **Maintain focus.** Encourage patients to stay on topic. You may say, "You were talking about. . . ."

>> **Make observations.** Tell patients what you think you see. For example, you may say, "I notice that you seem very uncomfortable."

>> **Offer general leads.** Encourage patients to continue discussing the topic. You may ask, "Why don't you tell me more about that?"

>> **Offer silence.** Give your patients time to think about themselves and their problems without any pressure or obligation to speak.

>> **Offer yourself.** Offer to provide comfort to patients through your presence. For example, you may tell a patient that you'll sit with her for a while. Manage your time accordingly so that you have time to develop a nurse-client relationship and create a safe and secure environment for each client.

>> **Reflect.** Direct patients' questions and statements back to them to encourage an expression of ideas and feelings. For example, if a client asks you, "Do you think I should have the surgery?" you may respond, "What are your thoughts about whether or not to have the surgery?"

>> **Restate.** Repeat what patients say to you. The patient may say, "I don't want to take this medicine." You may respond, "You don't want to take this medication?" to confirm that you understand him correctly and get more information.

>> **Use broad, opening statements and open-ended questions.** Encourage patients to introduce a topic of conversation, perhaps by asking, "What are you thinking about?" To gain more information, try questions such as "How are you feeling about . . .?" Don't use questions the client can answer with a yes or no.

Steering clear of nontherapeutic techniques

Nontherapeutic communication techniques effectively put up a wall between the nurse and the client — which is exactly what you don't want to do. The following is a list of nontherapeutic techniques with corresponding inappropriate responses:

>> **Advising:**
- "I think you should do this."
- "Why don't you do that?"

>> **Agreeing:**
- "That's right."
- "I agree."

>> **Challenging:**
- "You're not really the president of the United States!"
- "So if you're dead, why is your heart beating?"

>> **Changing the subject:** Client: "I want to die." Nurse: "So, are you having visitors this weekend?"

>> **Defending:**

- "This hospital has a great reputation."

- "Nobody here would lie to you."

>> **Disagreeing:**

- "That's wrong."

- "I definitely disagree with you on that."

- "I don't believe that could happen."

>> **Disapproving:** "Oh, that's bad."

>> **Making false reassurances:**

- "I wouldn't worry about that."

- "Everything is going to be fine."

>> **Giving approval (which is trite and not really listening):** "Okay, that's good."

>> **Interpreting:**

- "What you really mean is . . ."

- "So what you're really saying is . . ."

>> **Making stereotypical comments:**

- "Nice day today, huh?"

- "I'm good, how are you?"

- "This is for your own good."

- "Keep your chin up."

- "Do what the doctor tells you, and you'll be fine."

>> **Rejecting:**

- "Let's not discuss that."

- "I really don't want to hear about that."

>> **Requesting an explanation:**

- "Why do you think that?"

- "Why do you feel that way?"

REMEMBER

Your personal feelings and past experiences can negatively or positively affect your relationship with the client, so try to keep them separate from the relationship at all cost.

Nurses also can create barriers to communication with clients by

>> Failing to understand cultural differences

>> Rejecting the person, not the behavior

- » Blaming the environment or something else for the patient's situation

- » Disagreeing or arguing with family members

- » Pressuring the patient or the family member to explain a situation that the nurse may not need to know about

- » Giving one-word responses to questions and acting unconcerned about the patient

- » Using medical terminology or medical jargon without explaining it in the conversation with the patient and other family members

- » Being racist or culturally offensive, either intentionally or unintentionally

- » Minimizing a patient's concerns and/or the family's concerns

- » Choosing sides in interactions among clients, their family members, and staff

- » Offering advice about a situation that the nurse doesn't know much about

- » Using denial when discussing serious situations with patients or their families

- » Ignoring language deficits and not getting appropriate interpretation to understand the patient's needs

TIP

When behavioral, cultural, and/or language differences exist among the nurse, the patient, and the patient's family, the probability is much higher that the patient won't understand the nurse's instructions regarding nursing care. To prevent conflicts and misunderstandings, be sure that the message you send is the same message that the patient receives. This clarification is especially important when you face a language barrier, whether it's the case that you don't understand the patient or that the patient doesn't understand you.

Applying U.S. Nursing Know-How to the NCLEX-RN

Some questions on the NCLEX-RN may cause problems for you if you don't have a good understanding of accepted U.S. standards of therapeutic communication and relationships (see the preceding sections). Here are some questions to practice on:

EXAMPLE

A nursing student is working with an alcoholic client. Although the nurse has negative feelings toward people who abuse alcohol, she feels that her client is deserving of respect and attention regardless of her own feelings. This is an example of

(1) Unconditional positive regard

(2) Countertransference

(3) Partnership

(4) Genuineness

The correct answer is Choice (1). In this case, the nurse has put her own feelings aside. She isn't showing genuineness or developing a partnership, which are both responses that aren't part of the therapeutic relationship. *Countertransference* refers to transferring one's feelings onto the client, which isn't the correct answer in this case.

EXAMPLE

A new patient has been admitted to your unit. Which action is most effective in initiating the nurse-patient relationship?

(1) Introducing yourself and explaining the purpose and plan for the working relationship

(2) Describing your family and having the patient describe hers

(3) Waiting for the patient to be ready to talk

(4) Asking the patient why she was brought to the hospital

The correct answer is Choice (1). In this case, the patient needs an orientation to you (the nurse) and your purpose. Open, honest communication sets the tone for your relationship.

EXAMPLE

Which of the following statements by a nurse doesn't demonstrate a judgmental attitude?

(1) "People who are mentally ill have basically weak characters."

(2) "I think the nurse is exaggerating her feelings so she can leave work early."

(3) "Mental illness is, for the most part, all in people's heads and could be easily solved if people were forced to continue their daily activities instead of listening to their complaints."

(4) "Cindy has struggled with her life circumstance of living with a man who beats her, and she's trying very hard to make the changes necessary to help herself."

The correct answer is Choice (4). It's the only nonjudgmental answer of the four options. The others place judgment on the situation or the person. Passing judgment on someone normally isn't accepted in U.S. culture and sets up a block to communication when trying to establish the nurse-client relationship.

EXAMPLE

As the nurse begins pre-op teaching for open-heart surgery, the patient becomes more restless, avoids eye contact, and seems distracted by hospital sounds around the room and corridor. Which statement is most appropriate by the nurse?

(1) "Please settle down and pay attention. This is important."

(2) "You seem nervous about your surgery."

(3) "I know you're probably worried about the surgery; everyone feels that way."

(4) No response. The nurse should just ignore the reaction and go on with the teaching.

The correct answer is Choice (2). This response acknowledges the client, whereas Choice (1) belittles the client. Choice (3) is untruthful and closes the discussion, and Choice (4) denies the problem.

EXAMPLE

A client in labor asks the nurse about the labor's progress and how much longer it will be until her baby is born. What is the appropriate response by the nurse?

(1) "I understand your concern; your baby should be delivered in a few hours."

(2) "You shouldn't be concerned; we're here to help make you comfortable."

(3) "Each person's labor varies. Is there something I can do to make you more comfortable?"

(4) "You shouldn't be concerned; the first stage of labor takes longer, and you're making great progress."

The correct answer is Choice (3). This response is truthful and encourages the client to express her needs. Choice (1) closes the discussion and may be untrue. Choices (2) and (4) are false reassurances and close the discussion.

EXAMPLE

A patient really wants to become more assertive with her husband but fears that her husband will be upset or that it will be too much of a shock for him with his heart condition. The most appropriate response to the client is

(1) "I'm sure your husband would understand."

(2) "Tell me more about how you think your husband would respond."

(3) "He's under a lot of stress now. I'd wait until he's feeling better before you talk with him about this."

(4) "This really has nothing to do with him. You should only consider what's right for you."

The correct answer is Choice (2). This response encourages an exploration of the client's feelings, whereas Choice (1) is perhaps untruthful and doesn't relieve the patient's anxiety. Choice (3) ignores her feelings and puts off the discussion until a later time, and Choice (4) ends the discussion and may be untruthful as well.

EXAMPLE

One day during an interview in the psychiatric unit, a client says, "I have nothing to live for. I just can't go on." What is the best response by the nurse?

(1) "Are you thinking of suicide?"

(2) "What would your husband do without you?"

(3) "Don't talk that way. You can't mean that."

(4) No response. The nurse should just change the subject.

The correct answer is Choice (1). This response encourages the discussion and an expression of the client's feelings. In this particular case, even though it's a closed-ended question, it's important to ascertain the presence of the client's thoughts of committing suicide. Choice (2) changes the subject and ignores the client's original problem. Choice (3) closes the discussion and ignores the problem, and Choice (4) doesn't explore the client's feelings and closes the discussion, which in this case could be fatal.

EXAMPLE

If a pregnant woman expresses indecision about whether or not to breastfeed, which is the most appropriate response by the nurse?

(1) "Your baby will feel more loved and secure if you breastfeed."

(2) "Why don't you wait until after the baby is born to decide?"

(3) "There are advantages and disadvantages to all methods of feeding."

(4) "Breast milk is the best possible food for a baby, and you certainly should give the baby this advantage."

The correct answer is Choice (3). This response encourages discussion and client teaching. Choices (1) and (4) are untruthful and close the discussion. Choice (4) also doesn't take into account the cultural beliefs of the mother. Choice (2) closes the discussion.

EXAMPLE

During a one-on-one interaction with the nurse, the patient is silent for the last five minutes. Which response is most appropriate by the nurse?

(1) "Apparently, you don't want to talk to me. How have I made you angry?"

(2) "I notice you're not saying anything. Tell me what you've been thinking about."

(3) "If you don't want to talk, that's okay. We'll meet again tomorrow at the same time."

(4) "If you don't use this time to solve this problem, how is it ever going to get any better?"

The correct answer is Choice (2). This response states the facts and opens the door to further communication. Choice (1) ignores the problem and may end up shifting the topic to something else. Choice (3) actually closes the discussion, setting up barriers to further communication about the issue at hand. Choice (4) may make the client feel guilty and may shut him down completely.

EXAMPLE

A depressed client states, "I've done everything in the world for my family. Now I'm in the hospital, and they'll get along fine without me." Which is the nurse's best response in this situation?

(1) "I'm sure they'll miss all you've done for them."

(2) "Now is the time for you to rest after all your hard work."

(3) "You sound hurt that your family doesn't seem to need you."

(4) "I'll teach you some relaxation exercises."

The correct answer is Choice (3). This response is the most therapeutic because it's an open-ended statement designed to elicit more information from the client. Choice (1) gives false reassurance and doesn't deal with the underlying problems. Choice (2) avoids the issue, and Choice (4) is a diversion that moves the client's attention away from the discussion of the problem.

EXAMPLE

A small child is off the unit having some tests when the parents approach the nurse and say, "We're going home now." Identify the best nursing response.

(1) "Good night, I'll see you tomorrow."

(2) "Please wait to tell your child goodbye before you leave."

(3) "You can go; I'm sure your child won't mind."

(4) "I'll tell your child that you had to go."

The correct answer is Choice (2). It's important that the child and the parents have closure before the parents leave. Choices (1) and (4) ignore the client's needs and are inappropriate. Choice (3) is completely untruthful and ignores the situation.

EXAMPLE

A visiting nurse schedules a 9 a.m. appointment with a Hispanic client for a home visit following a hospital stay. The client asks the nurse whether her daughter and son can be present at the visit. The nurse knows

(1) That the client has a poor memory and wants them there to reinforce any teaching that will occur

(2) That Hispanics often have close extended family ties, and family members are often involved in health decisions

(3) That the client is old and will not remember anything about the visit

(4) That the client is fearful of the nurse

The correct answer is Choice (2). In Hispanic cultures, extended families are often involved in making healthcare decisions. Choices (1), (3), and (4), although possible, aren't the primary focus in this situation.

Appendix C
Glossary of Nursing Terms

abdominal hysterectomy: Removal of the uterus through the abdomen via a surgical incision

absorption: The way substances pass into tissue as nutrients from food move from the small intestine into the cells of the body

accessory digestive organs: Organs that help digestion but aren't part of the digestive tract. These organs include the tongue, glands in the mouth that make saliva, pancreas, liver, and gallbladder.

accommodation: The ability of the eye to focus

active immunity: Immunity acquired after being exposed to the infection or exposure to an antigen

activities of daily living (ADLs): Personal care activities necessary for everyday living, such as eating, bathing, grooming, dressing, and toileting; a term often used by healthcare professionals to assess the need and/or type of care a person may require

acute kidney injury: A sudden loss of kidney function after renal cell damage has occurred; causes are prerenal, intrarenal, or postrenal

adenocarcinoma: A cancer that develops in the lining or inner surface of an organ

adrenal cortex: The outer portion of the adrenal gland that secretes hormones that are vital to the body

agonist: A drug capable of combining with receptors to initiate an action that can be known in advance

akinesia: Loss of voluntary movement

alimentary canal: Digestive tube

alternative medicine: Any form of therapy used alone without recommended standard or conventional treatment

anesthetics: Medications that cause loss of awareness or sensation to pain

angiotensin-converting enzyme (ACE) inhibitor: A medication that lowers blood pressure. ACE inhibitors work by blocking the production of angiotensin II, a substance that narrows blood vessels and releases hormones such as aldosterone and norepinephrine, by inhibiting an enzyme called angiotensin converting enzyme. Angiotensin II, aldosterone, and norepinephrine all increase blood pressure and urine production by the kidneys. If levels of these three substances decrease in the body, this allows blood vessels to relax and dilate (widen), reducing both blood and kidney pressure.

anticholinergics: Medicines that calm muscle spasms in the intestine. A major side effect is dry mouth. Anticholinergics are medications that block the action of acetylcholine, a neurotransmitter (chemical messenger). Used to treat a variety of conditions, including urinary incontinence, overactive bladder, some poisonings, Parkinson's, chronic obstructive pulmonary disorder (COPD), among others.

antiemetic: A drug that prevents or relieves nausea and vomiting

antioxidant: Compounds that protect against cell damage inflicted by molecules called oxygen free radicals, which are a major cause of disease and aging

aphasia: Total or partial loss of the ability to use or understand language; usually caused by stroke, brain disease, or injury

apraxia: Inability to make a movement in spite of being able to demonstrate normal muscle function and desire to perform the task

arterioles: Small branches of arteries

arteriosclerosis: A thickening or hardening of the walls of blood vessels

arthralgia: Pain in a joint, usually due to arthritis or arthropathy

arthroplasty: Total joint replacement

atherosclerosis: A type of arteriosclerosis caused by a buildup of plaque in the inner lining of an artery

atrial flutter: Ineffective contractions of the heart muscle. The atrium contract too rapidly and are ineffective in pumping the blood into the ventricles.

atrioventricular block: An interruption of the electrical signal between the atria and ventricles in the heart

atrophy: A decline of a body part or tissue, usually a muscle, typically preceded by a period of disuse or immobility

atypical: Not usual; abnormal; often refers to the appearance of precancerous or cancerous cells

autoimmune process: A process in which the body's immune system attacks and destroys body tissue that it mistakes for foreign matter

autologous transplant: A procedure in which a patient's own blood or bone marrow is removed, treated with anticancer medication or radiation, and then returned to the patient

autonomic dysreflexia: A life-threatening condition, requiring immediate treatment, that can occur after a T6 or above spinal cord injury. The client may experience high blood pressure, headache, and excessive sweating after experiencing a noxious stimulus. The stimuli can be urinary retention, wrinkled sheets, or impacted rectum.

avulsion: When a muscle is forcefully stretched beyond its freely available range of motion, or when a muscle meets a sudden, unexpected resistance while contracting forcefully and tears free

balloon angioplasty: A procedure used to widen narrowed arteries. A catheter with a deflated balloon at the tip is inserted into the narrowed part of the artery, and the balloon is inflated, causing the artery to dilate.

Barium sulfate: A metallic, chalky, chemical liquid used to coat the inside of the esophagus, stomach, or intestines so that they show up on an X-ray

basal body temperature: Temperature of a person's body taken first thing in the morning after several hours of sleep and before any activity, including getting out of bed or talking; often charted to determine the time of ovulation

basal ganglia: Several large clusters of nerve cells, including the stratum and the substantia nigra, deep in the brain below the cerebral hemispheres

basal metabolic rate (BMR): A measurement of energy required to keep the body functioning at rest. Measured in calories, metabolic rates increase with exertion, stress, fear, and/or illness.

base of the lung: Bottom portion of lower lobes of the lungs, just above the diaphragm

beta blocker: A medication class that limits the activity of epinephrine. They're often used to reduce blood pressure and treat other heart conditions.

beta cells: Cells that make insulin, found in areas of the pancreas called the islets of Langerhans

bilateral: Affecting both sides of the body. For example, bilateral breast cancer is cancer occurring in both breasts at the same time (synchronous) or at different times (metachronous).

blood-brain barrier (BBB): A protective semipermeable border that separates solutes in circulating blood from brain cells

blood plasma: The fluid part of blood that contains nutrients, glucose, proteins, minerals, enzymes, and other substances

body mass index (BMI): A number, derived by using height and weight measurements, that gives a general indication of whether a person's weight falls within a healthy range

bone density test: A test that measures the strength and density of bones; often used to determine the risk of developing osteoporosis

bradycardia: Abnormally slow heart rate

brain attack: Stroke or cerebrovascular accident (CVA)

brain scan: An imaging method used to find abnormalities in the brain, including brain cancer and cancer that has spread to the brain from other places in the body

Braxton-Hicks contractions: Relatively brief, painless contractions of the uterus that may begin during the second half of pregnancy

bronchodilators: A group of medications that widen the airways in the lungs

Brudzinski's sign: An indicator of meningeal irritation; when a patient's neck is passively flexed, the hip and knee respond by an involuntary flexion

bundle branch block: A condition in which the heart's electrical system is completely or partially interrupted, after the atrioventricular (AR) node, inside the wall of the heart that leads to the two ventricles

calcium channel blocker: A medication used to treat heart conditions by decreasing the contractility and workload of the heart

calculi: Stones, often made of mineral salts, such as gallstones, that form in organs or ducts in the body

candidiasis: Infection caused by the Candida fungus, which lives naturally in the gastrointestinal tract. Infection occurs when a change in the body — for example, antibiotic use — causes the fungus to overgrow suddenly.

capillaries: Tiny blood vessels between arteries and veins that distribute oxygen-rich blood to the body

carcinogen: A substance known to cause cancer

cardiac output: Total amount of blood being pumped by the heart over one minute. It is reported in L/min.

cardiac ventricle: One of the two pumping chambers of the heart. The right ventricle receives unoxygenated blood from the right atrium and pumps it to the lungs through the pulmonary artery to the left ventricle, which receives oxygen-rich blood from the left atrium and pumps it to the body.

carotid arteries: The major arteries in the neck that supply blood to the brain

cartilage: A smooth material the covers bone ends of a joint to cushion the bone and allow the joint to move easily without pain

CAT scan: See *CT scan*

catheter: A flexible tube inserted into a body cavity, vessel, or duct, usually to allow for administration of fluids, medications, or gases, or to drain fluids or to provide access for surgical procedures. The most common catheter is the Foley catheter, which drains urine from the bladder.

cerebellum: A large structure consisting of two halves located in the lower part of the brain; responsible for the coordination of movement, posture, speech, and balance

cerebral embolism: A blood clot that travels via the bloodstream from one part of the body to the brain, where it blocks an artery

cerebrovascular: Pertaining to blood vessels in the brain

cerebrum: Consists of two parts (lobes), left and right, which form the largest and most developed part of the brain. Associated with intelligence and higher brain functions including logic, interpretation, and critical thinking, as well as the initiation of all voluntary movement. The basal ganglia are located immediately below the cerebrum.

cholecystitis: Inflammation of the gallbladder

cholelithiasis: A condition in which gallstones are present in the gallbladder

claudication: Pain and fatigue in the legs due to the poor supply of oxygen to the muscles

clostridium difficile (C. difficile): A fungal-like anaerobic bacteria that can be naturally present in the large intestine in small numbers. With overgrowth (from taking antibiotics or from contact transmission of the bacteria), serious infections such as pseudomembranous colitis can occur. It can't be eliminated with hand sanitizer and must be washed off.

colectomy: Partial or complete removal of the large bowel

computed tomography: see *CT scan*

corticosteroids: Potent anti-inflammatory hormones that are made naturally in the body or synthetically for use as medications. The most commonly prescribed medications of this type is prednisone.

crepitus: Grinding noise or sensation within a joint. It also can refer to air coming to the surface of the skin when a client has a pneumothorax. The area on the skin looks like bubbles under the skin.

CT scan: Noninvasive diagnostic imaging that takes cross-sectional images of bones, blood vessels, soft tissues or organs to detect any abnormalities that may not show up on an ordinary X-ray; also called a CAT scan or computed tomography

cyanosis: Bluish color to the skin due to insufficient oxygen levels in the blood

decerebrate posturing: Response to a brainstem injury in which the client extends both arms and legs

decorticate posturing: Response to damage to the nerve pathway in the midbrain between the brain and spinal cord in which the client brings the arms in toward the body core or chest and extends the legs

defibrillator: An electronic device used to establish a normal heartbeat when the heart has a dysrhythmia

delegation: Transfer of the actual care or task needed for a patient to another healthcare worker after ensuring the task is within the person's scope of practice

delusion: A condition in which the patient has lost touch with reality and may experience hallucinations and misperceptions

dialysis: Process used when kidneys are not functioning; can involve filtering the blood through an ultrafiltration system or placing fluid into the abdominal cavity and using osmosis through the peritoneum to remove waste from the body

diaphragm: Primary muscle used for respiration, located just below the base of the lungs

diastolic blood pressure: The lowest blood pressure in the arteries, which occurs between heartbeats

digestion: Process the body uses to break down food into simple substances for energy, growth, and tissue repair

distention: Bloating or swelling of the abdomen

diuretic: A medication that increases urine formation and is often used to lower blood pressure

diverticulosis: A condition that occurs when small pouches (diverticula) push outward through weak spots in the colon

dopamine: A chemical substance, a neurotransmitter, found in the brain that regulates motivation, reward, movement, balance, and walking

durable power of attorney: A legal document denoting another person to be able to act on their behalf in case one is unable to make decisions for oneself

dyskinesia: An involuntary movement such as athetosis or chorea

dyspepsia: Indigestion

dysphagia: Difficulty swallowing

dysplasia: An abnormality of growth

dyspnea: Shortness of breath

dysrhythmia: An abnormal heart rhythm

dystocia: Prolonged labor that is painful and difficult

dystonia: An abnormal muscle tone or extended spasm in a group of muscles

ECG: A test that records the electrical activity of the heart, shows abnormal rhythms (arrhythmias or dysrhythmias), and detects heart muscle damage

eczema: Inflammation of the skin that causes itching and sometimes crusting, scaling, or blisters

edema: Swelling due to fluid buildup

ejection fraction: The measurement, expressed as a percentage, of the blood pumped out of the ventricles with each contraction

EKG: See *ECG*

electrical cardioversion: The procedure of applying electrical shock to the heart through the chest and possibly the back to change an abnormal heartbeat into a normal one

electrocardiogram: See *ECG*

electromyogram (EMG): A test to evaluate nerve and muscle function

electrophysiological study (EPS): A cardiac catheterization to study electrical current of the heart in patients who have arrhythmias

embolus: The "wandering" blood clot

encephalitis: An inflammation of the brain usually due to an infection or allergic reaction

endocardium: The membrane that covers the inside surface of the heart

endometrium: Mucous membrane lining of the inner surface of the uterus; grows during each menstrual cycle and is shed in menstrual blood

endothelium: The layer of cells that line the heart, blood vessels, and other body cavities

enteral nutrition: Way to provide liquid nourishment through a tube inserted into the nose, stomach, or small intestine. A tube in the nose is called a *nasogastric* or *enteral tube*. A tube that goes through the skin into the stomach or small intestine is called a *gastrostomy* or *percutaneous endoscopic tube.*

enterostomy: A surgical procedure in which the small intestine is diverted to an opening in the abdominal wall or another part of the intestine. Can also be the artificial opening in the abdominal wall after the procedure.

epicardium: The membrane that covers the outside of the heart

epidural anesthetic: An anesthetic that's injected into the epidural space in the middle or lower back to numb the lower extremities

epinephrine: One of two chemicals (the other is norepinephrine) released by the adrenal gland that increases heart rate by forcing heart contractions and narrows blood vessels. Can also be produced synthetically and is used for cardiac conditions and allergic responses.

ergonomics: The study of how the workplace relates to human functions

erythrocyte sedimentation rate (ESR): Blood test that measures the speed at which red blood cells settle on the bottom of the test tube. High ESR signals a possible inflammatory disease.

estrogen: A hormone secreted by the ovaries that affects many aspects of the female body, including menstrual cycles and pregnancies

extrapyramidal system: System consisting of nerve cells, nerve tracts, and pathways that connect the cerebral cortex, basal ganglia, thalamus, cerebellum, reticular formation, and spinal neurons; concerned with the regulation of reflex movements such as balance and walking

fecal incontinence: Inability to hold stool in the colon and rectum

fetal heart rate variability: Changes in the fetal heart rate (FHR) baseline

fibrillation: Rapid contractions of the heart muscle

flexor muscle: Any muscle that causes the flexion of a limb or other body part

follicle-stimulating hormone (FSH): Hormone secreted by the pituitary gland in the brain that stimulates the growth and maturation of eggs in females and sperm in males as well as sex hormone production in both males and females

food intolerance: An adverse food-induced reaction that doesn't involve the immune system; an example is lactose intolerance

ganglion: A cluster of nerve cells

gas: Air that comes from a normal breakdown of food and passes out of the body through the rectum (flatus) or the mouth (belch)

gastric: Related to the stomach

gastroenteritis: Infection or irritation of the stomach and intestines, which may be caused by bacteria or parasites from spoiled food or unclean water, food that irritates the stomach lining, or emotional upset such as anger, fear, or stress

gastrointestinal (GI) tract: A large muscular tube that extends from the mouth to the anus; where the movement of muscles and release of hormones and enzymes digest food

general anesthetic: An anesthetic usually given during surgery that causes the patient to become unconscious

glucose: A simple sugar that's the body's main source of energy

gluteus maximus: The large superficial buttock muscle

glycogen: Converted glucose for storage; plays a role in controlling blood sugar levels

granuloma: A mass of granulation tissue usually due to infection, inflammation, or a foreign substance. In the GI tract, a massive red, irritated granuloma is found in Crohn's disease.

gray matter: The darker colored tissues of the central nervous system. In the brain, the gray matter includes the cerebral cortex, thalamus, basal ganglia, and outer layers of the cerebellum.

H2 blockers: Medicines that reduce the amount of acid the stomach produces by blocking histamine, which signals the stomach to make acid

halitosis: An oral health condition characterized by consistently malodorous breath

hamstrings: Muscles located in the posterior compartment of the thigh

headache, primary: Includes tension (muscular contraction), vascular (migraine), and cluster headaches not caused by other underlying medical conditions

heart block: Interrupted electrical impulse to the heart muscle

heart valve prolapse: A condition of the heart valve in which it's partially open when it should be closed

hemorrhage: Uncontrolled bleeding

high-density lipoprotein (HDL): The "good" cholesterol that promotes breakdown and removal of cholesterol from the body

histamine: A chemical present in cells throughout the body that's released during an injury or an allergic or inflammatory reaction

hormones: Chemical substances created by the body that control numerous body functions. Can also be produced synthetically.

human chorionic gonadotropin (HCG): Hormone produced by the placenta during early pregnancy

human papillomaviruses (HPV): A group of viruses that can cause warts. HPVs are sexually transmitted and can cause wart-like growths on the genitals. HPV is a major risk factor for cervical cancer.

hydrocortisone: A hormone secreted by the adrenal cortex, which affects metabolism and inflammation

hypercalcemia: High levels of calcium in the blood

hyperextension: Active or passive force that takes the joint beyond its normal physiological range of extension

hyperglycemia: High levels of glucose in the blood

hyperkalemia: High levels of potassium in the blood

hypermagnesemia: High levels of magnesium in the blood

hypernatremia: High levels of sodium in the blood

hyperphosphatemia: High levels of phosphorus in the blood

hypertrophy: An increase in size of tissue

hypocalcemia: Low levels of calcium in the blood

hypokalemia: Low levels of potassium in the blood

hypomagnesemia: Low levels of magnesium in the blood

hyponatremia: Low levels of sodium in the blood

hypophosphatemia: Low levels of phosphorus in the blood

hypotension: Abnormally low blood pressure

hypothalamus: Small structure at the base of the brain that regulates many body functions, including appetite and body temperature

hypoxia: Depletion of oxygen in the cells and tissues

idiopathic: Of unknown origin

ileostomy: An operation in which an opening is made in the abdomen and the bottom of the small intestine (ileum) is attached to it; makes it possible for stool to leave the body after the colon and rectum are removed

imaging: An evaluation procedure that produces pictures of areas inside the body

immune system: The complex network of specialized cells and organs that work together to defend the body against attacks by "foreign" invaders such as bacteria and viruses

immunoglobulins: Proteins in blood and tissue fluids that help destroy microorganisms such as bacteria

immunosuppressive medications: Medications to suppress the body's immune system; often used to minimize rejection of transplanted organs

immunotherapy: Treatment for allergies to substances such as pollens, house dust mites, fungi, and stinging insect venom; involves giving gradually increasing doses of the substance, or allergen, to which the person is allergic

impaction: Trapping of an object in a body passage, such as stones in the bile duct or hardened stool in the colon

in vitro fertilization: Treatment for infertility in which a woman's egg is fertilized outside her body with her partner's sperm or sperm from a donor

infection: The invasion of the body by microorganisms that cause disease

inferior vena cava: The large blood vessel that returns blood from the legs and abdomen to the heart

infiltration: Infusion of fluids into the tissues caused when the IV canula exits the vein. Patient's extremity affected are cool to the touch and pale and experience swelling or edema and pain.

inflammation: Characteristic reaction of tissues to injury or disease; marked by four signs: swelling, redness, heat, and pain

information security: Privacy of the patient's personal health information (PHI)

informed consent: A consent form signed by the patient prior to surgery that explains everything involved in the surgery, including its risks

inotropic medications: Medications that increase strength of the contractions of the heart

insulin: A hormone produced by the pancreas that affects the amount of glucose absorbed by the liver

intercostal muscles: Muscles lying between ribs; often injured by rotary stress of the thorax

intestinal flora: Bacteria, yeasts, and fungi that grow normally in the intestines

intolerance: Allergy or sensitivity to food, drug, or other substance

intravenous line: A thin plastic tube inserted into a vein through which a volume of fluid is injected into the bloodstream

ischemia: Decreased flow of oxygenated blood to an organ due to obstruction in an artery

ischemic heart disease: Coronary artery disease or coronary heart disease caused by narrowing of the coronary arteries and decreased blood flow to the heart

joint: Where the ends of two or more bones meet

jugular veins: Veins that carry blood from the head back to the heart

keratitis: Inflammation of the cornea

Kernig's sign: Indicator of meningeal irritation; a positive occurs if the client complains of pain around the spinal column when the hip and knee are flexed and then extended

ketoacidosis: High blood glucose; often caused by illness or taking too little insulin

ketone: Breakdown product of fat that accumulates in the blood as a result of inadequate insulin or inadequate caloric intake

labyrinth: Organ of balance that's located in the inner ear; consists of the cochlea, three semicircular canals, and the vestibule

lactase: Enzyme in the small intestine needed to digest milk sugar (lactose)

lactose: Sugar found in milk; broken down by the body into galactose and glucose

laminectomy: Surgical procedure that includes removal of a portion of the lamina to provide more room in the vertebral channel; usually performed to treat disc herniation or spinal canal stenosis

laparoscope: Thin tube with a tiny camera attached that's used to look inside the body and see the surface of an organ

larynx: Valve structure between the trachea and the pharynx; contains the vocal chords, the primary organ of voice production

lavage: The process of washing (cleaning) an organ such as the bowel or stomach

laxatives (cathartics): Medications to induce a bowel movement

lesion: Any injury or wound

levodopa: An effective anti-Parkinson drug that's changed into dopamine in the brain

ligament: A flexible band of fibrous tissue that connects the bones and binds the joints together

lipid: A fatty substance in the blood

lipoproteins: Transport fatty substances in the blood

liver: The largest organ in the body; performs important functions such as making bile, changing food into energy, and cleaning alcohol and poisons from the blood

living will: A legal document that states medical preferences for treatment and resuscitation in the event that one can no longer speak for oneself

low-density lipoprotein (LDL): The major carrier of "bad" cholesterol in the blood; high levels of LDL are associated with narrowing of the arteries and heart disease

lumpectomy: A surgical procedure in which only the tumor and a small area surrounding tissues is removed

lung volume: The amount of air that the lungs hold

lymph nodes: Small glands clustered throughout the body, for example in the neck, armpits, abdomen, and groin that supply cells to the bloodstream that fight infection and filter out bacteria and other antigens

lymphatic system: Tissues and organs, including bone marrow, spleen, thymus, and lymph nodes, that produce, store, and carry white blood cells to fight infection and disease

lymphocytes: Any one of the group of white blood cells of crucial importance to the adaptive part of the body's immune system

magnetic resonance imaging: See *MRI*

malabsorption syndromes: Occur when the small intestine can't absorb nutrients from foods

Maslow's hierarchy: Six-level pyramid ranking the importance of human needs; developed by Abraham Maslow

mastoid: The portion of the temporal bone behind the ear

mean blood pressure: Average blood pressure, counting the rise and fall that occurs with each heartbeat. It's often estimated by multiplying the diastolic pressure by two, adding the systolic pressure, and then dividing the sum by three.

median nerve: Large nerve comprising segments from the cervical spine that's involved in neural function of upper limbs; commonly entrapped in the carpal tunnel of the wrist to create carpal tunnel syndrome

melena: Blood in stool

meniscus: A crescent shaped cartilage in the knees and other joints

middle ear: Part of the ear that includes the ear drum and three tiny bones and ends in the round window that leads to the inner ear

miosis: Constriction of the pupil

mitral valve: The valve that controls blood flow between the left atrium and left ventricle in the heart

motility: Ability of an organism to move, or ability to move food through the digestive tract

MRI: A noninvasive procedure that produces two-dimensional views of an internal organ or structure, especially the brain and spinal cord

mucosal lining: Lining of the respiratory and GI tract organs that makes mucus

mucus: Clear liquid made by the respiratory tract and intestines that coats and protects tissues in the gastrointestinal tract

murmur: A blowing or rushing sound heard while listening to the heart, caused by increased turbulence; may or may not indicate problems within the heart or circulatory system

myocardial infarction: Also known as a heart attack; occurs when one or more regions of the heart muscle experience severe or prolonged decrease in oxygen supply caused by a blocked blood flow to the heart muscle that results in heart muscle injury

myocardial ischemia: Insufficient blood flow to any part of the heart

myocardium: Muscle wall of the heart

myoclonus: Jerking, involuntary movements of the arms and legs; may occur normally during sleep

nephrectomy: Surgical removal of the kidney

neural stimulation: To activate or energize a nerve through an external source

neuralgia: A painful condition of the nerves caused by disorders of the nervous system

neuritis: Inflammation of a nerve or nerves

neurogenic: Of nerve origin

neuron: A cell specialized to conduct and generate electrical impulses and to carry information from one part of the brain to another

neurotransmitters: Chemical substances that carry impulses from one nerve cell to another; found in the space (synapse) that separates the transmitting neurons terminal (axon) from the receiving neurons terminal (dendrites)

nonsteroidal anti-inflammatory drugs (NSAIDS): Medications that produce antipyridic, analgesic, and anti-inflammatory effects

norepinephrine: A neurotransmitter found mainly in areas of the brain that are involved in governing autonomic nervous system activity, especially blood pressure and heart rate

nuclear medicine: A specialized area of radiology that uses very small amounts of radioactive substances to examine organ function and structure

nutrients: Proteins, carbohydrates, fats, vitamins, and minerals provided by food and necessary for growth and the maintenance of life

occult: Disease or symptoms not readily detectable by physical examination

oropharynx: The part of the throat at the back of the mouth

orthostatic hypotension: A large decrease in blood pressure upon standing; may result in fainting

ototoxic drugs: Medications that can damage the hearing and balance organs located in the inner ear

ovaries: Pair of small glands, located on either side of the uterus, in which egg cells develop and are stored and the female sex hormones estrogen and progesterone are produced

pacemaker: An electronic device that's surgically implanted into the patient's heart and chest to regulate heartbeat; can also be combined as a pacemaker/defibrillator

palliative care: Therapy that relieves symptoms, such as pain, but doesn't alter the course of the disease; its primary purpose is to improve the quality of life

palpitations: Sensation of rapid heartbeats

palsy: Paralysis of a muscle or a group of muscles often accompanied by involuntary tremors

Parkinsonism: A group of disorders with similar characteristics, including four primary symptoms — tremor, rigidity, postural instability, and bradykinesia — that are the result of the loss of dopamine-producing brain cells

partial collectomy: The removal of part of the large intestine

pathology: Study of diseases

peak flow: The measure of how air flows from lungs in one "fast blast" to measure the ability to push air out of the lungs; used primarily to measure airflow of asthmatic patients

pepsin: Enzyme in the stomach that breaks down proteins

peptic ulcer: A sore in the lining of the esophagus, stomach, or duodenum usually caused by the bacterium Helicobacter pylori. An ulcer in the stomach is a gastric ulcer; an ulcer in the duodenum is a duodenal ulcer.

perfusion: Flow of blood or other fluid into organs or tissues

pericardium: Membrane that surrounds the heart

perineal: Related to the perineum

perineum: Area between the anus and the sex organs

peritoneum: Lining of the abdominal cavity

pharmacological cardioversion: The administering of antidysrhythmics to convert the heart back into normal rhythm

pharynx: The space behind the mouth that serves as a passage for food from the mouth to the esophagus and for air from the nose and mouth to the larynx

phlebitis: Inflammation of the veins from medications or mechanical irritation, potentially leading to clot formation. The site is red, warm, and painful, and a streak may form up the extremity.

photophobia: Sensitivity to light

pituitary gland: Gland at the base of the brain that secretes hormones and regulates and controls other hormone-secreting glands and many body processes, including reproduction

placenta: Organ that develops in the uterus during pregnancy; links the blood supplies of a pregnant woman and her fetus to provide nutrients to and remove waste products from the fetus

placental abruption: Premature detachment of the placenta from the wall of the uterus, causing severe bleeding; is life-threatening to both the pregnant woman and the fetus

plasma: The watery, straw-colored fluid that carries the cellular elements in the bloodstream

platelets: Type of cells used for blood clotting; found in the bloodstream

polyunsaturated fat: A type of fat found in nuts, seeds, and vegetable oils

portal hypertension: Abnormally high blood pressure in the portal vein, which supplies the liver with blood from the intestine

presbycusis: Loss of hearing that gradually occurs because of changes in the inner or middle ear as individuals grow older

preterm labor: Labor that begins before the 37th week of pregnancy

prioritization: Decision on what action or problem needs attention first, as determined by Maslow's hierarchy

progestin: Synthetic form of the female sex hormone progesterone

prognosis: A prediction of the course of the disease

prolapse: A condition that occurs when a body part slips from its normal position

prostate-specific antigen (PSA) blood test: A blood test used to help detect prostate cancer by measuring a substance called prostate-specific antigen produced by the prostate

pulmonary: Pertaining to the lungs and/or respiratory system

pulmonary artery: Blood vessel delivering unoxygenated blood from the right ventricle to the lungs

pulmonary vein: The vessel that carries newly oxygenated blood from the lungs to the heart; the only vein in the body that carries oxygenated blood

pyloric sphincter: Muscle between the stomach and the small intestine

pylorus: Opening from the stomach into the top of the small intestine (duodenum)

QRS complex: Combination of three graphic deflections that reflect the contraction of the ventricles on an EKG

quickening: The first fetal movement a pregnant woman feels; occurs around the 16th to 20th week

radiation: Use of high-energy radiation from X-rays, neutrons, and other sources to kill cancer cells and shrink tumors

radical mastectomy: Surgical removal of the entire breast, the pectoral muscles, and the ancillary lymph nodes

radiculopathy: Pinched nerves that usually result from a herniated, or slipped, disc; can cause pain, numbness, tingling, weakness, or a shooting pain often described as an electrical feeling

range of motion (ROM): Measurement of the extent to which a joint can go through all its normal movements

Recommended Daily Allowance (RDA): Recommendations for daily intake of specific nutrients as set by the Food and Nutrition Board of the National Academy of Sciences/National Research Council; recommendations are different for children, adults, males, and females

reflux: The flow of a fluid through a vessel valve that is in the opposite direction of normal. Condition that occurs when gastric juices or small amounts of food from the stomach flow back into the esophagus and mouth is called gastric reflux. This can also occur in the heart valves and other places in the body.

regional anesthetic: An anesthetic used to numb a portion of the body

rehabilitation: The process of attempting to restore a part of the body or a person to as near-normal as possible functioning after an injury or disease

residual: Gastric contents left from the previous enteral feeding

respiration: Gas exchange from air to the blood and from the blood to the body cells

retraction: Pulling in of the chest muscles between the ribs on inspiration; easier to see on children. Indicates difficulty breathing.

saturated fat: Fat found in animal meats and skin, dairy products, and some vegetables

secretin: A hormone made in the duodenum that controls the pH in the duodenum by regulating stomach acid secretion, the liver to make bile, and the pancreas to make bicarbonate and insulin

septal defect: A hole in the wall that separates the two sides of the heart (the septum)

septum: The muscle wall that divides the heart chambers

serum: A clear fluid that separates when blood clots

shunt: Connector that allows blood or fluid flow between two locations; can be congenital or acquired, biological or mechanical

sigmoid colon: A part of the colon that empties into the rectum

silent ischemia: Condition in which a decreased flow of oxygenated blood to an organ due to arterial obstruction (ischemia) isn't accompanied by any pain

sinus node: The cells that normally initiate the electrical impulses that cause the heart to contract

small intestine: The organ where most digestion occurs; measures about 20 feet and comprises the duodenum, jejunum, and ileum

smooth muscle: Muscle that performs automatic tasks, such as constricting blood vessels

soft tissue: Generally, this is soft tissue that connects, supports, or surrounds other structures/organs in the body including muscles, ligaments, fibrous tissues, tendons, fascia, nerves, fat, blood vessels, and synovial membranes

spasm: A condition in which a muscle or group of muscles involuntarily contract

sphincter: Ring-like band of muscle that opens and closes an opening of the body

spinal anesthetic: An anesthetic injected into the spinal canal fluid for surgery in the lower abdomen, pelvis, rectum, or other lower extremities

spleen: Organ lying between the stomach and diaphragm that stores red blood cells and filters blood

spondylosis: A condition of the spine involving a degenerative process of the discs and joints

stenosis: The narrowing or constricting of an opening or a blood vessel or a valve of the heart

stoma: An opening in the abdomen that's created by an operation (ostomy); must be covered by a bag to collect the stool or urine

streptokinase: A clot-dissolving medication

superior vena cava: A large vein that returns blood to the heart from the head and arms

synapse: Tiny gaps between the ends of nerve fibers across which nerve impulses pass from one neuron to another and cause the release of the neurotransmitter, which diffuses across the gap and triggers an electrical impulse in the next neuron

syncope: Fainting caused by insufficient blood supply to the brain

synovitis: Inflammation of the synovial membrane, the tissue that lines and protects the joint

systolic blood pressure: The highest pressure to which blood pressure rises with the contraction of the heart

tachycardia: Rapid heart beat

tendon: A chord that connects muscle to bone or other tissue

thoracotomy: Surgery to view the lungs or chest cavity; performed on patients with chest trauma to detect the source of bleeding

thrombolysis: The breaking up of a blood clot

tinnitus: Sensation of a ringing, roaring, or buzzing sound in the ears or head often associated with various forms of hearing impairment

tissue plasminogen activator (tPA): A medication used to dissolve blood clots

tocolytics: Medications that relax the uterus and slow the uterine activity

Tourette syndrome: Neurological disorder characterized by recurring involuntary movements and/or sounds (called tics)

transient ischemic attack (TIA): A stroke-like event that lasts for a short period of time; caused by a blocked or spasming blood vessel

tricuspid valve: The heart valve that controls blood flow from the right atrium into the right ventricle

trimester: Usually used to describe a three-month period during pregnancy

type 1 diabetes: An autoimmune condition in which the pancreas produces so little insulin that the body can't use blood glucose as energy; must be controlled with daily insulin injections

type 2 diabetes: A condition in which the pancreas produces a little insulin, but not enough to effectively use blood glucose as energy; can often be controlled through meal plans, physical activity plans, and a variety of diabetes pills. Insulin may be needed depending on advancement of the disease.

ulcer: Sore on the skin surface, mucosa, or in the stomach lining

unlicensed assistive personnel (UAP): Healthcare workers to whom nurses can delegate some tasks

ureters: Two tubes that carry urine from the kidneys to the bladder

urethra: Narrow channel through which urine passes from the bladder out of the body

urinary retention: The inability to empty the bladder

uterus: A hollow, pear-shaped organ located in a woman's lower abdomen, between the bladder and the rectum. If fertilization doesn't occur, the uterus sheds its lining each month during menstruation; if fertilization does occur, the fertilized egg implants in the uterus wall and grows into a fetus.

vagus nerve: The tenth cranial nerve that connects the brain to the thorax and abdomen. It plays a role in the regulation of the production of stomach acid.

varices: Stretched veins, such as those that form in the esophagus from cirrhosis

vascular: Pertaining to blood vessels

vasodilator: An agent that widens blood vessels

vein: A blood vessel that carries blood from the body back into the heart

vena cava syndrome: Hypotension occurring in pregnancy when the uterus compresses the vena cava while the patient lies supine. Lying on the left side alleviates the compression.

ventilation: Movement of air in and out of the lungs

ventricular fibrillation: A condition in which the ventricles contract in rapid and unsynchronized rhythms and can't pump blood to the body

viral hepatitis: Hepatitis caused by a virus. Five different viruses (A, B, C, D, and E) most commonly cause hepatitis, but other rare viruses may also cause hepatitis.

whole blood: Blood containing all of its components, including red and white blood cells and platelets

Index

Brunner and Suddarth's Textbook of Medical-Surgical Nursing (Hinkle et al.), 45

BSN (Bachelor of Science in Nursing), 17

Buck's traction, 219, 234, 259, 267

C

C vitamin, 135

CABG (coronary artery bypass graft), 210

caffeine, 115

California, 313

call bell system, 91

CAM (complementary and alternative modalities), 147–148, 162

Canada, 341

Candidate Performance Report (CPR), 291

canes, 149–150

carbachol eyedrops, 224, 261

carbohydrates, 135

carbon monoxide poisoning, 230, 265

cardiac catheterization, 186, 250, 280

cardiac strips, 201

cardiac transplant, 210

cardiopulmonary resuscitation (CPR), 86, 249, 279

cardiovascular system, 231–233, 265–266

  complications in, 188

  hemodynamics, 201–202

  practice exam

    answers, 274

    questions, 242

  tests, 183–184

  therapeutic procedures for, 190–191

care plans, 78–79, 112–116

  assessing patient's physical condition, 112–114

  screening tests, 116

  teaching patients, 114–115

caring, 8. *See also* management of care

case management, 80–81

case study questions, 41

CAT (computer adaptive testing) exam, 9–10, 290

catheters, 143, 164, 168–169, 201

cations, 196

CD4+ T cell count, 238, 271

central venous catheter (CVC), 168–169

cerebral angiography, 185, 186

cerebral infarct, 250, 280

cerebrospinal fluid (CSF), 184–185

cerebrovascular accident (CVA)

  answers to practice questions, 260, 262, 280

  practice questions, 223, 225, 251

certification examination, 8

CEUs (continuing education units), 310

CGFNS (Commission on Graduates of Foreign Nursing Schools) certificate, 338–340

chart/exhibit questions, 40–41

cheat sheet, for this book, 3

chemical abuse, 130

chemical bioterrorism, 95

chemical restraints, 101

chemotherapy, 210, 240, 272

chest x-ray, 182

chickenpox (Varicella), 99

child abuse, 112

child life specialist, 82

children. *See* pediatrics

Chinese Americans, 129

chlamydia trachomatis infection, 248, 278

cholesterol screening, 116, 252, 281

chronic illness, 208

chronic obstructive pulmonary disease, 237, 270

chronic renal failure, 218, 258

cirrhosis of the liver, 229–230, 264

civil law, 84–86

Class A/B/C/ABC fire extinguishers, 94

clean technique, 96

cleanliness, 343

P

Dedication

Rhoda L. Sommer: This book is dedicated to my husband of 25 years, Stephen, and our daughters, Wendie, Cindie, Becky, and Missy. Without their support, this book would not have happened.

A second thanks goes to the memory of my parents, Dr. Lee and Maxine Haines. Both had master's degrees and pushed my brother and me to learn. At an early age, my mother started showing me how to teach. I am forever grateful for the heritage my parents gave me in education, teaching, and most of all my love of my Lord Jesus Christ.

Dr. Patrick Coonan: This book is dedicated to my wife of over 40 years, Anita, and our four children, David, Lauren, Phillip, and Amy Coonan. My wife has enhanced my work life for as long as we've been married and has been incredibly supportive throughout my many career-direction changes and "dreams of what I want to be when I grow up." Well, maybe I've finally grown up . . . nah! My wife and our children have provided patience, understanding, and assistance while I put this book together as well as a curiosity as to how they may be able to do it too. Without their encouragement, this innovative, comprehensive, and informative book would not have been possible.

A second thanks goes to the memory of my "two fathers" — my father, George E. Coonan, and my father-in-law, Dr. Michael J. Vetere, Sr. — who through their lives gave me the gift and taught me what it is to be a teacher.

Authors' Acknowledgments

Rhoda L. Sommer: I couldn't have written this book without the assistance, knowledge, and encouragement of Dee Truax and Fawn Updike, who are coworkers and nurse educators themselves. They both, in their own ways, helped me become who I am as an educator, and I am so grateful.

Another person, Courtney Castagne-McCavit, my assistant at the office, has proven herself to be so valuable in researching information for the application process in each of the states and territories. Her persistence in finding the information on the different websites has made a huge difference in the information provided in this book. With a tutoring business that was full time and adding a book into the mix, Courtney has managed my schedule to give me time dedicated to writing.

I also want to give thanks to Lindsay Lefevere, executive editor, and Alissa Schwipps, project editor, at Wiley for their help and guidance in the process of writing.

Dr. Patrick Coonan: I couldn't have written this book without the assistance, knowledge, and writing contributions of four of my expert faculty members: Dr. Veronica Arikian, Dr. Maryann Forbes, Professor Jacqueline Brandwein, and Professor Pasqua Spinelli. Thank you's go to Veronica for all the questions and to Maryann, Jackie, and Pasqua for chapters in their areas of expertise and for putting up with all my emails about deadlines. We all found out how hard it is to write about something you think you know, stick to deadlines, and do all the other important things in your life simultaneously. I'd also like to acknowledge the faculty of the Adelphi University School of Nursing, who made me realize that this book needed to be written.

Additionally, I'd like to thank Kali Chan from the public relations department of Adelphi University for finding this opportunity for us, quite by accident. Finally, Wiley Publishing has to be commended for taking serious subject matter and a difficult examination and making it fun.

About the Authors

Rhoda L. Sommer owns and runs One on One NCLEX Tutoring, a tutoring business especially for nursing students. She has used her 39 years of RN and teaching experience to help nursing students succeed, whether that's before nursing school for the TEAS test, during nursing school for trouble with classes, or after graduating nursing school for preparing to take the NCLEX. Since she started the company in 2014, her students' pass rate for the NCLEX has been between 90 and 100 percent.

Rhoda received her bachelor's degree in nursing from Indiana Wesleyan University and worked as a nurse in various capacities: a staff nurse on med surg floors, ICU, and peds. After working in the hospital, she found her true passion: long-term care, where she was a staff nurse, in-service director, assistant director of nursing, and director of nursing. In 2012, Rhoda received her master's degree in nursing education from Indiana Wesleyan. Her academic experience includes fundamentals and med surg teaching at three nursing schools in Indianapolis, Indiana.

Since getting her MSN, Rhoda has helped many students at local nursing schools as well as in her tutoring business. She uses critical thinking and kinesthetic flashcards to help promote her students' success. Her students at One on One NCLEX Tutoring will tell you, "Rhoda is your biggest cheerleader. She will push you, but she will make sure you know that she is behind you all the way!"

Dr. Patrick Coonan is the former Dean of and Professor at the School of Nursing at Adelphi University in Garden City, New York, where he also went to nursing school, as he likes to say, "125 years ago." Throughout his career, Dr. Coonan has held senior patient care management positions at major medical centers in the New York metropolitan area. He was the Chief Nursing Officer in an academic medical center, a health system, and a teaching community hospital and was a fellow in the Johnson & Johnson–Wharton Fellows Program in Management for Nurse Executives at The Wharton School, University of Pennsylvania.

Dr. Coonan's academic experience includes administrative and teaching positions at other academic institutions in the New York area, where he developed technology-enhanced education programs and directed and taught informatics and critical care nursing as well as nursing leadership/management programs. Dr. Coonan received his EdD and MEd from Columbia University, a master's degree in Public Administration/Health Care Administration (MPA) from Long Island University, and a BS in Nursing from Adelphi University. He has consulted, written, and presented extensively on nursing management, leadership, nursing education, emergency service and response, as well as healthcare management.

His research interests are in the areas of health services research, including developing academic/service partnerships; improving patient outcomes; and measuring the impact of leadership, management, nursing care, and systems on traditional measures such as complications, costs, personnel, and work environment issues.

Dr. Coonan is board certified in Nursing Administration, Advanced from the American Nurses Association. His educational and consultative work has included leadership assessment and education, integrating technology into nursing management and educational systems, improving and developing educational delivery models, executive coaching, nursing systems assessment and improvement, and leadership development.

Publisher's Acknowledgments

Executive Editor: Lindsay Sandman Lefevere

Editorial Project Manager and Development Editor: Alissa Schwipps

Copy Editor: Megan Knoll

Technical Editor: Penelope F. Callaway DNP, APRN-BC, FNP-C

Production Editor: Tamilmani Varadharaj

Cover Photos: © SDI Productions/Getty Images

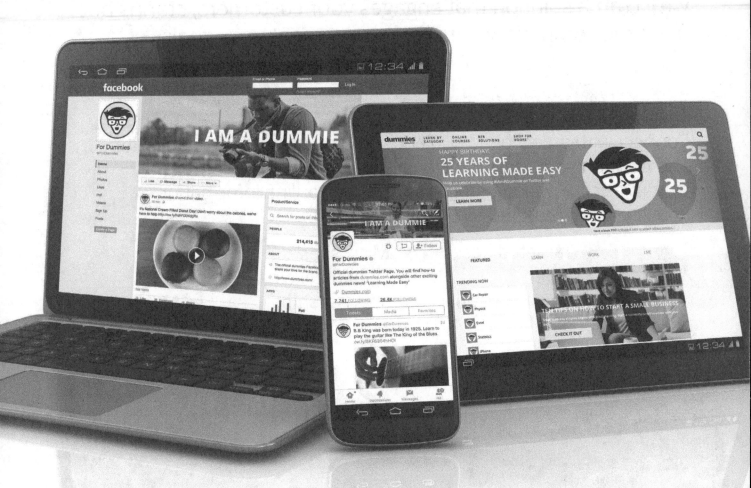
  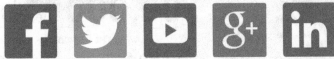
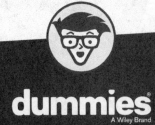

Leverage the power

Dummies is the global leader in the reference category and one of the most trusted and highly regarded brands in the world. No longer just focused on books, customers now have access to the dummies content they need in the format they want. Together we'll craft a solution that engages your customers, stands out from the competition, and helps you meet your goals.

Advertising & Sponsorships

Connect with an engaged audience on a powerful multimedia site, and position your message alongside expert how-to content. Dummies.com is a one-stop shop for free, online information and know-how curated by a team of experts.

- Targeted ads
- Video
- Email Marketing

- Microsites
- Sweepstakes sponsorship

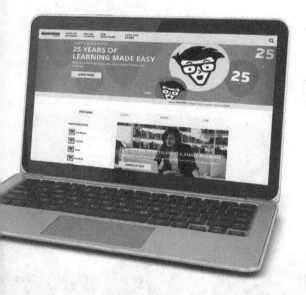

20 MILLION PAGE VIEWS **EVERY SINGLE MONTH**

15 MILLION UNIQUE VISITORS PER MONTH

43% OF ALL VISITORS ACCESS THE SITE VIA THEIR MOBILE DEVICES

700,000 NEWSLETTER SUBSCRIPTIONS

TO THE INBOXES OF

300,000 UNIQUE INDIVIDUALS EVERY WEEK

# of dummies

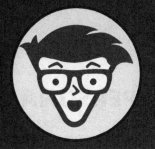

Custom Publishing

Reach a global audience in any language by creating a solution that will differentiate you from competitors, amplify your message, and encourage customers to make a buying decision.

- Apps
- Books
- eBooks
- Video
- Audio
- Webinars

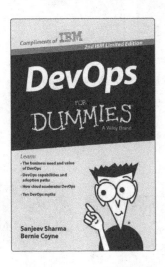

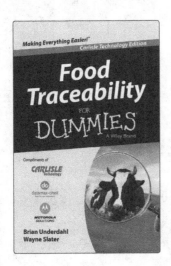

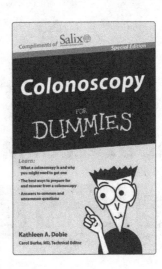

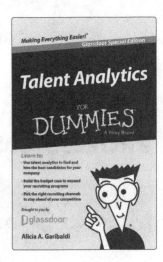

Brand Licensing & Content

Leverage the strength of the world's most popular reference brand to reach new audiences and channels of distribution.

For more information, visit **dummies.com/biz**

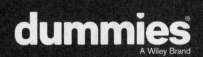

PERSONAL ENRICHMENT

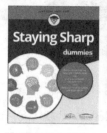 **Staying Sharp**
9781119187790
USA $26.00
CAN $31.99
UK £19.99

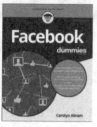 **Facebook**
9781119179030
USA $21.99
CAN $25.99
UK £16.99

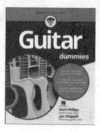 **Guitar**
9781119293354
USA $24.99
CAN $29.99
UK £17.99

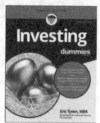 **Investing**
9781119293347
USA $22.99
CAN $27.99
UK £16.99

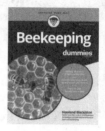 **Beekeeping**
9781119310068
USA $22.99
CAN $27.99
UK £16.99

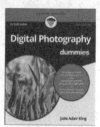 **Digital Photography**
9781119235606
USA $24.99
CAN $29.99
UK £17.99

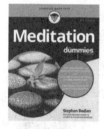 **Meditation**
9781119251163
USA $24.99
CAN $29.99
UK £17.99

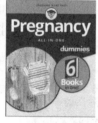 **Pregnancy**
9781119235491
USA $26.99
CAN $31.99
UK £19.99

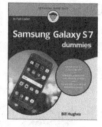 **Samsung Galaxy S7**
9781119279952
USA $24.99
CAN $29.99
UK £17.99

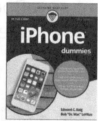 **iPhone**
9781119283133
USA $24.99
CAN $29.99
UK £17.99

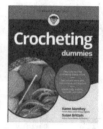 **Crocheting**
9781119287117
USA $24.99
CAN $29.99
UK £16.99

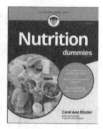 **Nutrition**
9781119130246
USA $22.99
CAN $27.99
UK £16.99

PROFESSIONAL DEVELOPMENT

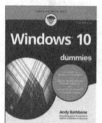 **Windows 10**
9781119311041
USA $24.99
CAN $29.99
UK £17.99

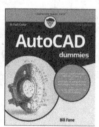 **AutoCAD**
9781119255796
USA $39.99
CAN $47.99
UK £27.99

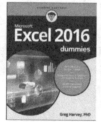 **Excel 2016**
9781119293439
USA $26.99
CAN $31.99
UK £19.99

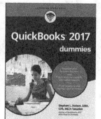 **QuickBooks 2017**
9781119281467
USA $26.99
CAN $31.99
UK £19.99

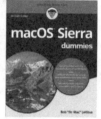 **macOS Sierra**
9781119280651
USA $29.99
CAN $35.99
UK £21.99

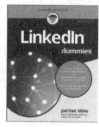 **LinkedIn**
9781119251132
USA $24.99
CAN $29.99
UK £17.99

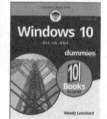 **Windows 10**
9781119310563
USA $34.00
CAN $41.99
UK £24.99

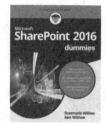 **SharePoint 2016**
9781119181705
USA $29.99
CAN $35.99
UK £21.99

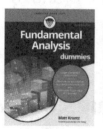 **Fundamental Analysis**
9781119263593
USA $26.99
CAN $31.99
UK £19.99

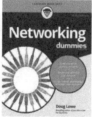 **Networking**
9781119257769
USA $29.99
CAN $35.99
UK £21.99

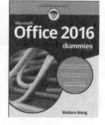 **Office 2016**
9781119293477
USA $26.99
CAN $31.99
UK £19.99

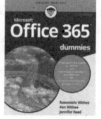 **Office 365**
9781119265313
USA $24.99
CAN $29.99
UK £17.99

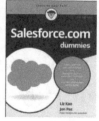 **Salesforce.com**
9781119239314
USA $29.99
CAN $35.99
UK £21.99

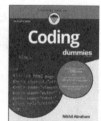 **Coding**
9781119293323
USA $29.99
CAN $35.99
UK £21.99

dummies.com

dummies®
A Wiley Brand

Learning Made Easy

ACADEMIC

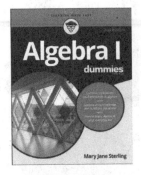

Algebra I dummies

Mary Jane Sterling

9781119293576
USA $19.99
CAN $23.99
UK £15.99

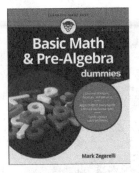

Basic Math & Pre-Algebra dummies

Mark Zegarelli

9781119293637
USA $19.99
CAN $23.99
UK £15.99

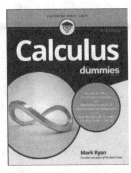

Calculus dummies

Mark Ryan

9781119293491
USA $19.99
CAN $23.99
UK £15.99

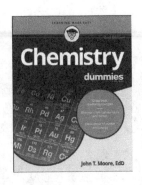

Chemistry dummies

John T. Moore, EdD

9781119293460
USA $19.99
CAN $23.99
UK £15.99

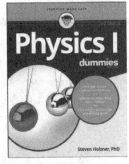

Physics I dummies

Steven Holzner, PhD

9781119293590
USA $19.99
CAN $23.99
UK £15.99

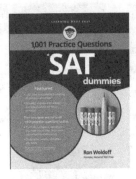

1,001 Practice Questions
SAT dummies

Ron Woldoff

9781119215844
USA $26.99
CAN $31.99
UK £19.99

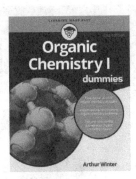

Organic Chemistry I dummies

Arthur Winter

9781119293378
USA $22.99
CAN $27.99
UK £16.99

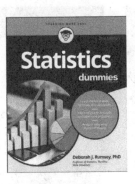

Statistics dummies

Deborah J. Rumsey, PhD

9781119293521
USA $19.99
CAN $23.99
UK £15.99

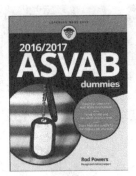

2016/2017
ASVAB dummies

Rod Powers

9781119239178
USA $18.99
CAN $22.99
UK £14.99

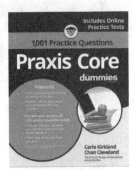

Includes Online Practice Tests
1,001 Practice Questions
Praxis Core dummies

*Carla Kirkland
Chan Cleveland*

9781119263883
USA $26.99
CAN $31.99
UK £19.99

Available Everywhere Books Are Sold

dummies.com

dummies
A Wiley Brand

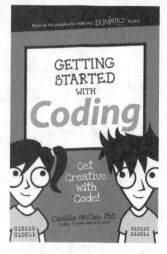
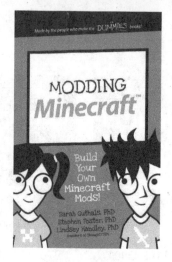
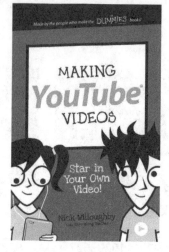
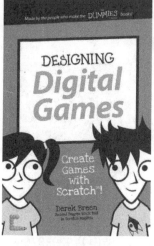
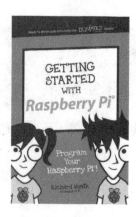
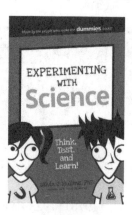
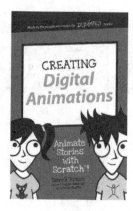
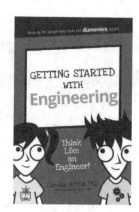
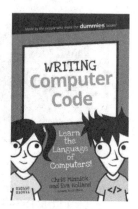